ORAL DIAGNOSIS

ORAL DIAGNOSIS

DONALD A. KERR, D.D.S., M.S.

Professor and Chairman, Department of Oral Pathology,
University of Michigan School of Dentistry;
Ann Arbor, Mich.

MAJOR M. ASH, Jr., D.D.S., M.S.

Professor and Chairman, Department of Occlusion,
University of Michigan School of Dentistry,
Ann Arbor, Mich.

H. DEAN MILLARD, D.D.S., M.S.

Professor of Dentistry and Chairman, Department of Oral Diagnosis,
University of Michigan School of Dentistry,
Ann Arbor, Mich.

FOURTH EDITION

With 746 illustrations

The C. V. Mosby Company

SAINT LOUIS   1974

FOURTH EDITION

Copyright © 1974 by The C. V. Mosby Company

All rights reserved. No part of this book may be reproduced in any manner without written permission of the publisher.

Previous editions copyrighted 1959, 1965, 1970

Printed in the United States of America

Distributed in Great Britain by Henry Kimpton, London

Library of Congress Cataloging in Publication Data

Kerr, Donald A
    Oral diagnosis.

    Includes bibliographies.
    1. Mouth—Diseases—Diagnosis. 2. Teeth—Diseases—
Diagnosis. I. Ash, Major M., joint author.
II. Millard, Herbert Dean, joint author. III. Title.
[DNLM: 1. Diagnosis, Oral. WU141 K41o 1974]
RK308.K4 1974   617′.522′075   73-11119
ISBN 0-8016-2659-5

VH/VH/VH 9 8 7 6 5 4 3 2

Preface

It is evident since the first edition was published that oral diagnosis has developed as a subject and discipline in a significant number of dental schools. The acceptance of the subject of oral diagnosis as a basic requirement of dental education demonstrates the concerted efforts of clinicians and educators who have been dedicated to the concept that oral diagnosis is the basis for the clinical science of dentistry.

Reviews of previous editions have been responsible for some of the changes in the present edition. We wish to thank the many reviewers for their constructive comments. Some ideas were a challenge that we endeavored to meet; others required changes in the text material or a shifting in emphasis that did not appear to be consistent with our goal in writing the book. As in the past every effort has been made to revise the material to include new and relevant topics in the field of oral diagnosis.

Although the format for the presentation of the material has been altered, it still adheres closely to that sequence followed in the clinical situation; that is, first the interview and case history, then the clinical examinations, and finally formulation of the diagnosis and treatment plan. For ease of teaching and learning, the book has been sectionalized and, where possible, extended topics have been divided into chapters. Since the changes reflect the desire of a number of teachers, we hope that this edition will meet better the needs of all teachers of oral diagnosis. As in prior editions, our goal for this edition is the presentation of a systematic and objective approach to the development of a diagnosis on which to base rational treatment.

Donald A. Kerr
Major M. Ash, Jr.
H. Dean Millard

Contents

SECTION I
INTRODUCTION

1 Scope of oral diagnosis **3**

Types of examinations 5
    Periodic health-maintenance examinations 6
    Screening examination 8
    Emergency or incomplete examination 10
Summary 11

② Signs and symptoms **13**

Cardinal manifestations of disease 14
    Pain 15
    Headache 20
    Weakness 20
    Dyspnea 21
    Other cardiovascular manifestations 21
    Alteration of weight 23
    Lesions 23

3 Case history **36**

Approach to the patient 37
Plan of history taking 38
    Chief complaint(s), symptom(s) 39
    Present illness 42
    Past history 43
    Family history 53
    Personal and social history 54
Systems review 54

4 Significance of drugs in oral diagnosis **71**

Drug-induced diseases 75

SECTION II
THE CLINICAL EXAMINATION

5 Principles of the clinical examination **79**

6 Clinical examination—general **84**

    General survey 84
    Head 88

Skin   98
Neck   107
Jaws   114

7   **Examination of soft tissues** **118**

General appraisal   118
Lips   120
Labial and buccal mucosa   125
Palate   139
Oropharynx   146
Floor of the mouth   148
Tongue   152

8   **Examination of the periodontium** **162**

Gingiva   162

9   **Examination of the teeth** **193**

10   **Examination of the occlusion** **214**

Developing occlusion   214
Adult occlusion   227

11   **Examination of the edentulous and partially edentulous mouth** **247**

Partially edentulous mouth   253

SECTION **III**
RADIOGRAPHIC AND SUPPLEMENTARY EXAMINATIONS

12   **Radiographic examination** **261**

Interpretation of normal radiographs   261
Normal landmarks—periapical radiographs   261
Method of radiographic examination   266
Radiographs of the complete mouth   266
Lamina dura—continuity and thickness   266
Periodontal spaces—variations in width   268
Level of the alveolar crest in relation to the cementoenamel junction   269
Periapical radiolucency   272
Pathologic conditions of the teeth   274
Pathologic conditions of the jaws   279
Osseous radiolucencies   279
Osseous radiopacities   285
Combination of osseous radiolucency and radiopacity   288
Other dental findings   290
Posterior bite-wing radiographs   291
Lamina dura continuity   291
Alveolar crest level   291
Crown shape and formative defects   291
Pulp size and pulpal calcification   292
Existing restorations   293
Location of calculus   293
Location of carious lesions   293

Supplemental radiographs 293
    Special radiographic procedures 297
Radiographs for children 297
Radiation hazards 298
Illustrative case 298
    Comment 301

13   Supplementary examination aids **302**

Bacteriologic studies 304
Blood studies 308
    Hematologic diagnosis associated with anemia and polycythemia 308
    Hematologic diagnosis associated with bleeding 309
    Hematologic diagnosis associated with infections 313
    Hematologic diagnosis associated with lymph node enlargement 313
    Hematologic diagnosis associated with leukemias 313
    Hematologic diagnosis associated with chemotherapy 314
    Serologic tests 314
Urine studies 318
Biochemical profiles 319
Contact sensitivity tests 319
Biopsy 322
Exfoliative cytology 326
Pulp vitality tests 328
Study casts 336
    Articulation of casts 337
Use of surveyor 344
Stomatomicroscope 345
Disclosing solution 345

14   Synopsis of diagnostic procedures **348**

    Significance of questions in health questionnaire 351

SECTION   **IV**
ELEMENTS OF THE DIAGNOSTIC METHOD AND TREATMENT PLANNING

15   Diagnosis and treatment planning **375**

Diagnosis 375
    Collecting the facts 375
    Analysis of the facts 376
    Synthesis of examination facts and of descriptive features of disease ... 378
    Making the diagnosis 379
    Diagnosis of neoplasms 380
    Prognosis 382
Diagnosis in dentistry 382
Treatment planning 382
    Rationale and outline for a treatment plan 382
    Systemic treatment 383
    Preparatory treatment 385
    Corrective treatment 387
    Periodic recall examinations and maintenance treatment 387
    Principles for outlining a treatment plan 388
Illustrative case 391

ORAL DIAGNOSIS

SECTION I
INTRODUCTION

Oral diagnosis as a subject consists of the fundamentals of the interview, principles and procedures of clinical examinations, methods of identifying oral disease, and the rationale for oral therapy. Oral diagnosis may also be defined as the identification of oral disease by interviewing, examining, and synthesizing the descriptive features of diseases and the facts obtained from the examination and interview. Finally, oral diagnosis is a systematic method of identifying oral disease.

The first principle of oral diagnosis is to observe and describe deviations from normal. It is the accurate and pointed description that enables a student to utilize reference material to the greatest advantage. It is impossible for a student or general practitioner to recognize all the various diseases that exist; nor is it expected that searching through voluminous reference books for an identical picture of the clinical manifestation of a disease will improve anything but an ability to thumb through reference books. It is true that this form of diagnosis brings fair results in matching clinical and textbook pictures, but it can never lead to a system of diagnosis that is not dependent on trial and error. Furthermore, the practitioner who is thoroughly trained in observation is apt to contribute to the scope of information already known about disease. Thus matching clinical with textbook pictures, either mentally or with the reference book at hand, is not a method of diagnosis to be desired. Not only does it consume valuable time, but all too often the patient's abnormality does not exactly match anything in the reference material because of the wide range of expression that any disease may present. This does not mean that reference books are not valuable in diagnosis; it does mean that they should be used efficiently and when necessary to substantiate a diagnosis. Thus the diagnostician should have a basic knowledge of disease and at least know where to look to verify his clinical impression of a disease without leafing through a reference book in hope of finding a "picture" that will match the one that presents the diagnostic problem.

The diagnostician must recognize that disease exists and must be able to describe it and to classify it within certain limits, namely, type of lesion, tissue involved, etiologic agent, or whether it represents a developmental disturbance. A diagnosis is not always apparent, but the acute observer pays attention to details and is systematic in his approach to the problem. "Spot" diagnoses that impress students usually are based on rapid, almost subconscious, but thorough observations. However, all too often an attempt is made to arrive at diagnoses without first considering all the items that may have a bearing on the diagnosis. If the facts are first collected by a definite procedure, little will be left to doubt regarding the rationale of the diagnosis.

This book provides a method of approach to the diagnosis of disease. Certain premises must be adhered to in presenting a systematized discipline. Note that, aside from any illustrative cases presented to show the pro-

1

cedures for arriving at a diagnosis, many of the photographs depict the normal and deviations within the range of normal. This is done for two reasons: (1) an appreciation for the normal is necessary before abnormal states can be detected, and (2) the illustrations of the procedures of a clinical examination are not subject to distraction by emphasis on pathologic states.

A section of illustrative cases is presented to bring out those analytic processes that are necessary for the final diagnosis of abnormal conditions. In general, those cases involving the most common diagnostic problems are presented. Inasmuch as this is not a textbook of dental medicine or oral pathology, no claim to complete coverage of all the diseases or their description is made. The systematic procedure for making a diagnosis that is presented herein will serve to make more efficient the use of descriptions of disease that may be obtained in textbooks and other reference material on dental medicine and oral pathology. Stated simply, the objective of this book is to answer the question of how a diagnosis is made. It is assumed that the reader has already acquired the fundamentals of the basic sciences and has had some training in the clinical sciences.

The following is an outline for considering the scope of oral diagnosis, signs and symptoms, history taking, and drugs in oral diagnosis:

Scope of oral diagnosis
    Types of examinations
        Complete
        Periodic health maintenance
        Screening
        Emergency or incomplete
Signs and symptoms
    Subjective symptoms
    Objective symptoms (signs of disease)
    Cardinal manifestations of disease
    Primary and secondary lesions
Case history
    Principles of the interview
    Contents of the history
        Complaints and related symptoms
        Evaluation of dental and general health
        Family, personal, and social histories
        Systems review
Drugs of diagnostic significance
    Drugs for treatment of disease
        Effect on diagnosis and treatment
    Drug-induced disease

1

Scope of oral diagnosis

The basis for modern therapy is diagnosis. This concept of diagnosis presupposes that the disease be identified first and then eliminated. The procedure by which the information needed to make a diagnosis is obtained is directly related to the success of a diagnosis since the diagnosis itself is based on a favorable interview and examination of the patient.

Probably the most important concept that a student must learn, whether in school or out, is the importance of an efficient discipline for collecting the material necessary to make a diagnosis. Sometimes students and even some teachers think that much of the information gathered about patients in a dental school clinic is unnecessary and far removed from the practical aspects of a dental office. At times a student is impressed by the apparent ability of a teacher or practitioner to arrive at a diagnosis rather quickly. Such a quick diagnosis does not necessarily represent snap judgment but reflects the examiner's ability to reduce the history to a minimum while at the same time covering the necessary field of inquiry and examination. A history that is brief but good represents the product of adequate training and practice in the subject of oral diagnosis; it does not represent any special innate ability of the clinician to "pull a diagnosis out of thin air." This is especially true in dealing with pain and soft tissue lesions in the oral region.

In addition to being able to reduce the detail of a history to a great degree, a "busy" general practitioner has very few new complete histories to take because much of the time is spent in caring for those individuals who have been his patients for years. In view of these considerations, objections to teaching a procedure that in itself may seem too detailed for practical application in a dental office appear to be unjustified.

Since most students can learn in school only a small part of what they need to know about diagnosis, and since much of what is learned is forgotten, it is necessary that they be taught a systematic approach to diagnosis that is simple enough to learn yet so rational as to be difficult to forget. It should supply the foundation that best fits the student not only to start practicing dentistry, but also to improve continually his diagnostic ability.

Only a few observations will lead to original descriptions of disease. However, to describe the wide variations in disease that exist and to apply facts and ideas to new situations, a practitioner must be able to grasp broad principles and use a method of thought and action that will enable him to meet such a variety of situations. The Hippocratic method of systematic observation and description is the foundation of oral diagnosis. Practice in observation and description is necessary even though the approach is logical and systematic. Sound reasoning is hard to attain, but training and practice in a rational discipline of thinking promote this faculty.

The study and practice of dentistry today must take into consideration not only changes in management of disease, but also changes in its prevention. The more effec-

3

tive control of dental caries by fluoridation, diet, and therapeutic dentifrices presents new problems for which the dentist is responsible. The dental practitioner is confronted with a changing set of demands upon his services and skill not only because of the changes in therapy, but also because of the increasing number of persons in the older age groups. Because of the remarkable control that has been established over acute and communicable diseases and the decrease in infant mortality, people are living to an older age.

Although the efforts of dentists today are directed toward the restoration of carious teeth, the changing scene of dental practice would indicate that the prevention and early detection of periodontal disease will play an important role in the future. Traditionally, people have come to the dentist with the complaint of a toothache; but now, because of health education and control of caries, patients see the dentist for a periodic examination and assistance in the prevention of dental and periodontal disease. With this change in attitude the dentist is faced not only with the treatment of oral disease, but also with the examination of patients who are ostensibly well. This is especially true of children whose parents are concerned with their welfare and desire them to be examined at periodic intervals to be sure development is normal. With this trend established in childhood, the demand for periodic examination will carry on into adult life, increasing the demand for quality and quantity in oral diagnosis. The changing pattern of dental care does not mean that the restoration of carious teeth will be a minor part of dental practice but means that in the future more time will have to be spent in the prevention of oral disease. To carry out the early detection of disease effectively, it will be necessary for the examiner not only to attend properly to signs when they first appear, but also to give repeated examinations before symptoms and signs develop. The dental practi-

tioner who is adapted to the changing scene must be interested in the health as well as the illnesses of his patients, and he must be adequately prepared in the technics of clinical examination. This means that he must develop not only his ability to carry out the technical aspects of restorative procedures, but also his acuity of observation so that he may recognize incipient disease.

The dental profession has done exceedingly well in educating the public about oral health; this advice to the public has either implied or explicitly suggested that to consult one's dentist regularly will maintain his health and prevent disease. It is not by chance that industry and large universities are particularly demanding of preventive medicine and dentistry. These demands are not simply altruistic, since the prevention of disease pays off in terms of healthier workers, less loss of valuable personnel because of sickness, and less absenteeism. There can be no doubt that periodic examination of the mouth by the general practitioner who is prepared to thoroughly examine his patients will do much toward the prevention of disease. The accumulating body of information being gathered from surveys of ostensibly well people indicates that a high incidence of diseases are present that could have been prevented by periodic examination.

Several obstacles are encountered in the practice of preventive dentistry even though everyone knows that prevention of disease is a worthy aim. The changes in man brought about by his living to an older age and by changes in his environment have resulted in a relative increase in some diseases and a relative decrease in others. These changes usually occur faster than the dentist and his scientific collaborators can provide therapeutic measures to control them. Thus, while inroads are being made in the prevention of dental caries in children, a larger population is reaching the age at which disease of the supporting structure becomes paramount. The lapse of time before scientific knowledge can be widely and effectively applied is well known. For example, chlorination of drinking water was not effectively utilized for many generations after its discovery even though its effectiveness in the prevention of disease was known. There can be no question that fluoridation will be impeded by the same lack of interest on the part of the dental profession and the public.

Another obstacle is exemplified by the lack of interest in the periodic examination of the apparently well patient; the tendency of the majority of patients is to wait and pay only for delayed therapy. People are far more ready to pay for the treatment of oral disease than they are to pay for preventive services. Some of this enigma has developed because of the availability of relatively cheap over-the-counter medications, such as certain toothpastes that are widely proclaimed in advertising media to prevent all kinds of oral disease. To the prospective patient this alternative appears to be far less unpleasant in terms of cost and time than making and keeping an appointment with a dentist.

Still another obstacle lies in our formal dental education, in which little or no stress is laid upon the prevention of disease. This state of affairs may be aptly defined by paraphrasing Vines: the academic blunder of the divorce of preventive from clinical dentistry and its forced marriage to public health dentistry has led to the subsequent relegation of the unhappy pair to the isolation of a faintly depressed specialism. For this mistake there is much to answer; through it, generations of dentists have been trained in the belief that preventive dentistry is inseparably linked with fluoridation, special city and county pedodontic clinics, and the supervision of campaigns to make dental health a national habit.

It is hoped that the present trend in dental education to institute courses in preventive dentistry and oral diagnosis will do much to place these fields of endeavor into their proper perspective. The place of oral diagnosis in preventive dentistry can be readily appreciated since the prevention of disease is based upon a thorough examination of all patients. Thus the disciplines of an examination as taught in oral diagnosis must be directed not only to the examination and diagnosis of obvious disease, but also to an examination that will stress the normal development of children and the range of normal in the adult. With this concept in mind, it is to be expected that the dental practitioner will broaden his interest in the diagnosis and care of disease and encourage his patients in the maintenance of good health.

Many practitioners integrate an appreciable amount of preventive dentistry into their practice; however, many find it difficult to spend any time in the examination of the well patient for the prevention of disease since the benefits of this type of examination are usually much less prompt, less obvious, and less appreciated. Many individuals without obvious symptoms of disease benefit from a thorough examination because previously known but neglected conditions may be re-evaluated. It must be emphasized that the examination of the supposedly healthy mouth must be thorough and careful, since the early detection of disease demands that minute and inconspicuous deviations from the normal be carefully evaluated. There can be no doubt that there is a greater likelihood of a favorable eventual outcome from a disease when it is discovered in relatively early stages. This is true not only for neoplasms but also for dental caries, periodontal disease, malocclusion, and other abnormalities in the mouth and adjacent structures.

TYPES OF EXAMINATIONS

From a practical standpoint it appears that at least three types of examination procedures should be employed in a general practice: (1) a thorough and *complete* examination, utilizing all the skills of interviewing, physical examination, and supplementary diagnostic aids; (2) a *screening* type of examination, utilizing a dental modification of the Cornell Medical Index Health Questionnaire, a brief clinical examination of the teeth and supporting structures and mouth, and limited x-ray examination utilizing posterior bite-wing radiographs; and (3) the emergency or *limited* type of examination necessary for the diagnosis and management of acute and emergency conditions.

The latter two forms of examination represent a practical compromise with a more complete form of examination; however, they should be used only when indicated. From the standpoint of being indicated, the routine examination of the teeth with a pulp tester in those patients complaining of toothaches hardly seems less indicated than a bite-wing radiographic examination of the teeth when the patient complains of the same symptom. It is apparent that the findings of both forms of examination are sufficient to constitute an indication for their performance. While the complete testing of the teeth (by a pulp tester or by thermal tests) is considered to be a part of a more complete examination than a screening examination, this arbitrary assignment of examination procedures to a particular form of examination is not sufficient justification for the exclusion of one or the other, since both forms may be indicated in any particular instance. A thorough and complete examination should include all the commonly accepted diagnostic and examination procedures.

Periodic health-maintenance examinations

A periodic health-maintenance examination must necessarily be initiated by a complete and thorough examination of the patient; the results are then used in subsequent examinations to measure what deviations might have occurred during the interval. When health-maintenance examinations are repeated on the same individuals after varying intervals of time, significant changes are likely to be encountered. Many factors such as age, sex, and initial examination findings influence the interval of time between examinations. Although the ideal time interval between thorough examinations of supposedly healthy individuals free of disease would appear to be from 6 months to a year, it is apparent that certain individuals might be able to go as long as 2 years between thorough periodic health-maintenance examinations. In such instances the use of a screening type of examination in the interval between complete examinations should be considered. A thorough examination should include the following (see also Chapters 3 and 4 for details):

1. Case history
   Patient's chief complaint, present illness, past history, and systems review
2. Clinical examination
   a. General appraisal of the patient
   b. Detailed oral examination
   c. Supplementary examination and special tests when indicated
3. Diagnosis
   a. Summary of the nature of the abnormality, its etiology and significance
   b. Prognosis
4. Treatment plan
   a. Ideal
   b. Alternate

The extent of the screening examination depends largely upon the yield of positive findings that may be expected from a particular examination procedure and its relationship to the cost of testing in terms of time, patience, and expense. The examination for acute and emergency conditions depend upon the nature of the disease and whether the disease is local or systemic in origin. Obviously the localization, examination, and diagnosis of a toothache will utilize those examination procedures necessary to make a diagnosis in order that prompt therapeutic measures may be instituted. In certain instances it is conceivable that acute or emergency conditions may require an examination as thorough as any that can be devised. At other times a screening type of examination may be necessary to rule out contraindications for the particular type of therapy that is to be used in the treatment of patients with acute or emergency conditions. Thus, although certain basic forms of examination procedures might be outlined for differing purposes, one must recognize that from a practical standpoint the diagnosis of any disease, regardless of its nature, may require the most extensive form of examination. The majority of patients who have a thorough examination will be found to have some type of periodontal disease of which they are totally unaware. The high prevalence of incipient periodontal disease and incipient caries found during a health-maintenance examination alone justifies the performance of this type of examination.

An analysis of the complete dental examinations carried out at the University Health Service of the University of Michigan as a part of the periodic health appraisal program of the faculty reveals that the yield for a complete examination is significantly high. As a part of a total health appraisal program, its value to the patient warrants the small amount of time required to carry it out. The findings from the history of those examined reflect its value:

History of rheumatic fever	8%
Sensitivity to drugs used in dental therapy	14%
Past history of significant systemic disease	12%
History of periodontal therapy	14%
History of necrotizing gingivitis	5%

The frequency of rheumatic fever, sensitivity to drugs, and systemic disorders such as hypertension and diabetes mellitus emphasizes the necessity of obtaining this information before beginning treatment.

The findings in the following list are of significance in view of the fact that 60 percent of those examined visited their own dentist at periodic intervals of 6 months or 1 year, and 32 percent visited their dentist regularly at greater than 1-year intervals. Only a small percentage showed complete lack of oral health and dental care:

Simple gingivitis	11%
Necrotizing gingivitis—acute, subacute, and recurrent	4%
Periodontitis—incipient	
Unknown to patient	7%
Periodontitis—moderate	
Known to patient	5%
Unknown to patient	14%
Periodontitis—advanced	
Known to patient	7%
Unknown to patient	5%
Dental caries (% of individuals having incipient to moderate carious lesions)	80%
Advanced dental caries	9%

The findings from radiographic examination of the teeth and periodontium show the need for complete mouth radiographs, as well as posterior bite-wings, periodically. The findings in 261 patients examined in a 1-year period are given in the following list:

Nonvital teeth (not including those endodontically treated)	27
Periapical radiolucencies	36
Retained root tips	5
Impactions	11
Radicular cysts	3

These findings indicate that even patients who are obviously well cared for need periodic complete and thorough dental examinations. The prevalence of disease might well be expected to be considerably higher in a general population group that is not as interested in oral health as the faculty members of a university. Thus a complete and thorough examination of a general population group should show even a greater yield of disease than do the results of the survey given here.

It is obvious that the clinical examination and radiographic examination are probably responsible for the discovery of more asymptomatic phases of disease than is the case history. Although the interview of the patient appears to be of relatively less value in preventive dentistry than in emergency and acute disease, the value of a history that is taken in the examination of ostensibly well people should not be underestimated, since the diagnosis of many important disorders depends upon the history obtained from the patient. This does suggest, however, that where circumstances do not permit extensive history taking by the dentist, a questionnaire to be completed by the patient should be used, provided that the dentist elaborates on the positive and significant negative answers to the questions on the questionnaire. The type of questions and the number of questions included in a health questionnaire will depend upon the yield in a form of positive findings. In order that the questionnaire not be too extensive and filled with questions whose yield does not present statistically proved evidence of their value, only those questions that may be expected to effectively uncover the cardinal manifestations of the most common forms of disease should be used. The accompanying health questionnaire is utilized for the purpose of supplementing the case history. It is basically a system review and is not intended to determine the patient's complaints or to describe his disease. It is a practical method of evaluating a patient's general health and serves to alert the examiner's attention to a departure from good health that may have a bearing on the presence and treatment of oral disease.

A health questionnaire should obtain certain vital statistics about the patient such as the name, age, height, weight, occupation, marital status, and the name of the patient's physician. Introductory statements should be made relative to how the questionnaire is to be answered, and some reassurance should be given on the questionnaire that the answers to the questions will be held confidential. Furthermore, the questions contained in the questionnaire all have some direct or indirect bearing on the diagnosis of the patient's condition and may be significant in providing treatment for him comfortably and safely. The questions should be so stated that only the affirmative answers require further interview for the purpose of obtaining details. The significance of affirmative answers to the questions may be found at the end of this chapter.

Screening examination

A screening examination is one that attempts to compromise between a thorough and complete examination and a less extensive one because of the practical aspects of reduced time, costs, and skill involved in a shorter type of examination. The degree of compromise of course depends upon the decrease in potential yield in the form of positive findings that the examiner wishes to allow. Although the yield from a screening type of examination and a more thorough complete type of examination may be the same in some instances, both the dentist and physician should be aware of their potential difference. Obviously the yield of certain forms of screening examinations directed toward a particular lesion or disease may compare favorably with that of a more extensive examination, since the procedures used may be the same. For example, the use of posterior bite-wing radiographs for the detection of carious lesions is used both in the complete examination and the screening examination. The posterior bite-wing radiographic examination may be expected to yield about 75 percent or more of the carious lesions present; however, a more complete examination utilizing periapical radiographs and a sharp explorer and mouth mirror may raise the yield to 100 percent. Thus the yield from bite-wing radiographs compares somewhat favorably with the extensive form of examination in yield of carious lesions. One must remember that other lesions of the supporting structures and of the apices of the teeth may show additional disease that would not be indicated by posterior bite-wing radiographs. Thus the examiner must take into consideration those factors for which he is screening, the efficiency of the screening procedure, and the scope of the screening process. The scope of the screening examination must necessarily be determined by the examiner with regard to time available, number of patients to be screened, purpose of the screening, facilities available, economic considerations, skill of the examiner, and desires of the patient. The following screening examination outline is presented as one form of this type of examination that might be used routinely to yield a fairly high percentage of potential positive findings either in the office of a general practitioner or a dental clinic.

1. Chief complaint—an apparently well patient may or may not have a significant complaint, but the chance to express one should be given
2. Health questionnaire
3. Posterior bite-wing radiographs
4. Gross appraisal for decay; missing and filled teeth
5. General appraisal of the gingiva for alteration of color and form
6. Gross appraisal of the soft tissues for the presence of lesions
7. Brief appraisal of oral hygiene
8. Brief appraisal of occlusion

This form of general screening examination may be expected to yield a significant amount of disease in unselected patients and will provide a certain degree of coverage in a health-maintenance examination. As has been previously stated, this form of examination may well be utilized to bridge the gap between more extensive and thorough examinations and thus is more successfully used as an adjunct to an initial thorough periodic health-maintenance examination. This form of examination may also be used as a precursor to a more thorough examination. In fact, it may well serve to point out the necessity for a more thorough examination. Probably the mini-

mum type of screening examination includes posterior bite-wing radiographs and a series of questions to reveal whether or not a patient has or has had some type of disease that contraindicates a proposed dental treatment. Such questions as: Are you now under the care of a physician? Have you ever had rheumatic fever? Do you have difficulty with bleeding? and Are you sensitive to any drug such as penicillin, iodine, and so on? are representative of the type that may be used. More often than not a brief type of screening examination is carried out by a simple study of posterior bite-wing radiographs. Further examination is solely for the purpose of confirming clinically the presence of carious lesions that are manifest in the radiographs. Evidently there is as much variation in the contents of a screening examination as there is in a more thorough and complete type of examination. Irrespective of the type of examination used, there can be no doubt that the more detailed the examination, the greater the yield of positive findings from the performance of the examination. Generally the omission of any portion of the thorough examination in favor of a screening examination will compromise any examiner's effectiveness, but the adverse effect on the yield of the examination is necessarily dependent upon the scope and demand on the examination. In respect to the shorter screening type of examination, the following general rules should apply: *No patient should be given a short or screening type of examination unless there is an awareness of its limitations.* Awareness includes both that of the examiner and the patient. When patients are told of having chronic destructive periodontal disease that has been present for many years, they will complain, all too often, of having had many examinations in the past without being told of this condition. This dilemma can be avoided by a thorough examination of the mouth, including an analysis of the supporting structures of the teeth, and by telling the patient of potential and existing disease. The responsibility of the examiner lies not only in the discovery of carious lesions, which he may expect and treat, but also in the discovery of any latent or other disease in the mouth requiring treatment or referral; this is what a patient should receive when coming to a dentist for an examination. When anything less than a thorough examination has been made, the patient should be told. There is a place for a screening type of examination in the general practitioner's office, but it is not meant to exclude or take the place of a more thorough and complete examination of the mouth as it relates to the rest of the body. As previously mentioned, a screening type of examination may be used:

1. To indicate gross disease in broad surveys
2. To indicate the necessity for a complete and thorough examination where screening of ostensibly well patients is being undertaken
3. To allow practical extension of the interval of time between thorough periodic health-maintenance examinations
4. To take the place of a thorough type of examination when time, cost, and skill prevent its use

Emergency or incomplete examination

An emergency type of examination is limited to those procedures that obviously appear related to the complaint of the patient. The history and examination of the complaint are initially sharply limited to the signs and symptoms of the disease and its causative agent. In certain instances the problem may be broad enough in scope to tax the ingenuity of the examiner and demand all his diagnostic acumen.

The simplest form of emergency examination may consist only of the patient opening his mouth and the examiner observing the disease, for example, a fractured tooth. The history will consist solely of the time of occurrence, the manner in which the accident occurred, the presence or absence of associated signs and symptoms, and the presence or absence of systemic disease of immediate importance to therapy. The clinical examination would consist of inspecting the fracture to determine involvement of the pulp and testing the pulp to determine its vitality. The radiographic examination would include periapical radiographs to determine the possibility of root fracture, bone fracture, and apical involvement.

This type of examination is minimal and for obvious reasons cannot be utilized for a screening or periodic health examination. For expediency the emphasis is placed upon the evaluation of acute and known complaints and their relief. In those instances in which the diagnosis may not be easily obtained, this type of examination may well serve to provide the examiner with sufficient information to institute treatment of the symptoms. Once again it should be pointed out that this type of examination does not take the place of a more thorough examination, and the relief of a symptom itself, without due regard for the determination of the cause and its eradication, cannot be considered as a logical approach to therapy. This does not mean that the relief of symptoms does not have a place in the practice of dentistry. All too often the location of the offending tooth causing severe pain cannot be immediately determined and the treatment of the symptoms becomes of primary concern to the dentist. In the emergency type of examination the dentist has no routine or set pattern of procedures; the circumstances that exist determine the trend of the examination. The success of the emergency examination is directly related to the ability of the examiner to effectively utilize the basic principles of oral diagnosis (interviewing, clinical examination, and formulation of a diagnosis).

SUMMARY

It is not our intent to list all the possible diseases and their cardinal manifestations. The objectives of this book are to (1) present an outline for the systematic collection of subjective information alluding to the cardinal manifestations of disease, (2) give the actual procedure for determining the presence of cardinal manifestations of disease, (3) show by illustrative cases how to make a differential diagnosis, and (4) show how a clinical history, examination, and diagnosis are utilized in the practice of dentistry. The pertinent content of preclinical sciences will be integrated with clinical dentistry. No attempt will be made to incorporate all of the physiologic bases for disorders of structure and psychology since such material can be found elsewhere.

When cardinal manifestions of disease exist in a patient, the dentist should be aware of their basic mechanisms for the purpose of establishing a basis for initiating further diagnostic and therapeutic procedures. While taking the clinical history, the examiner may find that a patient has one of the cardinal manifestations of disease such as pain. Before appropriate measures for its relief can be instituted, it is necessary that he be aware of the physiologic basis for pain and know its causes. For example, he may know that certain manifestations of pain may be related to angina of effort, but he may not know that this condition is caused by arteriosclerosis that, in some manner, sensitizes the coronary arteries to the effects of increased demands on the heart and reacts by spasms of the coronary arteries at a time when increased myocardial circulation is required. A spasm of the coronary artery produces myocardial hypoxia, which causes the pain. The examiner will have established that the precipitating cause of the pain is effort and in a general way is related to heart disease. However, he can in no way establish a rational basis for treatment unless he is aware that the basic cause of the pain is arteriosclerosis and that the functional cause is a spasm of the coronary arteries. In this particular instance the basic cause of the pain is not treatable; however, in other instances the cause of pain may be of primary consideration. In this and in some other cases, pain must be treated by removal of the precipitating cause or by treatment of the functional cause of the disease.

Another example where the concept involved in the proper evaluation and treatment of disease may be readily appreciated concerns the diagnosis of pain associated with dysfunction of the temporomandibular joint. The examiner may determine from the clinical history that the patient is in distress when functional movements of the temporomandibular joint are made. If he is unaware of the underlying basic pathologic disturbances responsible for the production of pain in the region of the joint, he may be satisfied to treat only the symptom or the precipitating cause of the symptom. In this case the precipitating cause would be the movement of the jaw. Thus his treatment might be directed toward palliation of pain by injection of hydrocortisone or sclerosing solution into the joint or even by surgical removal of the disk. Or he may attempt to treat the precipitating cause by complete immobilization of the mandible by wiring or by reducing the function of the mandible by Hawley retainers or splints. Such treatment implies a lack of knowledge of the functional ultimate cause of the pain—occlusal trauma. This does not imply that all pain associated with the temporomandibular joint has its origin in occlusal trauma. Though this is probably the most frequent cause of pain in the temporomandibular joint, other conditions may also produce pain in this area. These are discussed in more detail elsewhere.

The practical approach to oral diagnosis requires that the diagnostician utilize a systematic method for determining the subjective manifestations of disease. This is best initiated by the proper taking of a case history. The facts gathered in a case history should orient the examiner's thinking to the basic mechanisms responsible for the symptoms that have been elicited in the case history, and this orientation should direct the examiner to certain areas of emphasis in the general appraisal of the patient. This step-by-step discipline will expedite the examination and serve to gain the patient's confidence. The use of such a procedure allows the complete evaluation of all the possible ramifications that disease may present. Even when the procedure is reduced to a minimum for the simplest and most obvious cases, it will assure the examiner that he has not overlooked some significant and latent aspect of the patient's complaint.

REFERENCES

Barr, J. H.: Trends in the development of courses in oral diagnosis, J. Dent. Educ. **18**:25-29, 1954.

Bodecker, C. F.: Oral diagnosis, J. Dent. Educ. **8**:244-256, 1944.

Easton, G. S.: The place of systemic studies in undergraduate instruction in oral diagnosis, J. Dent. Educ. **18**:40-45, 1954.

Editorial: The dentist and the medical patient, J.A.D.A. **56**:253-254, 1958.

Hubbard, J. P. (editor): The early detection and prevention of disease, New York, 1957, McGraw-Hill Book Company.

Koch, R. W.: Thoroughness in oral diagnosis, Washington Univ. Dent. J. **31**:2-7, June, 1965.

Levin, M. L.: Detection of chronic disease, J.A.M.A. **146**:1397-1401, 1951.

Millard, H. D., and Tupper, C. J.: The role of oral diagnosis in periodic health appraisal examinations, Oral Surg. **121**:1273-1278, 1959.

Muhler, J. C., Hine, M. K., and Day, H. G.: Preventive dentistry, St. Louis, 1954, The C. V. Mosby Co.

Petrie, L. M., Bowdoin, C. D., and McLoughlin, C. J.: Voluntary multiple health tests, J.A.M.A. **148**:1022-1024, 1952.

Reynolds, R. L.: Recent trends in oral diagnosis, Michigan Dent. A. J. **48**:312-314, Sept., 1966.

Smith, R. M.: Diagnosis and treatment planning; the keystone, Amer. Col. Dent. J. **31**:233-238, Oct., 1964.

Tarsitano, J. J.: Never treat a stranger, J.A.D.A. **73**:856-862, Oct. 1966.

Vines, H. W. C.: To make preventive medicine a clinical reality, we must overcome our obsession with beds, Mod. Hosp. **81**:51-54, 106-108, 1953.

Ziskin, D. E., Burket, L. W., and Blevins, G. C.: Teaching oral diagnosis to dental students, J. Dent. Educ. **10**:61-82, 1945.

2
Signs and symptoms

It is obvious to almost everyone commencing the study of oral diagnosis that several of the symptoms of one disease are also the symptoms of some other disease. Many diseases have numerous symptoms in common because the external conditions are actually secondary or nonspecific reactions. These conditions are the result of biologic variations from individual to individual, variations within the same individual, and variations in the causative agents. Thus the manifestations of disease are many and varied.

Applied symptomatology of disease may be considered to be the descriptive knowledge of the subjective and objective manifestations of disease necessary to carry out the process of oral diagnosis. Lest the examiner become confused with the wide variety of symptoms that may be presented to him during the examination, it is necessary that some useful grouping of manifestations of disease be utilized.

The cardinal signs of inflammation as one group are an example of a symptomatologic classification that aids in identifying tissue alteration and disease. Manifestations of disease may also be classified on an anatomic or system basis whereby symptoms are grouped according to the part of the body or system involved. Symptomatology may also be based on morphologic alteration of the tissues which gives rise to characteristic types of lesions; these are divided into so-called elementary or *primary* lesions and *secondary* lesions, which occur consecutively in consequence to the primary lesions. It must be remembered, however,

that all classifications are artificial and are made by emphasizing certain differences and neglecting certain resemblances. The examiner should not let any arbitrary division of symptoms detract from the evaluation of the whole individual, since the process of analyzing and interpreting symptoms cannot be based on the description of an isolated symptom relative to a classification but must be based upon the orientation of the symptoms not only to the classification, but also to the whole body as a physiologic and psychologic unit. The most common classification in symptomatology is the division of symptoms into objective and subjective manifestations of disease.

Subjective symptoms are those that may be discerned by the patient and are obtained by inquiry during the case history. In most instances the subjective symptoms are the ones that bring the patient to the dentist. In some instances the symptoms will present the picture that will largely establish the diagnosis regardless of the outcome of the clinical or laboratory examinations. The subjective symptoms usually determine the line of inquiry that the examiner must take to determine the various causes for the symptoms. Although subjective symptoms may be related entirely to local disturbances of the mouth, they may also be expressions of general or systemic disease. Thus, the examiner must be aware not only of subjective manifestations of disease of the mouth, but also of subjective symptoms outside this area that will complete the pattern or clinical picture of the patient's departure from good health. The subjective oral manifestations of disease, or complaints of the patient referable to the mouth, are various types of pain, alteration of taste, foul breath, inability to masticate food, esthetic and psychogenic complaints, dryness of the mouth, swelling, speech problems, and a sense of an unclean mouth. Obviously these same symptoms will rarely be described in the same way by all patients. Not infrequently patients will present without obvious subjective symptoms of disease because of their adaptation to the distress or discomfort or because of indifferent effects on the body or its functions. Today, with periodic dental examinations being made on presumably well people, the dentist has an additional obligation to seek out those manifestations of latent disease or potential sources of disability.

Objective symptoms or signs of disease are those which produce functional and structural changes that may be seen by the naked eye of the patient or the examiner. Generally, alteration of structure and function may be manifested by changes in shape, size, color, form, density, number, position, and relationship. The clinical evaluation of the alterations of form and structure is carried out by inspection, palpation, percussion, and auscultation. Although these technics are used in examination of the entire body, their application varies with the part of the body being investigated. Thus examination of the mucous membrane entails chiefly inspection and palpation, whereas examination of the teeth, jaws, and temporomandibular joint entails inspection, palpation, percussion, and auscultation. Radiographic examination may be considered as an extension of the visual examination.

From the foregoing it may be readily seen that subjective manifestations of disease are elicited by inquiry and that objective manifestations of disease are found by clinical examination. The basis for modern therapy is diagnosis; this proposes that the

cause of the disease be identified and eliminated. Though this is a modern approach to treatment, it is not always feasible, since many situations will arise in which the relief of symptoms becomes an important adjunct in caring for the patient. The relief of symptoms is important to the patient and may provide positive benefits in the treatment of the disease provided that the symptom relief does not interfere with the diagnosis of the disease. For example, it is necessary to make a differential diagnosis between herpetic gingivostomatitis and acute necrotizing ulcerative gingivitis, but the basis for therapy is not directed toward elimination of the disease in both instances. Inasmuch as herpetic gingivostomatitis is a self-limiting disease, therapy is generally directed toward relief of symptoms associated with this condition. The symptomatic relief of acute necrotizing ulcerative gingivitis is contraindicated since the cause of the disease or predisposing factors in the causation of the disease have not been eliminated. Symptomatic relief in the treatment of acute necrotizing gingivitis should be considered only as an adjunct to formal therapy. Symptomatic treatment of patients after gingivectomy, endodontics, oral surgery, and operative dental procedures is advocated only when the cause of the symptoms has been taken into proper consideration. Therefore, the examiner should institute symptomatic therapy only after he has identified the cause of the symptoms. Thus, he should evaluate the symptoms of a patient in terms of the previous treatment of the patient and what complication or unfavorable sequela may have arisen as the result of such treatment.

CARDINAL MANIFESTATIONS OF DISEASE

Just as the cardinal signs of inflammation are heat, redness, swelling, and pain, the cardinal manifestations of systemic disease are pain, fever, weakness, shortness of breath, circulatory disturbances, indigestion, jaundice, polyuria, oliguria, edema, alteration of weight, anemia, bleeding, and lymphadenopathy. In rendering a health service the dental practitioner has a professional, legal, and moral obligation to learn as much as possible about the health of his patient before beginning treatment, since the knowledge gained may be a basic consideration in the clinical examination and in the determination of treatment. The emphasis on the clinical manifestations of systemic disease should be directed toward the correlation of signs and symptoms of disease in all areas of the body that may be related or possibly related to oral disease. The purpose of the evaluation of the clinical manifestations of systemic disease is not to establish a medical diagnosis but to make an evaluation of the health of the patient that will allow the examiner (1) to consider the presence of systemic disease and its relation to dental treatment, (2) to take prophylactic or precautionary measures for the good of the examiner and the patient, (3) to determine the best treatment possible in the presence of systemic disease, (4) to establish a sound basis for medical consultation when indicated, and (5) to give the dentist a better idea of what to expect in the way of prognosis.

It is obvious that the indications for the evaluation of the cardinal manifestations of systemic disease will depend upon the character of the disease and the therapeutic procedures that are to be instituted. Since the relationship of oral disease to systemic disease is not always obvious and the need for systemic evaluation is not always apparent, the oral examination of any patient should include a basic screening discipline to uncover any systemic disease that may be present. The proper rationale for oral therapy demands that the examiner (1) consider the constitutional status of the patient (with emphasis on nutrition, metabolism, and hormonal balance) and (2) recognize systemic disease that may modify the therapeutic procedures (rheumatic or

congenital heart insufficiencies, blood dyscrasias, and contagious diseases). The recognition of the clinical manifestations of systemic disease should not be considered as usurping the province of the physician. It is not intended that the dental practitioner be as proficient as a physician in the recognition of all the signs and symptoms of systemic disease but rather that he be proficient in the recognition of systemic disease that might have a bearing on oral diagnosis and therapy.

The following presentation of the cardinal manifestations of systemic disease is not intended to be all inclusive, since coverage of this material may be found in textbooks of internal medicine and oral medicine.

Pain

Pain is a specific sensory experience mediated through nerve structures separate from those that mediate other sensations such as touch, pressure, heat, and cold. Pain cannot be considered as being desirable; however, it is an important warning of the presence of noxious stimuli, although pain itself does not appear to be essential to a suitable biologic adjustment since many persons without ability to experience pain are able to adjust themselves to their environment. Pain may produce a protective adaptive reaction to noxious stimulation that causes significant impairment of bodily function or actual tissue damage. Adaptive or protective reactions may become especially significant when an individual reacts to any stimulus that has been previously associated with dangerous situations or injuries. These reactions to symbols of danger are the same as those that might be expected from actual tissue damage but are initiated by nonpainful stimuli.

Whereas the threshold for perception of pain is the lowest intensity of stimulus that may be recognized and is approximately the same in all normal individuals, the threshold at which patients react to pain varies considerably. Emotionally disturbed patients and those who already have some degree of pain generally show a lower threshold of reaction than do normal individuals. A person's reaction to pain depends considerably upon the association that the individual makes in the higher brain centers between painful stimuli and the interpretation of pain. Inasmuch as the reaction to pain includes not only voluntary reactions, but also those mediated through the autonomic nervous system, it may readily be appreciated that pain has a large emotional, as well as a purely physical, component. This dual aspect of pain makes it somewhat difficult for the examiner to differentiate completely the pain sensation from the reaction of the patient to pain.

Pain is subjective in character, and the examiner must depend upon what the patient relates to him in terms of quality, time of occurrence, location, intensity, and reaction to the pain. It is essential that he attempt to get the patient to be objective in his description of his discomfort to the end that his reactions to the pain will be completely divorced from his description of actual pain sensations. When this is accomplished, the examiner will be able to more fully evaluate the precise nature and location of the pain. Thus the patient who is able to tell the examiner that he has pain associated with the lower first molar when he bites on that tooth rather than describing all of his reaction to the pain makes it much easier for the examiner to arrive at a diagnosis. In evaluating symptoms of a painful nature, it is essential that the examiner assist the patient in discriminating between pain itself and his reaction to pain.

The diagnosis of the sensations of pain must be based on anatomic, physiologic, and psychologic considerations. Pain impulses set up by noxious stimuli are received by specific receptors known as free nerve endings, which are scattered throughout the skin, mucous membranes, subcutaneous structures, and viscera. The impulses are carried through groups of myelinated and unmyelinated nerve fibers of various sizes at various speeds either directly to the posterior root ganglia in somatic nerves or indirectly in sympathetic trunks and through sympathetic ganglia to the posterior root ganglia via the white rami communicantes. The cell bodies of the sensory nerves, including those passing through the sympathetic chain, are located in the posterior root ganglia. From this area the dendrites or neurons enter the cord and penetrate to the region of the posterior horn. Here the impulses are shunted to a second neuron whose cell body is in the posterior horn. Pain impulses then cross to the opposite side of the cord and ascend to the lateral spinothalamic tract to the thalamus. These impulses then travel along additional neurons that extend to the postcentral area of the cerebral cortex.

Of special interest to the dentist is the transmission of sensory impulses by the peripheral branches of the trigeminal nerve. Pain impulses arising from pain-sensitive structures served by the peripheral branches of the trigeminal nerve are carried to the gasserian ganglion into the pons. In the pons the central fibers from the gasserian ganglion divide into short ascending and long descending branches. The long descending branches form the spinal tract of the trigeminal nerve and mediate all pain and temperature sensations. These branches terminate in the nucleus of the spinal tract in the medulla. Pain impulses are relayed from here to the thalamus and then to the sensory facial area from the postcentral gyrus of the cerebral cortex. The localization of perceived pain is most highly developed in the cerebral cortex, whereas the hypothalamus dictates the autonomic response and attitude of the patient to the noxious stimulant. Thus in the simplest conduction of the pain impulse, the spinal ganglionic, spinothalamic, and thalamocortical neurons take part. The cerebral cortex is necessary for the localization and evaluation of the intensity of the impulses, and the thalamus is important in the integration of pain.

Although all pain fibers enter the spinal cord through the dorsal root ganglion, the two varieties of pain known as superficial pain and deep pain have different routes of conduction by sensory fibers. Pain impulses from the surface of the body are generally carried in the somatic nerves and enter the spinal cord through the dorsal routes. This pathway is much more simple than that of the deep pain impulses, which are conducted to the cerebral nervous system by a variety of routes. Since deep-seated pain impulses may be carried by fibers attached to the blood vessels that join the autonomic nervous system, deep-seated pain may travel in association with autonomic nerves or with somatic nerves.

The quality of painful sensation depends to a large extent upon the origin of the stimulus. Several different clinically distinguishable qualities of pain have been found to exist: a bright, pricking pain, a burning pain, and a deeper-felt aching pain. The bright, pricking and burning pains have been associated with noxious stimulation of body surfaces. The bright, pricking pain is thought to be carried in thick, rapidly conducting myelinated fibers, whereas burning pain is thought to be carried by slower conducting fibers of a smaller size. Pricking of the gingiva with a sharp explorer usually gives rise to an initial sharp pain of abrupt onset with a pricking quality and is then followed by a pain of slower onset that has a burning quality. Not only may the quality of pain vary, but also its intensity. The quality of pain from the deeper tissues differs from that of cutaneous or superficial areas in that it is more diffuse and long lasting and may tend to radiate. It is also more likely to be associated with nausea, slowing of the pulse, and a fall in blood pressure. Whereas superficial pain is fairly well localized, deep pain with its duller aching nature is more diffuse in character and is less accurately perceived. Localiza-

tion of superficial pain varies according to the region, the number of sense organs present, and the frequency with which the organs are stimulated. Localization is highly developed in the hands, the lips, and tongue because of the abundance of sense organs and the amount of cortical training that has resulted from the identification of many objects. Localization of pain is poor in those areas in which there are but few sense organs and in which the cortical training necessary for the identification of objects is not well developed.

The localization of deep pain is likely to be poor and, in many instances, may be referred to a surface area of the body. Thus, pain from the teeth, jaws, temporomandibular joints, and other deep structures may be falsely localized and referred to the surface of the face. The exact mechanism of how this referral occurs is not well understood. The skin and mucous membranes may become abnormally sensitive to noxious stiimuli because of a lowering of the pain threshold or because of an alteration of the excitability of central pain pathways so that various stimuli evoke a more intense sensation. Hyperalgesia of the skin and mucous membranes associated with a lowering of the pain threshold may be seen with inflammation. Hyperalgesia associated with alteration of the excitability of the central pain pathways supplying the skin and mucous membranes is sometimes seen in association with referred pain.

The diagnosis of superficial pain is based upon its quality, cause, intensity, localization, site, distribution, and duration. Two types of superficial pain may be recognized: a rapidly conducted pricking sensation that is bright and sharply localized and a slowly conducted burning sensation that is less sharp but fairly well localized. Deep pain is characterized by its quality, poor localization, and spread, and by associated phenomena such as hyperalgesia, hyperesthesia, and tenderness. Deep pains are dull and aching in quality and are usually poorly localized. They have a tendency to spread to areas other than those that are stimulated. This spread may involve deep or superficial pathways or both and may give rise to "referred pain."

Two other types of pain that should be mentioned are central pain and psychogenic pain. "Central pain" arises in patients suffering from lesions of the thalamus or spinothalamic tracts. This type of pain is constant or recurrent in nature and is usually not well localized, and dysesthesia is readily elicited. Occasionally a patient will complain of pain for which no organic cause can be found. One must remember, however, that pain may be facilitated since perceptive centers in the brain may become hypersensitive after repeated stimulation. The patient who has had a pulpitis and still has the typical pain after the tooth has been removed presents an occasional problem to the dentist. The cortical threshold may be lower generally, as well as locally, and the effects of this may be seen in such individuals as neurasthenics who may be hypersensitive to any type of painful stimulus. One must also remember that psychoneurotic patients usually have a lower threshold of reaction to pain than do normal individuals.

Pain may arise from any of the pain-sensitive structures of the mouth and adjacent structures. Whether pain is produced is dependent upon the type of noxious stimulus and the pain sensitivity of the structures involved. A stimulus that may cause pain in the mucous membranes or skin may not produce pain in the muscles. The pain produced by a needle puncture of muscles is generally slight; however, it is severe in the presence of vascular disease or when the noxious stimulus is caused by injection of a hypertonic solution. Pain is produced in muscles when a spasm, such as trismus, or in muscular cramps such as might be produced by tetany. Subcutaneous fat gives little pain when pierced by a needle or when it is cut, but if cutaneous

nerves passing through the fat are injured, considerable pain may be perceived. Needle puncture of deep fascia is always painful. Tendons and the periosteum are sensitive to needle pricks or hypertonic solutions, and pain is a prominent feature of periostitis. Compact bone may be cut without pain, but pain may be produced when cancellous bone is cut. Joints are insensitive to a needle prick, knife cut, or cautery, but the synovial membrane is sensitive to inflammation, hypertonic solutions, and needle pricks. The arteries and veins may react painfully to needle puncture.

No pain sensations can be elicited from the enamel, but the dentin is somewhat sensitive, and the pulp is extremely sensitive to noxious stimuli. Free nerve endings are the only nerve receptors found in the pulp, and for this reason the pulp registers only pain regardless of the stimulus. Other complex receptors that register touch, cold, heat, pressure, and position sense are found throughout the oral mucosa, periodontal membrane, muscles, and adjacent structures. Pain associated with pulpitis is difficult to localize and may be referred to almost any area on the same side of the face supplied by the trigeminal nerve. Where pulpitis has involved the apical area of the tooth, localization of the area of involvement will be possible because of the stimulation of the other complex receptors in the periodontal membrane. Even in these instances the ability to localize pain varies considerably from one individual to another. Unfortunately, the lack of localization of a diseased pulp has led to the extraction of many healthy teeth. Inasmuch as pain may be referred from other regions to the teeth, jaws, and temporomandibular joints, patients may come to the dentist or be referred to the dentist under the misconception that the teeth must be at fault. Thus it is not uncommon for a patient to insist upon the extraction of a particular tooth upon which a fixation has been made when in reality the pain is referred from

may also produce purpuric areas in the mouth.

Frank bleeding associated with scaling procedures and extractions may be related to defects in those factors concerned with the coagulation of blood. This may be related to a qualitative deficiency or a quantitative deficiency of blood platelets, a deficiency of platelet thromboplastin, a lack of vitamin K, liver damage, drug intoxications, a decrease in fibrinogen, and an anticoagulant in the blood. This last occurs frequently as the result of anticoagulant therapy in the treatment and prevention of coronary thrombosis. The patient's history is the most useful instrument in the prevention of hemorrhagic accidents from dental procedure. A past history of excessive bleeding should alert the examiner to an appraisal of a bleeding tendency. In the absence of a history of bleeding, the examiner must rely on the signs and symptoms of disorders that point to a hemorrhagic tendency. If these are found, an examination of the blood is indicated. Examination of the blood should show coagulation time, prothrombin time, bleeding time, platelet count, and clot retraction. The tourniquet test is also important. These tests may be carried out by qualified personnel in the dental office or by a physician to whom the patient is referred. In most instances the referral procedure will be the most expedient for a general dental practitioner.

Alteration of weight

Excessive gain or loss of weight, especially of recent origin, is of more importance to the dentist than whether a patient meets the optimum for height, build, and age. Any deviation from normal as expressed in terms of recent gain or loss of weight suggests the introduction of a new factor in the life of the patient. This may be the manifestation of disease or of physiologic adaptation to the individual's environment.

The most common cause of an increase in weight in childhood is that of normal growth and development. Pregnancy is another cause of physiologic increase in weight. Overeating is another factor in weight increase that must be considered in evaluating deviations from normal. Of considerable significance are those increases in weight caused by metabolic and hormonal disturbances. Renal disturbances (nephrotic syndrome), congestive heart failure with water and salt retention, and glandular disturbances may bear an important relationship to increases in weight. Hormonal disturbances that may be responsible for excessive weight include hypothyroidism, hypogonadism, pituitary or adrenal disease, and adiposogenital dystrophy.

Recent weight loss may be digestive, hormonal, neoplastic, anorectic, pharmacologic, or psychogenic in origin. Digestive causes include vitamin deficiencies, diarrhea, vomiting, disturbances in mastication and deglutition, and dietary fads. Neoplastic disease of the digestive tract or of other areas may affect digestion with a resultant loss of weight. Hormonal disturbances include hyperthyroidism, diabetes mellitus, Addison's disease, and Simmonds' disease. Loss of appetite may accompany anxiety, pain, anorexigenic drugs, and excessive smoking and alcoholism. Loss of weight may also result from drug therapy.

Lesions

Objective signs of disease include those morphologic alterations of the soft tissues that are characteristic enough to be classified as specific lesions. Most lesions may be grouped into certain categories because of their rather consistent similar morphology, pattern of distribution, time of occurrence, duration, and presence of associated symptoms. The alteration in morphology of the tissue is so characteristic in many lesions that they may be classified as basic or *primary* types of lesions. Primary lesions may not retain their initial appearance and may be altered by trauma, mastication, maceration, movement of the tissues, and time itself. Those lesions that appear consecutively to the primary lesions are known as *secondary* lesions.

The diagnosis of many oral diseases is based upon the recognition of primary lesions. Because of the character of the oral mucosa, the primary lesions are not always as clear cut as those appearing on the skin. In many instances, however, the oral lesions will be a part of the overall skin picture, and a referral to the skin will assist in making a more reliable evaluation of the oral lesions. Because of the rapid changes that occur to the initial primary lesions, secondary lesions are the most common lesions observed in the mouth. In an evaluation of any lesion in the mouth, the examiner must keep in mind those factors that might produce alteration in the primary lesions. An adequate history of the lesions may serve to indicate to the examiner what the initial lesion might have been.

Primary lesions. There are at least eight types of primary lesions that may occur in the mouth and on the skin in disease: macules, papules, nodules, vesicles, bullae, tumors, keratoses, and wheals.

Macules are flat, circumscribed alterations of tissue that may vary in size, color, and shape. The size varies from that of a pinhead to several centimeters. The color may vary from red and brown to white. Those of vascular origin are red to brown-red in color and may be called erythematous macules. Macules resulting from blood pigment (petechiae and ecchymoses) give

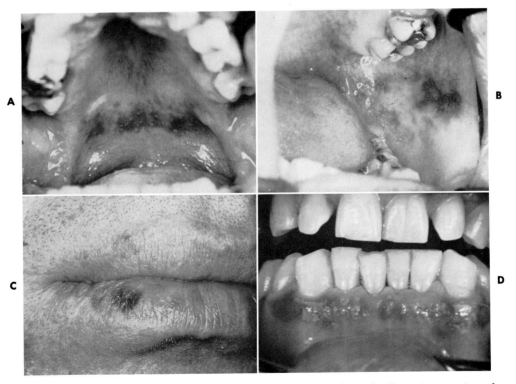

Fig. 2-1. *Macules.* **A,** Ecchymosis associated with constant coughing. **B,** Hyperpigmentation of buccal mucosa in Addison's disease. **C,** Hyperpigmentation associated with chronic trauma. **D,** Physiologic pigmentation of the gingiva (melanosis gingivae).

rise to varying colors of red to brown in the oral mucosa. The erythematous macule represents simple erythema and is caused by a localized congestion in the vascular bed; the color will fade on pressure. Petechiae and ecchymoses result from hemorrhage into the tissues; the color will not disappear on pressure. Pigmentary macules are brown to black in color and may be physiologic or pathologic in character. Examples of physiologic pigmentation are ephelides (freckles) and melanosis (melanoplakia); pathologic pigmentation may be seen in Addison's disease and in intestinal polyposis (Peutz-Jeghers syndrome). Macules may be transitory or permanent in character and vary in shape from circular, polygonal, and linear to polymorphous forms (Fig. 2-1).

Papules are circumscribed superficial elevated areas varying in size from a pinhead to about 5 mm. in area. They may be flat, conical, circular, and pointed to umbilicated. They vary in color from red, yellow, and white to bluish-red. The shape of the base may vary from round to more or less polygonal. The most common papule found in the mouth is that of lichen planus. Both the papule and the macule may provoke itching, burning sensations, or pain, or they may produce no symptoms at all either on the skin or on the mucous membrane. The

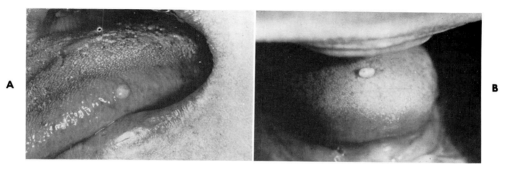

Fig. 2-2. *Papules.* **A,** Small raised lesion on the tongue caused by accidental biting. **B,** Traumatic hyperplasia of a fungiform papilla.

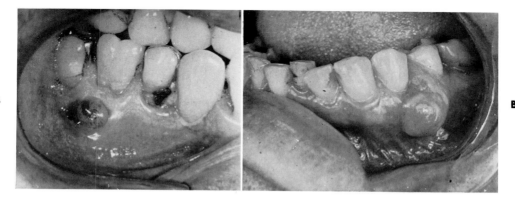

Fig. 2-3. *Nodules.* **A,** Resolving granuloma pyogenicum; other similar lesions of varying sizes include reactive lesions such as fibroid epulis, traumatic fibroma, and fibroepithelial papilloma. **B,** Parulis or so-called gumboil associated with pulpitis of the maxillary first molar.

surface may be eroded or overlaid with moist epithelial desquamations (Fig. 2-2).

Nodules are enlarged papules that are usually deep seated and involve the submucosa or lower dermis in the skin. They may also be slightly elevated above the surrounding mucosa. They may be traumatic in origin or may be associated with rheumatoid arthritis, leprosy, and syphilis (Fig. 2-3).

Vesicles are circumscribed single or grouped elevations of epithelium of the skin or mucous membrane beneath or within which are collections of serum, plasma, or blood. The surface may be flat, globoid, or umbilicated and may be tense or flaccid in character. Where vesicles have not rup-

tured spontaneously or as the result of trauma, they may be seen characteristically in primary herpetic stomatitis, herpes simplex, herpes zoster, and varicella (Fig. 2-4).

Pustules are vesicles that predominantly contain pus (for example, impetigo).

Bullae or blebs are similar to vesicles except that bullae are larger and more deep seated and the roof of the cavity is more resistant to rupture than the vesicle (Fig. 2-5). For this reason they are seen somewhat more frequently as primary lesions than vesicles. Bullae may be seen in pemphigus, Behçet's syndrome, and Stevens-Johnson syndrome or as the sequelae of trauma. The oral mucosa is commonly the first site to be

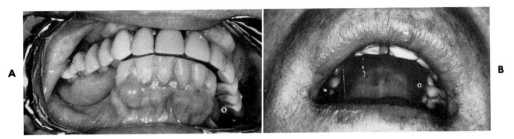

Fig. 2-4. *Vesicles.* **A,** Note the large vesicle located on the gingiva adjacent to the mandibular right cuspid. Its rupture will leave an ulcer like that seen in Fig. 2-11, *D;* its size approaches that of a bulla, and it is filled with a somewhat cloudy fluid. **B,** Small vesicle located on the upper lip characteristic of those seen in the early stages of primary herpetic stomatitis.

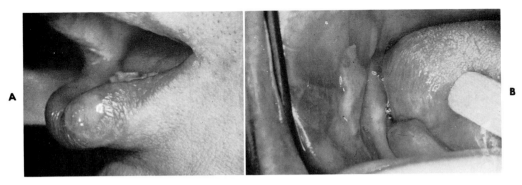

Fig. 2-5. *Bullae.* **A,** Bulla on the lower lip resulting from thermal injury; the character of the lesion differentiates it from a mucous retention cyst. **B,** Like most vesicles or bullae seen in the oral cavity, the one shown here has the collapsed roof; because of the deep involvement, the roof of a bulla tends to remain intact.

involved in certain types of pemphigus even though the skin may be completely normal. Consequently it may be the alert dentist who may make the original diagnosis. The bullae of pemphigus, unlike the bullae of other disorders such as erythema multiforme, usually do not have an erythematous areola at the border of the lesion. Rubbing a nonvesiculated area may result in the formation of a vesicle or denudation of the mucosa or epidermis (Nikolsky's sign).

"Tumor," "cyst," "epulis," "exostosis," "torus," "papilloma," and "polyp" are terms used to describe variously sized and shaped growths that have the common clinical characteristics of tumescence (Fig. 2-6). These lesions may be reactive or neoplastic in character. Etymologically the term "tumor" merely means swelling; however, its

present-day widespread usage to mean neoplasm or inflammatory enlargement has led to some confusion. More often than not the term is used to mean neoplastic disease. In view of the many blastomatoid, reactive, or nonneoplastic inflammatory enlargements that are present in the mouth, the use of the term "tumor" to describe these lesions does not appear to be justified. Although many lesions that are generally nonneoplastic in character are characterized by tumescence, their clinical classification as tumors should be reserved until microscopic examination reveals their true identity. The examination of lesions that are characterized by tumescence should be directed toward the history of the lesion and its clinical features.

Thus one may speak of a lesion clinically in terms of tumescence, shape, size, base,

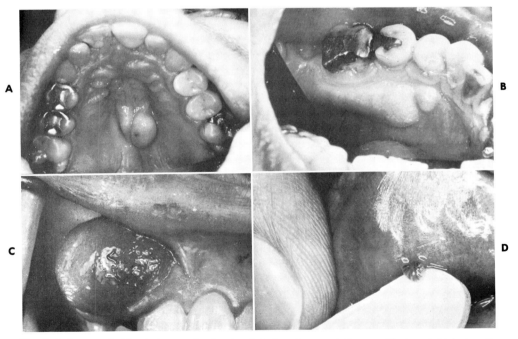

Fig. 2-6. *Tumors.* **A,** The lesion on the hard palate is a torus palatinus, a blastomatoid lesion. **B,** The same type of bony tumescence on the mandible is called a torus mandibularis. **C,** A large soft tissue mass involving the alveolar mucosa and attached gingiva. The true nature of this type of lesion can only be determined by biopsy; its size clearly denotes its designation as a tumor. **D,** A small fibroepithelial papilloma.

surface texture, and the form it may resemble. Tumefaction or tumidity refers to a swelling or the state of being swollen or edematous. The base of the lesion may be sessile, pedunculated, or stalked; "sessile" means attached by a broad base; "pedunculated" means that the lesion is provided with a peduncle, pedicle, or a stem; "polypoid" merely means that the morbid enlargement resembles a "polypus," which is a broad descriptive term for a smooth and pedunculated epithelial tumor arising from a mucous surface.

The term "papilloma" refers to a small nipple-shaped epithelial tumor in which the cells cover fingerlike processes of stroma. "Papillomatous" refers to a morbid enlargement resembling a papilloma. Though the terms "polyp" and "papilloma" have rather specific microscopic connotations and usually imply tumor in a neoplastic sense, the terms "polypoid" and "papillomatous" are somewhat less specific and may be used for clinical description of lesions regardless of their true nature. In general, a polypoid mass is attached by a more or less narrow peduncle and is rather spherical in shape; the attachment of a papillomatous mass is of the same dimensions as the mass itself, which is usually longer than it is wide. The clinical use of "polypoid" or "papillomatoid" (papillomatous) should in no way suggest the microscopic diagnosis of polyp or papilloma. The use of the term "papillomatous" or "papillomatoid" eliminates the necessity for referring to those nonneoplas-

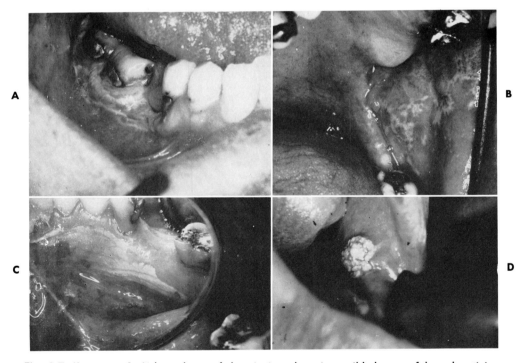

Fig. 2-7. *Keratoses.* **A,** Lichen planus of the gingiva; there is a mild degree of hyperkeratinization present. **B,** Lichen planus of the buccal mucosa; the lacelike network is rather characteristic; only slight hyperkeratinization is present. **C,** Diffuse hyperkeratosis on lingual aspects of the mandible with raised and somewhat smooth surface; this is characteristic of early leukoplakia. **D,** Focal hyperkeratotic lesion presenting a verrucous surface. The malignant possibilities of this type of lesion are obvious; this type of lesion should be biopsied (excisional).

tic inflammatory enlargements as "papillomas," which implies a neoplastic character.

The surface of a lesion may be warty (verruciform or verrucous), papillate (filiform or fungiform), keratotic, ulcerated, fissured, or desquamated or flat, pointed, or horny, and the base of a lesion may be sessile or pedunculated.

Keratosis refers to an abnormal thickening of the outer layers of the epithelium of the mucous membrane or the skin. Keratinization of the mucous membranes usually takes place only on the gingiva in the mouth and never reaches the proportion that may be seen on the skin except in pathologic conditions (Fig. 2-7). Keratotic lesions of the mouth may vary in color from grayish-white to white or brown, depending upon the amount of extrinsic pigmentation present. Hyperkeratinization of the mucous membrane may be localized, circumscribed, focal, or diffuse in character. Common kera-

totic lesions of the mouth include focal hyperkeratosis, nicotine stomatitis, lichen planus, and leukoplakia. Chronic cheek biting, focal hyperkeratosis, and nicotine stomatitis are probably the most common forms of hyperkeratotic lesions in the mouth. Keratosis may be primary in origin, as in lichen planus, or secondary to trauma, as in nicotine stomatitis. The latter type of keratinization may be considered as a secondary lesion (Fig. 2-8).

Secondary lesions. These lesions are the most common found in the oral cavity and include erosions (excoriations), ulcers, fissures, cicatrices, and desquamations.

Erosions. Erosions are a kind of ulceration or loss of substance such as that produced on the skin or mucous membrane by trauma or as a sequel to primary lesions. They are usually superficial in nature and may be circumscribed, punctate, linear, or irregular in form. These lesions involve a

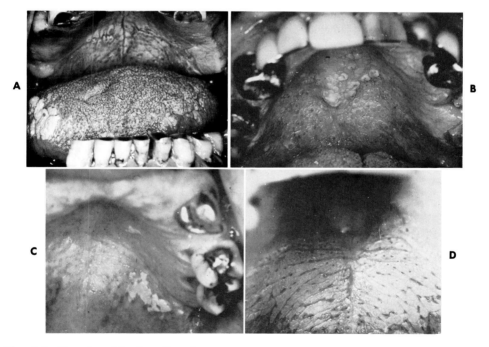

Fig. 2-8. *Hyperkeratinization.* Hyperkeratinization associated with nicotine stomatitis. **B,** The raised, punctate orifices of the mucous glands.

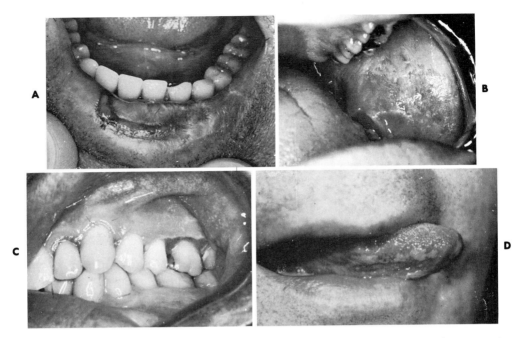

Fig. 2-9. *Erosions.* **A,** Solar cheilitis with linear-shaped erosion. **B,** Maceration and erosion of buccal mucosa caused by cheek chewing. **C,** Erosion of gingiva around first molar caused by overzealous use of a rubber tip stimulator. **D,** Erosion secondary to drug reaction (codeine).

loss of the outer layers of the mucosa and leave no scar on healing. Erosions in the mouth are usually moist in character and represent the necrosis and loss of the outer layers of the mucous membrane. Thus, moist erosions may be seen secondary to the collapse of vesicles and blebs or after the necrosis of the outer layers of the mucous membrane as in erosive lichen planus, desquamative gingivitis, or after traumatic wounds (Fig. 2-9).

Fissures. Fissures are any clefts or grooves in the tissue that are normal or pathologically present. They may be superficial or deep, linear, radiating, longitudinal, or transverse. It is not unusual for these cracks or fissures to become inflamed. They occur frequently at the mucocutaneous junction of the mouth where extensibility of the tissue is essential to accomplish the necessary movements of the tissue (Fig. 2-10). Fissuring of the surface of the tongue

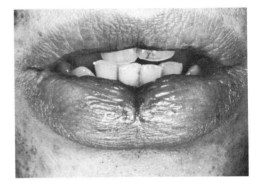

Fig. 2-10. *Fissure.* Developmental fissure with chronic ulceration.

is seen frequently and is not accompanied with inflammatory change unless the grooves are quite deep and accumulations of debris and bacteria occur. Scrotal tongue angular cheilitis, and syphilitic rhagades show fissuring.

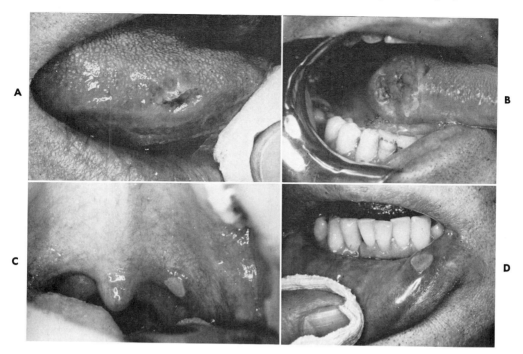

Fig. 2-11. *Ulcers.* **A,** Traumatic ulcer from biting the tongue—healing stage. **B,** Persistent traumatic ulcer with superimposed pyogenic infection. **C** and **D,** Recurrent herpetic ulcers.

Ulcers. Ulcers are defects of the skin or mucous membrane that are deeper than erosions or excoriations in that they extend to the tissue beneath the epithelium. Ulcers should be examined for their size, depth, contour, base, edge, floor, secretion, duration, pain, evolution, and involution. The edges of an ulcer may be ragged, punched out in appearance, undermined, or everted. The base may be soft or indurated and its floor smooth, granular, glazed, pus covered, or hemorrhagic. Ulcers may be acute or chronic in nature and may be shallow or deep in character. The outline of the ulcer may be circular, serpiginous, ovoid, crescentic, or irregular. Ulcers may result from physical agents such as heat or cold, chemical agents such as acids or alkalies, traumatic agents such as sharp teeth, dry toast, toothbrush bristles, or foreign objects in the mouth. They may appear secondarily to primary lesions or as a result of disease,

either local or systemic in origin. Ulcers may be painless or indolent, or they may be extremely sensitive. Ulcers in the mouth are seen most commonly in association with acute necrotizing ulcerative gingivitis, herpetic gingivostomatitis, and herpes simplex and as a result of traumatic agents (Figs. 2-11 to 2-13).

Pseudomembranes. Pseudomembranes may form on the mucosal surfaces as a result of pseudomembranous inflammation. The formation of a false membrane is a response of the mucous surfaces to a necrotizing agent. Because of the loss of surface epithelium, plasma exudes from the vessels and spreads on the eroded surface where it coagulates, enclosing necrotic epithelium in its fibrinous network. This occurs in acute necrotizing ulcerative gingivostomatitis; it may also be seen in diphtheria (Fig. 2-12, *C* and *D*).

Eschars. Eschars are masses of dead tis-

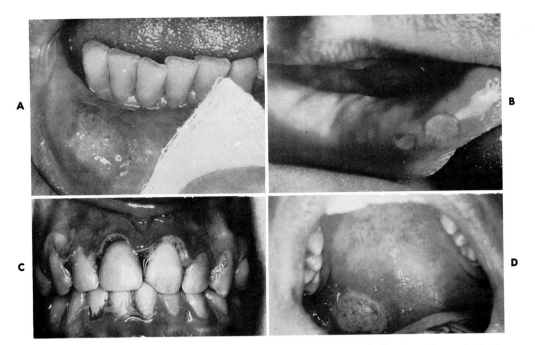

Fig. 2-12. *Ulcers.* **A,** Periadenitis mucosae necrotica recurrens—early healing phase. **B,** Periadenitis—late healing phase. **C,** Acute necrotizing ulcerative gingivostomatitis. **D,** Acute necrotizing ulcerative gingivostomatitis—palatal lesion.

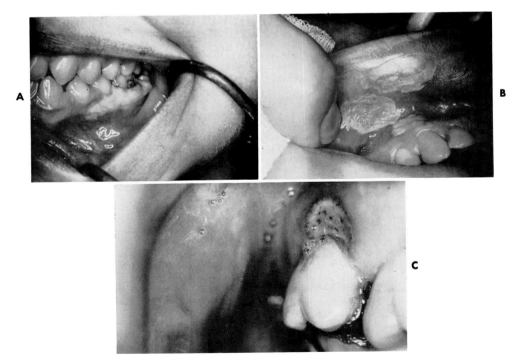

Fig. 2-13. *Eschars.* **A,** Coagulation of buccal gingiva by phenol. **B,** Aspirin-induced mucosal necrosis; note two areas of contact, one on gingiva and one on buccal mucosa. **C,** Herpetic ulcer with secondary slough produced by silver nitrate.

sue or sloughs produced by burning or chemical corrosives. Phenol and cresol may cause a firm, thick, dull-gray to brown eschar. "Aspirin burn" and phenol eschar appear white initially. Loss of the necrotic tissue leads to an ulcer. The laying down of fibin on the injured surfaces may lead to a pseudomembrane. Phenol and "aspirin" eschars are the most common type seen in the mouth (Fig. 2-13, *A* and *B*).

Desquamation. Desquamation is a shedding of epithelial elements in scales or sheets that vary in size and shape and that may or may not cover an erosion. In general, scales occur as a result of inflammation. In the mouth, scales do not tend to accumulate as on the skin but are lost because of the continual wetting by the saliva. However, certain lesions such as leukoplakia and focal hyperkeratosis accumulate thick shiny masses of scales that give the lesion a grayish white color (Fig. 2-14).

Crusts are the dry products of exudates from lesions occurring on the skin and lips. They do not usually appear in the mouth because of the maceration by saliva; however, they may be associated with scales and are termed moist desquamations. Crusts of the skin and lips are composed of pus, blood, dried serum, epithelial debris, and extraneous matter. The color varies according to the composition of the crust and may be yellowish to brown, depending upon the amount of pus or blood present. Crusts on the skin may be deep seated or superficial, whereas those of the lips tend to be superficial in character. Crusting appears most often on the lips of individuals exposed to the weather. Constant drying leads to crusting of lesions present on the

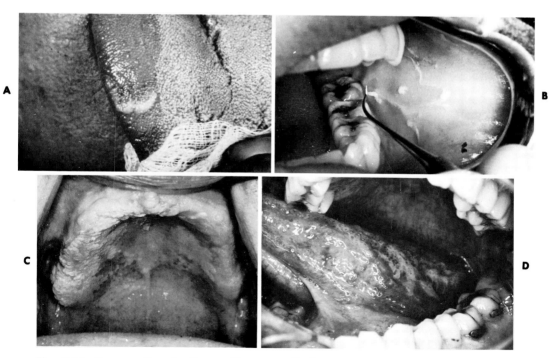

Fig. 2-14. *Desquamation.* **A,** Geographic tongue. **B,** Desquamation in dentifrice stomatitis. **C,** Desquamative hyperkeratosis associated with heavy smoking. **D,** Desquamation of tongue secondary to irradiation.

lips. Such crusts tend to crack, fissure, and bleed because of the constant trauma associated with speaking and mastication. Crusts are seen commonly at the mucocutaneous junction of the lips in angular cheilitis, vesicular and bullous lesions, traumatic ulcers, and carcinomas (Fig. 2-15).

Crusts form only if conditions permit drying of coagulated blood, tissue fluids, and debris. Crusting does not occur on the moist surfaces of the mucous membranes; however, if the blood, serum, and debris become coagulated and entrapped in a fibrinous meshwork, a moist membranelike mass may cover an eroded surface. This may generally be scraped away to leave a bleeding surface. The surfaces of vesicles and bullae may collapse and cover the underlying tissue; they may be adherent or slough off in a short period of time. When the membranous covering is lost, bleeding occurs, and a new pseudomembrane is formed (Fig. 2-13, *C*).

In addition to having an abstract descriptive knowledge of primary and secondary lesions, an examiner should also be able to detect and describe any lesion present in the mouth. Before a lesion can be related to one of the primary or secondary types of lesions, a systematic examination of the lesion must be made. First, one must determine whether the present appearance of the lesion represents a lesion in its pure form (natural history) or if it is the result of involution or additional complications such as scratching, treatment, or injury, and whether multiple lesions are generalized or local in character. In addition, the color, shape, size, arrangement, base, and consistency of lesions should be noted carefully. When the objective symptoms are described, it is then possible to identify a lesion as a primary or secondary type of lesion. When the student becomes aware of basic differences in lesions of the oral cavity and is able to describe those lesions that are present, he will be able to utilize effectively the subjective information collected from the history and those facts collected in the clinical examination so that little difficulty will be experienced in arriving at a diagnosis. A knowledge of the type of presenting lesion does not unequivocally designate a specific disease. However, it does serve to orient the examiner to a particular field of inquiry that may in itself be narrow enough to permit a relatively easy differential diagnosis. For example, when an examiner identifies the presence of a predominating vesicular or bullous eruption, he knows in a broad sense that he may be dealing with a virus infection. Many diseases of viral origin can be named, but it is not our purpose here to do so since these can be found in almost any text of oral medicine or internal medicine; rather it is

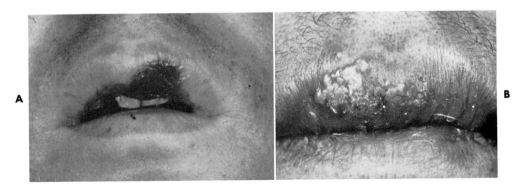

Fig. 2-15. *Crusts.* **A,** Syphilitic chancre; note deformity of the lip and serosanguineous crust. **B,** Crusted herpes labialis; note the conglomerate character of the lesion.

suggested that the examiner should at this time analyze his subjective and objective findings. Thus it might have been said that examples of virus infections are chicken pox, smallpox, herpes zoster, herpes labialis, and other distributions of herpetic eruptions. However, one must remember that physical agents such as poison ivy, poison, metals, or other irritative allergenic agents may also produce vesicles. Further, local parasites, infections such as impetigo, vesicular eczema, and scabies may also produce vesicular lesions. It is not expected that the student of oral diagnosis will be familiar with all possible diseases that may have vesicular eruptions, nor is it necessary to expect it since effective and efficient use of reference material allows a diagnosis to be made and at the same time enhances the training of the examiner.

REFERENCES

Adson, A. W.: Neuralgias of the face; diagnosis and treatment, J. Int. Coll. Surg. 11:1-8, 1948.

Agnew, R. G., and others: Pain problems in the practice of dentistry: a symposium, J.A.D.A. 53:528-542, 1956.

Allen, A. C.: The skin; a clinicopathologic treatise, ed. 2, New York, 1967, Grune & Stratton Inc., pp. 1182, viii.

Alling, C. C. (editor): Facial pain, Philadelphia, 1968, Lea & Febiger.

Barison, H. L., and Wang, S. C.: Physiology and pharmacology of vomiting, Pharmacol. Rev. 5: 193, 1953.

Bondy, P. K.: Gain and loss of weight. In Harrison, T. R. (editor): Principles of internal medicine, New York, 1954, McGraw-Hill Book Co., Chap. 24.

Bonica, J. J.: Management of pain, Philadelphia, 1953, Lea & Febiger.

Christie, R. V.: Dyspnea: a review, Quart. J. Med. 7:421, 1938.

Cushing, H.: The major trigeminal neuralgias: the varieties of facial neuralgia, Amer. J. Med. Sci. 160:157, 1920.

DuBois, E. F.: Fever and regulation of body temperature, Springfield, Ill., 1948, Charles C Thomas, Publisher.

Engel, G. L.: Fainting, J. Mount Sinai Hosp. N. Y. 12:170, 1945.

Friedman, M.: Functional cardiovascular disease, Baltimore, 1947, The Williams & Wilkins Co.

Harrison, T. R. (editor): Principles of internal medicine. Part II, Cardinal manifestations of disease, New York, 1954, McGraw-Hill Book Co.

Judge, R. D., and Zuidema, G. D.: Physical diagnosis; a physiologic approach to the clinical examination, ed. 2, Boston, 1968, Little, Brown & Co., pp. 465 xiv.

Lozner, E. L.: Differential diagnosis, pathogenesis, and treatment of thrombocytopenic purpuras, Amer. J. Med. 14:459, 1953.

McAuliff, G. W., Goodell, H., and Wolff, H. G.: Experimental studies on headache; pain from the nasal and paranasal structures, Proc. Ass. Res. Nerv. Ment. Dis. 23:185, 1943.

Robertson, S., Goodell, H., and Wolff, H. G.: Headache: The teeth as a source of headache and other pain, Arch. Neurol. Psychiat. 57:277, 1947.

Stead, E. A.: Fainting, Amer. J. Med. 13:387, 1952.

Tumulty, P. A.: The patient with fever of undetermined origin; a diagnostic challenge, Johns Hopkins Med. J. 120:95-106, Feb., 1967.

Ungerleider, H. E., and Gubner, R.: Extrasystoles and the mechanism of palpitation, Trans. Amer. Therap. Soc. 41:1, 1941.

Wolff, H. G.: Headache and other head pain, New York, 1948, Oxford University Press, Inc.

Wolff, H. G., and Wolf, S.: Pain, Springfield, Ill., 1948, Charles C Thomas, Publisher.

3

Case history

Taking a history is probably one of the most important parts of the examination of a patient, yet it is generally the least understood and most undervalued prerequisite to the process of formulating a diagnosis that exists today in the practice and teaching of clinical dentistry. The case history constitutes the foundation not only for an intelligent approach to diagnosis, but also for the establishment of a successful patient-dentist relationship. Only from an accurately taken and carefully interpreted history can diverse symptoms of disease be grouped into a meaningful pattern. All too often a diagnosis or the chance to prevent gross pathologic alterations by disease is missed because the examiner fails to uncover the earliest and detectable clues to disease. This may be largely avoided if the subjective sensations of the patient are brought out in a history. To attempt to make a diagnosis without systemically utilizing the patient's knowledge of the disease is not unlike the proverbial stories about a ship without a rudder.

There are occasions when it appears that a diagnosis is plainly evident by inspection alone; however, three important considerations are likely to be overlooked without at least a brief history: (1) coexistent disease may be present that will go undetected unless the patient is allowed to express his complaints, (2) the attitude of the patient, which is so important to the establishment of rapport, is often disregarded, and (3) all too often a diagnosis may appear to be obvious, yet it may be masking a serious and extensive disease.

A case history need not be extensive; it may consist of only a few questions if adequate coverage is thereby provided. However, it must be pointed out that the art of taking a history entails a knowledge of how extensive a history should be for any given occasion. This ability requires practice, and the diagnostic acumen of a clinician is generally directly related to his ability as a historian. There are at least two instances when a case history should be extensive, detailed, and arranged not only to cover the patient's immediate complaint, but also to include all historical facts relating to the patient's oral and systemic health: (1) all case histories taken by a student for training in oral diagnosis should be as complete as possible until such time as he demonstrates his ability to reduce the length and coverage, yet still have an adequate history, and (2) a case history that is to be the basis for periodic follow-up health examinations should initially be as thorough and complete as possible irrespective of lack of apparent relationship to the patient's complaint.

The approach to the patient is as important to the case history as the interpretation of the findings, since the information obtained is dependent upon the proper rapport between the patient and the clinician. Obtaining a case history is a procedure that requires the utilization of all the knowledge and experience a dentist has accumulated from his basic science and clinical training. This history is often called the subjective examination of the patient since it contains information that the patient tells the historian. Each case history presents the dentist with circumstances that are unlike any of his other cases, yet similarity between cases is often the basis for sound judgment and diagnosis. Obtaining a history provides the dentist with an opportunity to hear the patient's complaints and symptoms and also to determine his general health and well-being. It provides clues to diagnosis, focuses attention to specific areas in need of comprehensive evaluation, and alerts the dentist to the need of special precautions he must use in carrying out treatment procedures.

A case history should be brief and concise, yet it should contain all of the information required by a given situation. Unfortunately, no shortcut is available for the inexperienced historian to assure brevity and accuracy; however, a uniform procedure will ensure the inclusion of all the necessary details. The historian must direct the patient toward the subject at hand at all times, condensing and sorting the pertinent information from the irrelevant. A history that is lengthy and poorly organized is a time-wasting procedure and usually discourages further efforts.

The procedure is primarily a diagnostic effort; however, most patients will be favorably impressed with the interest shown in their health by the dentist. The confidence of the patient is often won during the first meeting with the patient, and since the history is usually taken on the patient's first visit to the dentist, it provides the dentist with an adequate opportunity to develop proper rapport with his patient. Though primarily a diagnostic procedure, a thorough, well-written case history often serves as evidence of professional competence in medicolegal cases. Errors of treatment by the dentist vary from those which cause minor inconvenience to the patient to those of a very serious nature; most of the errors may be predicted from information in the case history.

There should be no necessity for justifying history taking. As a diagnostic procedure it is invaluable, as a legal aid it is important, and as a factor in the improvement of patient relations it is most satisfying.

A clear understanding of the objectives of a case history will guide and improve the efforts of any practitioner (1) to arrive at a tentative diagnosis of the patient's chief complaint, (2) to determine any systemic factor that might affect the formulation of a diagnosis, and (3) to determine any systemic condition that requires special precaution prior to or during dental procedures to protect the health and life of the patient. Advantages of obtaining a case history include establishment of a written record that will serve as a diagnostic instrument, protection of the dentist from possible disease contact, establishment of a basis for future reference, and provision of a document that will serve as legal evidence of professional competence.

The basic method for history taking is that of the direct interview with the patient. In the direct interview the historian questions the patient in an orderly fashion, following a basic pattern of questions. He makes notes during the interview and afterward compiles the important information he has obtained. Other methods have been devised that are intended to decrease the time needed for the interview. Two such timesaving methods are the use of a printed questionnaire and the use of a printed checklist of information. Whatever the method used, it must serve the purpose of obtaining important information.

APPROACH TO THE PATIENT

The technic of history taking involves the dentist's initial behavior with the patient and the development of rapport with the patient. The interview should be more than the mere recording of answers to a set of questions; it must establish confidence and induce the patient to reveal eventually all the details relative to his or her illness. The attitude of the examiner must impart to his patient that he is not hurried and that he is completely interested in the patient's welfare. To establish confidence, the examiner must be patient and sympathetic and explain all the factors relative to any question he is asking; he must never express surprise or shock at anything the patient may reveal, and he must be able to talk in terms that the patient will understand and with which he will feel at ease. If the patient appears to be embarrassed, shows evidence of emotion, or hesitates to answer a question, it is obvious that the question touches strongly on the patient's emotional life and probably will have to be delayed until a later time. The examiner should sympathetically endeavor to have the patient express his complaints in simple language unadorned by a self-diagnosis derived from past experiences of friends.

To examine children, one needs to gain their confidence. Initially, too much attention should not be given to the child; it helps to place children at ease in the dental office if the dentist appears busy. Questions of a general nature may be asked first to establish the interest of the child, and then later, when this has been accomplished, questions relating to the history may be asked more effectively. Questions regarding the chief complaint and the present illness are better answered by the child, whereas questions regarding past history, family history, and social history are best answered in cooperation with a parent.

PLAN OF HISTORY TAKING

The taking of a history should be systematic and should follow a definite outline. Following a definite order either mentally or with a written outline tends to prevent the omission of pertinent information that might otherwise be forgotten. By placing the patient's complaint first, the patient is permitted to recount the complaint and symptoms that brought him to the examiner. The following outline is one commonly used in taking a history:

Chief complaint
Usually the answer to the question, What prompted you to seek dental treatment? should be limited to a word, phrase, or sentence

Present illness
Chronologic account of the patient's chief complaint and related symptoms; should include all relevant material since the time of onset of the complaint

Past history
All material of a nature to reveal the patient's dental and general health prior to the onset of the present illness; should include constitutional diseases, serious illnesses, manifestations of allergic states, and accident or operations

Family history
General health of family, history of mental disease, cause of death of parents if deceased, history of chronic infectious diseases in the family, history of dental problems in the family, etc.

Personal and social history
Marital status: Duration, health of partners, pregnancies, number of children, etc.
Habits: Use of drugs and medicines, tobacco, biting habits, and other oral habits
Occupation: Exposure to occupational hazards, working schedule as related to dental appointments, type of work, etc.
Personality: Moody, inclined to worry, complaining, meticulous, sociable easygoing, etc.
Weight: Recent loss or gain of weight with possible causes

Systems review
Head:
  Headache
  Eyes: Vision, diplopia, inflammatory disease
  Ears: Hearing, tinnitus, vertigo
  Nose: Obstruction, epistaxis, frequent "colds"
  Throat: Hoarseness, tonsillitis, sore throat
Cardiorespiratory: Chest pain, dyspnea, orthopnea, angina, palpitations, murmurs, hemoptysis, cough, night sweats, rheumatic fever
Gastrointestinal: Digestion, mastication, sore tongue, sore gums, saliva, occlusion, toothaches, devitalization of teeth, extractions, appliances, pyorrhea, nausea, vomiting, diarrhea, and abdominal pain
Genitourinary: Dysuria, nocturia, hematuria, oliguria, polyuria, edema
Catamenia: Menopause, menorrhagia, metrorrhagia, dysmenorrhea, menarche
Neuromuscular: Paresthesia, anesthesia, paralysis convulsions, neuralgias, arthritis, joint pains, limitation of motion, tremors, luxation and subluxation of mandible, centric relation, centric occlusion, closure pattern

The case history should follow this or a

similar outline so that the examiner covers a certain minimum field of information that in itself may call attention to the patient's symptoms and significant items of past history as well as facilitate the oral interview and establish rapport with the patient. The following elaboration of the outline has for its objective the presentation of all the facts that may have influenced the patient's health up to the time of the interview.

Chief complaint(s), symptom(s)

The chief complaint is a symptom or symptoms described by the patient in his own words relating to the presence of an abnormal condition. It is not necessarily answered by the question, Why did you come to the dental clinic? because the patient's answer may be, I need a checkup, I want a bridge, or My dentist told me to come. These should not be used as chief complaints because they are not symptoms. There is usually a reason *why* a patient believes he needs a checkup, a filling, or a bridge, or a reason *why* he has been referred by a dentist or physician. The chief complaint(s) is subjective in nature and is related to an uncomfortable or abnormal sensation. It is necessary that the chief complaint be a symptom because complaints expressed as symptoms leave no room for doubt regarding the patient's problem. Using expressions of desire or discontent for the chief complaint allows the patient to assume that the examiner knows why he wants a filling or a new plate, and also allows the patient to establish his own diagnosis and treatment plan. If the patient attempts to use the statement, I came for a checkup, the examiner is faced with the enigma of analyzing the chief complaint in terms of date of onset, type of onset, location, character, and related symptoms. A chief complaint is the patient's expression of disease, and that disease is what is to be treated—not the patient's diagnosis or desire.

It is quite possible that the patient has no chief complaint. This is a significant finding and should be recorded. However, a complaint may not be easily elicited or easily described, or it may not be of such magnitude that it can be localized by the patient, since people vary in their ability to accommodate for abnormal conditions. Such conditions as bleeding gums, bad taste, rough teeth, or vague pain which may have been troublesome to the patient at first may later became unapparent as he becomes accustomed to the symptoms. Symptoms of toothache and periodontal abscesses may be foremost in the patient's complaint, yet mask the symptoms of a more generalized disease. It is possible to overlook a chief complaint because the patient is not familiar with diagnosis or treatment procedures and is under the misconception that the examiner is aware of the condition causing his trouble.

Shaping the complaint. Since the patient does not express his discomfort or distress in terms of scientific symptomatology, many times it takes insight and ability on the part of the examiner to analyze the complaint; he may be called on to use all his skill to arrive at the exact nature of the symptom. When a complaint lacks the scientific details of formal symptom terminology, it has to be interpreted scientifically and accurately by the dentist if he is to find a rational basis for a diagnosis. The interpretation of the complaint and its conversion into more precise usable information are salient features of making a diagnosis.

The complaint that a patient makes to the dentist may be invested with special meanings and associations above and beyond the meaning given to more scientific definitions. It may be shaped by past experiences and by cultural and circumstantial forces. If a patient has had past experience with a symptom occurring in a particular disease, similar symptoms will cause the patient's complaint to be unconsciously molded by the comparative situation.

For a patient to have a complaint, he

must be aware of some abnormal disturbance. This awareness varies from individual to another. At what intensity of distress the patient will make his complaint known to the dentist depends upon the individual and upon many other factors such as age, stress, preoccupation, health, fatigue, social custom, perception, and past experience. A complaint may be couched in terms of location, dysfunction, or the extent of incapacitation that results from the disturbance. Either consciously or unconsciously many patients will try to fool not only themselves, but also their dentists in regard to complaints for fear that some disturbance will be found that is greater than they are prepared to accept. One must remember that patients' complaints are usually not objective; they are almost always colored by biased opinions.

The reaction of a patient to a particular symptom may vary with his mental attitude or preoccupation. For example, a toothache during a student's examination period may cause considerable distraction, whereas the same toothache may produce very little distraction at a time when he is enjoying himself, or he may be able to tolerate the pain well during the examination period but become quite distraught when required to wait a short time for treatment. The perception of a symptom may be acute for one patient, yet a symptom of the same intensity may be of no importance to another.

Another factor that may shape the complaint is the inability of the patient to communicate his abnormal experience to the examiner. This may be caused by the patient's lack of ability to express himself or to the fact that he has never experienced such symptoms previously and lacks terminology for an adequate description of his symptoms or complaint. Although it is true that the lay and dental vocabulary are different, the dentist may give considerable help to the patient by assisting in the proper use of comparisons. However, the tendency to lead a patient to an incorrect

history must be guarded against. Many times patients will complain of poorly defined sensations, for example, a vague sensation in the back part of the mouth, pressure on the chest, a feeling that one side of the mouth is higher than the other, and the like. In these instances the dentist should help the patient by suggesting the proper descriptive terms. Gestures, facial expressions, bodily attitudes, and physical demonstrations by the patient represent his inability to express himself, but they are actually a part of his means of communication.

One should remember that the complaint is also shaped by the memory of the patient Many times he forgets the symptom itself and recalls only his reaction to it. This is probably because the psychic component of distress is often so much more upsetting than any physiologic manifestation of disease. The complaint may be complicated by the fact that some individuals feel that to complain about anything even in the most diminutive fashion will brand them as a coward or as a malingerer. Many patients feel that a vist to the dentist for anything except the most dire toothache is to be avoided; as far as they are concerned, a visit to the dentist is only a step toward a full denture.

The age of the patient apparently influences the quality of the complaint. Young children are usually more concerned about what is gong to happen to them than they are about any particular discomfort they may have. Other patients, though they may be concerned about their discomfort, are probably more concerned with the significance of the symptoms. It would appear that adolescents are more concerned with their activities, such as examinations, classes, dates, and ball games, than with describing any discomfort unless it is of an acute nature. Even in acute problems they are usually more concerned with what is going to be done than with relating their problem. Although it is usually true that younger patients have keener symptom perception than do older people, they are less able to describe their symptoms. On the other hand, though elderly patients may be dulled in their mental processes, they are must better able to tell the dentist about their troubles because of experience in expressing themselves and past experience with symptoms.

The prestige of the dentist and his demeanor may also shape the quality of the complaint. It is not uncommon for patients to assume that the dentist is well aware of their complaint and will need but a minimum of information from them. Many times older patients are reluctant to give a young examiner anything but a cursory review of their disturbance, especially in a system review if they do not understand its intent. On the other hand, many patients feel that a young examiner does not have much experience and needs all the assistance they can give him. Some persons feel that gray hair and age are expressions of experience and ability and that no help from them is needed by a sage to make a diagnosis of their ailments.

The examiner must be quick to assess the feelings of the patient regarding his approach to them and must be ready to adjust to the type of patient-dentist relationship and examination that will establish the greatest harmonious relation. The dentist who rigidly approaches all patients in the same way will be successful only with those who appreciate his particular personality and methods.

The complaint may be shaped in one direction if the patient finds that his examiner is sympathetic; but it may be shaped in an entirely different way if he finds there is no expression of sympathy. However, an overly sympathetic examiner may have to listen to much irrelevant material. Some patients do not resent a matter-of-fact approach to their initial complaint, whereas others deeply resist this approach and seek to channel their complaints to a more receptive mood on the part of the examiner.

Many patients seek confirmation of their complaints and an authoritative acquiescence from the examiner and, when these are not forthcoming, choose another complaint in the hope that the new complaint will be confirmed.

When a patient knows a disease exists and has had some experience with it in the past, he is likely to interpret all his symptoms in terms of this known disease. Thus a patient who has a knowledge of an impacted asymptomatic molar may attribute any symptom relative to his teeth or jaws to the impaction and shape his complaint in terms of his abnormality. The patient who has been told at some time that he has heart disease is likely to be especially reactive to palpitations and to describe them in terms all out of proportion to their significance and severity.

The publicity given to certain diseases for the purpose of educating the public in the early recognition of the disease may also affect the complaint. It is not infrequent for patients to become aware of an innocuous lesion of the mouth such as lichen planus and to attribute imaginary changes in the lesion to cancer simply because they are afraid of cancer. Since such diseases as pyorrhea, syphilis, gonorrhea, and tuberculosis are not considered to be socially acceptable, many patients are reluctant to couch their complaint in terms that might draw attention to these diseases; instead, they let the examiner find out for himself a history or symptoms of these diseases. Also, many patients steer clear of all symptoms that might suggest a serious or hopeless significance. It may be only after a great interval of time or until the distress has become acute that the patient is willing to make known his complaints. In many instances in which a particular diagnosis is feared, a patient may attempt to hide or disguise the salient symptoms (symptoms such as dysphagia associated with cancer phobia) or present them in such a way as to keep the examiner from making the feared diagnosis. Some patients apparently nurture symptoms that are more attractive to them, and at the same time they tend to minimize in their mind symptoms less acceptable to them even though they know them to be more significant. For example, there are patients who believe that the esthetic result of a particular appliance is not in keeping with their own views, yet, in the opinion of the experienced prosthodontist, the results obtained are the best possible for that patient. Such patients may complain severely of malfitting dentures with the hope that their continued distress and complaint will force the prosthodontist to remake an appliance with the esthetic result they think is more suitable to them. Not infrequently, older patients with full dentures think they should have "white pearly teeth" like those of young movie stars.

The duration of the complaint is of considerable significance. The time it takes for a disease process to develop affects the complaint expressed to the examiner at the time of the examination. The patient has difficulty in remembering early symptoms and is concerned with more recent symptoms, which may be of a more severe nature. His inability to locate the symptoms is also significant. Those symptoms that are well localized usually tend to be well defined by the patient. On the other hand, those that are diffuse, radiating, and seem to travel are difficult for him to define clearly. One must remember that poorly defined symptoms may be organic or psychogenic in origin. A patient may complain of an uncomfortable feeling in his teeth and about gnashing of the teeth (bruxism) and yet be completely unaware of other symptoms of psychogenic origin.

Educated complaints are difficult to assess. Those patients who have a knowledge of the symptoms of a particular disease may shape their complaint to correspond with the symptoms of that disease. This occurs frequently with self-diagnosis and when a friend has had the same symptoms. The frequency, duration, and magnitude of symptoms appreciably affect the complaint given to the examiner. For example, an occasional mild pain of short duration in a tooth is often considered inconsequential, whereas continuous pain of the same intensity that interferes with working, sleeping, or pleasure is considered consequential.

It is necessary to determine the patient's chief complaint because it is his immediate and chief concern. It is also the basis for determining the remainder of the history and the treatment plan. The chief complaint is not necessarily the patient's latest complaint and is never a diagnosis. An analysis of one or more chief complaints and their mode, time of onset, course of development, character, and related symptoms constitute that part of the history termed "present illness."

Present illness

The present illness is a chronologic account of the chief complaint and associated symptoms from the time of onset to the time the history is taken. New complaints in the order of their appearance and relation to the chief complaint should be recorded. When possible, quantitative statements should be made, for example, "pain of toothache severe enough to keep patient from sleeping, from eating, from working"; "dyspnea after climbing one flight of stairs though previous climbing brought no onset of symptoms"; "pain sharp and lancinating in character, constant, and associated with chewing food."

The first statement should be a brief account of the date of onset of the chief complaint, type of onset, character, location, relation to other activities such as moving, eating, sleeping, cold, heat, reading, and so on, and association with the complications.

Each symptom should be expanded by detailed inquiry concerning development and relation to other symptoms in the same system in which the complaint lies; for example, if sore tongue is a symptom, an attempt should be made to determine whether there are present any symptoms associated with this disorder that may be suggestive of systemic disease such as pernicious anemia. One may suspect congenital syphilis when the patient complains of the poor esthetic quality of a notched incisor, but the presence of other associated signs and symptoms such as mulberry molars, interstitial keratitis, deafness, mouth rhagades, saddle nose, and family history should be investigated before suggesting a diagnosis of syphilis.

Negative as well as positive symptoms should be listed to more fully establish the identity and severity of disease. For example, a tooth that has previously reacted painfully to cold and then to heat and then reacts neither to heat nor to cold suggests pulp necrosis. If diabetes mellitus is considered an associated factor, other positive signs and symptoms such as polyphagia, polydipsia, polyuria, predisposition to pyogenic infections, periodontal abscesses, and decreased salivation should be investigated. The present illness record should include the patient's personal reaction to a disease. When the life of the patient is not at stake, he may not view the disease with any great concern. The treatment of such persons sometimes presents a problem because of the lack of cooperation. The treatment plan and prognosis may have to be modified to meet the existing conditions. The present illness record should also include constitutional symptoms such as recent loss or gain of weight, fatigue, fever, night sweats, and a statement from the patient as to the probable cause.

Previous diagnoses, medications, and treatment related to the chief complaint should be described as to form, intended purpose when known, and apparent effect. Just as the existence of a previous diagnosis and treatment of tuberculosis of the lung have a bearing on chest surgery, the previous diagnosis and treatment of Vincent's infection will have a bearing on the diagnosis and treatment of existing periodontal disease. The patient's adjustment to his environment and the effect of his disease on personal relationships should be mentioned briefly in the present illness and expanded in the social history. It is important to know why the patient came to you, why he was referred, what he had been told to expect, and what he believes to be the cause of his chief complaint.

A comprehensive and valuable write-up of the present illness necessitates a good basic knowledge of diseases of the oral cavity so that the interviewer is able to trace out leads given him by the patient during the interview. In many cases the historian will have considered some possibilities of the diagnosis during the interview that will direct his questioning. The possibilities considered must be both from the standpoint of elimination as a diagnosis and from the standpoint of requiring further investigation. Since the present illness deals with the details of the chief complaint, adequate time and careful questioning at this point in obtaining the history may save time and disappointment.

Past history

For the purpose of simplicity it is well for the dentist to consider the past history in two parts: the past dental history and the past medical history.

Dental history. The past dental history, or a patient's past history of dental treatment, often provides the dentist with valuable prognostic, as well as diagnostic, information. In obtaining such a history, the historian must always be aware of how the patient is presenting the story. Patients who have been dissatisfied with dental treatment in the past often distort a history and lead the historian to believe that they have been victims of a series of incompetent dentists when in reality they have been indifferent and neglectful toward their dental health. In most cases patients will be willing and cooperative at this point in the interview, since it is their opportunity to tell of their dental experiences. It is also an excellent opportunity for the dentist to determine the reactions of patients to dentistry in general and more specifically to the procedures they have experienced in the past.

The following is a list of details that should be investigated in the past dental history:

1. Frequency of visits to a dentist
2. Frequency of dental prophylaxis
3. Past experience during and after local anesthesia
4. Past experience during and after extractions
5. Past periodontal therapy, the condition that required the therapy, and the type of treatment that was given (scaling, occlusal adjustment, subgingival curettage, gingivectomy, and drug application)
6. Past orthodontic treatment: a positive history should include the condition that was treated, the length of time of active treatment, the nature of the appliances used in treatment, and whether a retainer is still required
7. Dental appliance history: length of time appliance worn, whether or not modified such as rebase or addition of teeth, personal care of appliance
8. Fixed bridges: length of service, comfort, modifications
9. Root canal fillings: length of time present, apicoectomy
10. Surgical procedures in and about the mouth other than extractions, nature of the tissue removed, manner in which it was removed, recurrences

The frequency with which a patient is accustomed to visiting a dentist provides the historian with information regarding the interest of the patient in his dental health. The frequency of dental prophylaxis may be a valuable guide in evaluating periodontal conditions that are present and provides the dentist with prognostic information. A knowledge of a patient's past experience during and after the administration of a local anesthetic may alert the dentist to the necessity for investigation into possible allergy to the anesthetic agent, or such information may allow him to anticipate possible syncope during the administration of local anesthetics in future appointments.

Patients who have had extractions must always be questioned regarding the healing process and whether they experienced any excessive hemorrhage after the extraction. Of particular interest are those individuals who have experienced prolonged bleeding and infections after extractions. In such patients one may need to obtain further systemic evaluation before proceeding with additional extractions.

A patient who gives a history of periodontal therapy should be questioned regarding the type of treatment and the time in the past it was received. The particulars of the type of treatment should be obtained so that the present status of the periodontal structures can be adequately evaluated. The patient should be questioned specifically about whether or not the treatment included complete scaling, occlusal adjustment, or surgery. In many cases it will be found that treatment consisted only of drug applications; insofar as possible, the type of drug used should be determined. The planning of future periodontal treatment for a patient who gives a history of previous treatment may depend largely upon the type of treatment the patient states he has received previously and the present clinical status of his periodontal tissues.

A patient giving a history of orthodontic treatment may present clinical findings that will be explained on the basis of the past treatment. An example of such a clinical

remote, and, if the history of diabetes is known prior to the dental treatment, proper precautions can be taken to prevent serious complications. Oral infections should be treated vigorously and promptly. This is particularly true in the patient with so-called "brittle" or juvenile diabetes. Any infection in the body, whether in the foot or in the oral cavity, upsets the insulin requirements of the diabetic patient. When an oral infection exists, it must be treated promptly and the patient must be advised to see his physician regarding readjustment of insulin requirements. The increased susceptibility to infection, combined with the effects of infection on insulin requirements, demands that the diabetic patient maintain good oral health at all times.

Injuries. Injuries to the face often involve the maxillary and mandibular bones, the teeth, and the temporomandibular joints. If a history of injury exists, it is necessary to determine its extent, the area involved, and the time it was received. A history of injury may seem insignificant to a patient, but occasionally an acute temporomandibular arthritis may develop any time from days to months after the injury. Initially an injury might not be severe enough to produce symptoms of acute temporomandibular joint arthritis; however, subsequent chronic minor trauma from occlusal irregularities may be sufficient to precipitate an acute traumatic temporomandibular joint arthritis.

When teeth are present in an area that has been injured, radiographic examination and vitality tests of the teeth in the associated area are indicated. The vitality of teeth should be determined in the arch involved in the injury, in the opposing arch, and in areas beyond the area of injury. Occasionally radiographic radiolucencies may be explained on the basis of previous injury to an area of bone. In questioning a patient relative to injuries he may have received, such things as auto accidents, accidental falls, and contact sports should be

considered as possible sources of injury to the face.

Operations. Any surgical procedure that has been performed on a patient may be potentially important to the dentist. The date of operation and the results reported to the patient by the surgeon should be determined. In the case of operation for neoplastic disease, the type of neoplasm and the area from which it was removed should be indicated in the history. Special consideration should be given to those neoplasms that have a tendency to metastasize to bone, especially the jaws. Although metastatic neoplasms are not commonly seen in the jaws, they nevertheless do occur. Operations involving the head, neck, and facial regions should receive particular attention from the historian since it may become the duty of the dentist to provide follow-up examinations for patients who have received surgical treatment for a variety of conditions involving the mouth and jaws.

Irradiation. Radiation therapy is being used effectively and extensively in the modern treatment of cancer, and certain immediate and long-range effects of this type of therapy are of concern to the dentist. The immediate effects are primarily related to an extremely sore mouth; this reaction to irradiation subsides in a period of from 4 to 6 weeks. The long-range effects are of more significance to the dentist in that they dictate certain precautionary measures for him to observe. When neoplasms in the mouth are irradiated, frequently the bone of the jaws is also subject to the radiation. This may result in a change in the vascularity of bone to such a degree that recovery from even minor trauma may be inhibited. Thus, in many instances, a past history of irradiation of the bone around the teeth contraindicates the extraction of the teeth in this area for the lifetime of the patient. In addition to the bones being irradiated, the salivary glands are frequently in the path of ionizing radiation. This may result in a loss of function of salivary gland tissue with a complete cessation or considerable decrease in salivary flow. Without the normal deteregnt action of adequate salivary flow, patients frequently develop rampant dental caries and progressive periodontal disease.

All forms of ionizing radiation have a similar effect on bone and salivary gland tissue whether the irradiation be from x-rays, radium, or radon. Whenever a patient gives a history of irradiation, it is wise to consult with the radiologist who rendered the treatment and discuss with him the extent of dental treatment that may be carried out without risking the possibility of osteoradionecrosis.

Allergy. A history of allergy, drug intolerance, and drug reaction is important to the dentist because of the relationship of the manifestations of these conditions to oral diagnosis and treatment. It is well known that dental procedures and dental drugs may elicit allergic or allergy-like manifestations. It is also true that patients present themselves for diagnosis of oral lesions that are manifestations of a reaction to a drug. Thus it is imperative that the dentist be aware (1) of the possibilities that a particular oral manifestation may have an allergic basis, (2) that a past history of an unfavorable reaction to a drug that is to be used in dental treatment may require careful consideration before it is used again, if at all, and (3) that although satisfactory evidence is still lacking that those patients with the so-called atopic diseases (hay fever, asthma, eczema, or hives) actually develop allergic reactions to drugs more often than those without them, nevertheless, clinical experience clearly shows that when allergic reactions do occur in this group, they tend to be more severe than in the nonallergic group.

Every dentist should be well acquainted with the basic concepts of allergy and hypersensitivity and with the various manifestations of allergy. Since it is not unusual for a patient who is allergic to one allergen to be allergic to several, a history of any type of allergy may be of the utmost importance. Since a wide range of allergens may produce allergic changes in the oral cavity, the dentist must know a variety of allergens and must be able to recognize allergic reactions in the mouth. At times when an allergic reaction in the mouth is suspected, it may be necessary for the dentist to carry out a detailed account of the patient's history of allergies and, in some cases, to request the patient to keep a diary of daily activities in order to determine the allergen.

Another important phase of the history of allergy is related to the administration of drugs in the dental office. With the wide variety of drugs available, there is an accompanying wide variety of allergic responses to these drugs. It is possible for the dentist to avoid producing an uncomfortable and perhaps incapacitating or even fatal allergic reaction to the drug he prescribes by obtaining a careful history regarding allergy to various drugs prior to their administration. Indiscriminate use of valuable drugs, particularly antibiotics, should be avoided in order to lessen the possibility of sensitizing the patient unnecessarily. The dentist should avoid dispensing drugs without first determining whether the patient is allergic to the contents of those drugs. This is particularly true of the patient who is given "pain pills" by the dentist and assumes that they are some potent analgesic and not aspirin. Patients who are allergic to aspirin show a particularly severe asthmatic type of reaction to the drug and may die in an acute asthmatic attack after its ingestion (Walton and Bottomley). An increasing number of untoward reactions to penicillin are being seen, and, although few in number, they are most generally severe and occasionally fatal. The serum sickness type of reaction to penicillin, which occurs from a week to 10 days after the drug is given, often incapacitates a patient for a period of 10 days and requires vigorous care for relief.

Clinical reactions to drugs may appear as true allergic responses to proteins, as a dermatitis, or as reactions not characteristics of allergy to proteins (Carr). Those reactions to drugs that are seen in allergy to proteins include systemic anaphylaxis, asthma, allergic conjunctivitis, rhinitis, urticaria, angioedema, serum sickness syndrome, and polyarteritis nodosa. Those reactions to drugs not characteristic of allergy to protein include deleterious effects to the blood and drug fever.

Anaphylactic shock is a term used primarily to designate a reaction in experimental animals, but a group of clinical signs and symptoms resembling anaphylaxis may be seen in human beings. The manifestations of anaphylaxis have been seen after the administration of penicillin. Systemic anaphylaxis is characterized by sudden onset, asthmatic dyspnea, urticaria, angioedema, weakness, nausea, vomiting, fall in blood pressure, syncope, respiratory failure, and death. These reactions may result rapidly in death or may not occur at all. It does not necessarily follow that all of the foregoing reactions will occur. Of special significance are the multiple reaction, including anaphylactic shock, which may accompany iodism. More cases of iodism have been attributed to contrast media than to any other cause (Alexander). Thus the use of a contrast media for outlining cysts and periodontal pockets or for other uses such as in disclosing solution, should always be preceded by questions regarding possible allergy to iodine. Reactions to iodine include direct chemical burns, generalized dermatitis related to external use on small areas, and urticaria, purpura, and dermatitis.

Bronchial asthma is an expression of drug hypersensitivity. It may occur alone or in association with urticaria, rhinitis, or hay fever. It differs from the alveolar congestion and bronchospasm of anaphylactic shock. Although aspirin is one of the most common causes of bronchial asthma, many other drugs may induce it.

Conjunctivitis may be seen after topical or systemic administration of drugs. It is often a prominent feature of the Stevens-Johnson syndrome. Conjunctival suffusion may be seen in conjunction with hay fever and with vasomotor rhinitis.

Urticaria refers to the phenomenon of whealing and is one of the most common reactions to drugs. It may occur as angioedema of the lips in penicillin hypersensitivity, as angioedema and bullous eruptions in iodine reactions, and in reactions to tannic acid, streptomycin, sulfonamides, and vitamin B_{12} concentrate.

Urticaria, sneezing, rhinitis, migraine, hay fever, and gastrointestinal upsets should also be considered. Positive statements should be included as to the patient's reaction to dust, pollen, food, sunlight, and drugs like aspirin, penicillin, local anesthesia, oil of cloves, mercury, sulfonamides, and iodine. Occupational diseases, metal intolerances, herpes simplex, hives, and so on should be considered in the past history and included in the record of the present illness where applicable.

Urticarial manifestations appearing after administration of antibiotics such as penicillin, chlortetracycline (Aureomycin), oxytetracycline (Terramycin), and chloramphenicol (Chloromycetin) may be present in patients who present an immediate type of allergic sensitivity. Penicillin or the involved antibiotic acts as a haptene and conjugates with a body protein to yield the complete antigen. Another reaction to the antibiotics may be an erythema of the ninth-day type that is characterized by a generalized macular, maculopapular, morbilliform, rubelliform, or scarlatiniform eruption usually accompanied by mild or almost absent constitutional symptoms; it appears from 7 to 10 days after administration of the antibiotic. Still another type of reaction to the antibiotics, more especially penicillin and chlortetracycline, is the "id" type of reaction characterized by eczematoid, erythematovesicular, and desquamating eruptions affecting more generally the feet, hands, and groin. Associated symptoms are not usually constitutional in nature. The onset is early in the course of treatment, usually within 24 hours. Urticaria caused by penicillin may subside while the drug is being used, may fail to recur when the drug is readministered, or may reappear periodically for many weeks after its use has been stopped.

Many drugs may produce systemic reactions similar to those described for the allergic reaction to therapeutic antiserum. As in serum sickness, symptoms appear between the first and second week after administration of the drug. The syndrome of fever, urticaria, arthralgia, and lymphadenopathy is known as the serum sickness pattern or syndrome. Peripheral neuritis and renal manifestations may also be a part of the drug reaction.

Periarteritis nodosa may be induced in susceptible individuals by iodides, hydantoins, sulfonamides, and serums.

Dermatologic manifestations of drug hypersensitivity must be differentiated from physical trauma and irritation. Sensitization of the skin does not necessarily imply that the mucous membranes are sensitized (Rostenberg). The most common dermatologic manifestations of drug hypersensitivity are allergic contact-type dermatitis, urticaria, and the exanthematous eruptions. Denture-sore mouth, polypoid hyperplasia of the palate, and black hairy tongue associated with overgrowth of yeast or fungus organisms should not be considered generally as allergic phenomena. Denture-sore mouth, characterized by erythema and at times hyperplasia, is more often than not the result of trauma rather than true sensitivity to the acrylic resins (Nyquist). It is possible, though rare, that poorly or inadequately processed acrylics will contain sufficient monomer to produce an untoward

reaction of the mucosa. Erythema multiforme refers to a multiplicity of lesions (macules, papules, vesicles, and bullae) that may occur as the result of drug hypersensitivity. The salicylates and sulfonamides are the most frequent offenders; however, these lesions may occur with serum sickness and penicillin, barbiturates, and other medication.

"Fixed" drug reactions may occur with the use of the antibiotics as well as with the usual drugs causing this type of reaction, for example, phenolphthalein and sulfonilamide. Clinically the eruptions consist of circumscribed areas of erythema, edema, and scaling that slowly subside when the antibiotic is withdrawn. Such lesions usually leave a residual pigmentation. Readministration of the drug brings about a recrudescence of the lesions in the same area.

Local anesthetics are not infrequently the cause of contact dermatitis. They may also cause death but probably not through true allergy or immune mechanisms. Local anesthetics may be divided into two groups: those that are chemically related to one another and whose basic structure permits cross-reaction and those that are not chemically related and do not cross-react (Alexander). Thus, when an unfavorable reaction to one of the local anesthetics in the first group occurs, an anesthetic should be selected from the second group whose members are not chemically related. A complete listing of the members of each group may be found elsewhere (Alexander). Briefly, the first group includes those local anesthetics containing procaine hydrochloride and the second group includes lidocaine (Xylocaine) and others.

Local anesthetics may product contact dermatitis, serum sickness syndrome, and asthma. Gilman classified the reactions to local anesthetics as follows: (1) manifestations caused by toxic influences such as excitement, delirium, convulsions, and respiratory failure; (2) an immediate type of reaction arising from a disturbance of the circulatory system, consisting of pallor, increased pulse rate, fall in blood pressure, and syncope; and (3) an allergic reaction manifested by asthma.

Diagnosis of allergy to drugs is generally based on the information obtained from a history. Patch testing for contact dermatitis should be done by one experienced in their application and interpretation since they may occasionally cause severe and distressing local reactions. Skin tests are of no value in the diagnosis of other allergies, and it is possible to elicit a true positive response with the development of a severe systemic reaction.

Blood dyscrasias may be produced by drugs through destruction of circulating blood elements or depression of the bone marrow. Such disorders may be produced by mechanisms other than hypersensitivity. Blood changes produced by drugs include granulocytopenia, thrombocytopenic purpura, and aplastic anemia.

Antihistaminic drugs may also frequently give rise to drug reactions. The more common side reactions are drowsiness, sleepiness, dizziness, headache, insomnia, nervousness, nausea, vomiting, constipation, diarrhea, and dryness of the mouth. Severe and rather bizarre reactions include delirium, narcolepsy, shocklike states, labyrinthitis, cardiospasm, urinary retention, fever, syncope, and dermatitis. These reactions have been thought to occur more commonly in allergic persons. Allergic reactions such as asthma and contact eczema, as well as arthralgia and urticaria, have also resulted from the use of antihistamines.

Potentiation of analgesic agents has been reported for many of the ataractic drugs. A history of the use of these tranquilizing agents should alert the dentist to the possibility of potentiation of narcotic analgesics that he may be prescribing. Since the tranquilizers do not have an analgesic property, the effect of potentiation is a true one and not one of summation. Adverse reactions, side effects, and toxicity, as well as habituation and addiction to the ataractic drugs have been reported (Hughes).

The importance of an adequate history concerning drugs to be used for a patient in the treatment of disease by a dentist cannot be overemphasized. Since an allergy to a drug generally does not occur spontaneously, a previous single exposure to a drug does not assure the dentist that an untoward reaction will not result from his administration of a drug. However, an adequate history of a previous reaction to a drug may well prevent the occurrence of an unfavorable reaction. To further emphasize the need for a history, one only has to consider the widespread use of aspirin, the most common drug in use, which causes severe allergic reaction; yet the knowledge of this fact is not widespread among the members of the dental profession or the laity. Although the number of cases of aspirin sensitivity is small in relation to its very extensive use, the untoward effects are often striking and dangerous to the patient and therefore should not be treated lightly. The dermatologic manifestations of an allergy to aspirin include urticaria and extensive angioneurotic edema involving the face, tongue, and palate. Systemic manifestations include bronchial asthma and constitutional or anaphylactic shock. Since in many instances there is a record of antecedent allergy, asthmatic patients should always be asked about previous use of aspirin and whether or not any untoward reaction occurred from its ingestion. Although sensitivity to aspirin may be mild and go undetected, such a sensitivity may become more severe with subsequent administration.

Family history

The family history should include the most important conditions that have tendencies to be inherited as well as an indication of the possibility of infective contact as in tuberculosis. Diabetes mellitus, cancer, allergy, and nervous and mental disorders are important. The record of an illness with unusual hereditary tendencies, such as hemophilia, should contain information concerning relatives more distant than the immediate family. Information regarding ages of living parents or ages at time of death and also cause of death is useful in determining familial patterns. Hereditary and familial patterns are important in primary erythroblastic anemia, osteogenesis imperfecta, hemorrhagic telangiectasia, hereditary opalescent dentin, hereditary cranifacial dysostosis, supernumerary teeth, missing teeth, malocclusion, and other disturbances.

Personal and social history

The personal and social history should include a brief summary of the patient's marital status, occupation, financial status, type of personality, habits, and religion. The excessive use of alcohol is an important consideration in general anesthesia and is important in the nutritional status of the patient. Cirrhosis of the liver and vitamin B complex–deficiency states may arise from alcoholism. Excessive use of alcohol may at times result in poor patient cooperation.

Tobacco is important because of its relationship to leukoplakia and verrucous carcinoma of the oral mucosa, oral hygiene, and nicotine stomatitis. Habits such as nail biting, tongue thrusting, pipestem chewing, pencil chewing, thread biting, tooth tapping and jiggling, and improper use of toothpicks should also be recorded if they have important relationships to abnormality in the mouth.

Problems imposed by illness, treatment schedules, financial arrangements, care of children, unemployment, time off from work, distance from the office, and the likelihood of the patient having to move to another area before completion of the treatment should be considered.

Personal hygiene may sometimes indicate what to expect in the way of home care. Education and intelligence are factors that must be considered when determining treatment to be carried on at home. The methods of toothbrushing and the home care the patient has been using, as well as the number of times daily he may carry out these procedures, are important. The manner in which the patient takes care of his toothbrush should also be indicated.

Systems review

The systems review permits organization of some of the apparently unrelated symptoms. It also decreases the possibility of overlooking important symptoms by including other areas of the body and giving the examiner logical sequence for a complete review of the patient's history. Negative statements should never be used as the answers to questions concerning the various systems. Positive statements leave no doubt as to their meaning and indicate that the subject has been covered with the patient. The rote one-breath question, Have you had

a cough, hemoptysis, edema, night sweats, cardiac trouble, loose teeth, pyorrhea, measles, mumps, or rheumatic fever? is to be avoided. Questions in the system review should be directed toward the signs and symptoms that have not been brought out in the record of the present illness and should give the examiner a better idea of the patient's health.

Head. Although the structures of the head are a part of the respiratory, gastrointestinal, nervous, and other systems and could be made a part of those respective systems under this systems review, the functional and anatomic integration of the eye, ear, nose, and throat suggest their grouping and review together.

Headache. The presence or absence of headaches or past head injuries should be recorded. Headaches fall into two major categories according to their origin: those that arise mainly as the result of stimulation of intercranial structures and those that occur on stimulation of tissues outside of and adjacent to the skull. The headaches of major concern to the dentist are migraine, hypertension, temporal arteritis, eye, sinus, and those associated with teeth, temporomandibular joint, or muscles of the head and neck. Diffuse headaches associated with disease of the teeth or pain in the teeth if prolonged may also be increased by severe sustained contraction of the muscles of the head and neck. The most commonly encountered headaches are migraine and those of sustained muscle contraction associated with anxiety and emotional tension. The teeth do not remain obscure as a cause of neuralgia or other facial pain. Dental pulpitis and pain associated with exposed dentin may be the cause of local pain or referred pain, but it is doubtful from clinical experience that such conditions are the source of headaches. Thus impulses arising from the teeth and associated with headache, although clinically important, are not a common cause of headache.

Usually a headache associated with a diseased tooth or teeth may be evaluated by the use of a local anesthetic around the tooth in question, since anesthetizing the diseased tooth will eliminate headache and other pain. However, generally in such instances tenderness and ache in the muscles of the neck and back of the head are still present. Headaches with intervals of complete freedom from pain do not have their origin in diseased teeth. The extraction of diseased teeth for the relief of such headaches is not justified. The rationale for treatment should be directed toward the alleviation of the disease of the teeth; if, in the course of treatment and restitution of the tooth, the neuralgia, headache, or other facial pain is eliminated, then the tooth can be considered responsible for the headache. However, teeth should never be extracted solely for the purpose of determining by exclusion the cause of the headache.

As previously stated, when noxious stimuli arise from the teeth, the infiltration of a local anesthetic about the source of noxious stimuli will eliminate the headache. However, pain and tenderness associated with noxious stimuli arising in the muscles of the head and neck usually remain for several hours. In the case of noxious stimuli arising from the teeth, the sustained muscle contraction is found in the masseter and temporalis muscles, in addition to the muscles of the occiput and neck. Therefore, headaches from sustained contractions of the muscles of the face, head, and neck are secondary to noxious impulses arising from the teeth. Some instances of extreme headache and toothache may result from traumatic occlusion. In addition to the headache, there may be associated pain of the face or temporomandibular joint. The patient may be indirectly aware of this association and may attempt to hold the jaw in a particular manner, thus inducing sustained contractions of the muscles of mastication and of the face, head, and neck. In these instances, the headache is probably caused primarily by sustained contractions of these muscles.

Eyes. The patient should be questioned concerning inflammation and pain in the eyes. A certain amount of information may be gained by asking questions relating to spectacles. Pertinent conditions associated with defective vision, yet showing little or no evidence of ocular affection, include squinting eyes, nystagmus, toxic states caused by renal disease, alcohol, tobacco, lead, and quinine, migraine, diseases of the visual cortex, severe hemorrhage, and so on. At times photophobia is associated with any headache experienced chiefly in the front or on the top of the head. It is commonly noted in patients with migraine headaches, nasal and paranasal disease, and muscular spasm headaches. (Any reaction to light by the eye must be interpreted in relation to the intensity of the light used. No one can be expected to stand the dental unit light shining directly into his eyes, and this should not be used as a criterion of photophobia.)

Occasionally after extractions of teeth and other dental operations, there may be lacrimation and slight reddening of the conjunctiva on the side of involvement. There also may be erythema on that particular side. The skin over the painful area may be hyperalgesic and accompanied by extensive motor reactions. Afferent impulses from injured periodontal tissues of an extraction site may produce a diffuse headache caused by noxious impulses arising from these injured tissues. These impulses give rise to excitatory processes in the brainstem that spread to exert their effects on many trigeminal structures.

Ears. The presence or absence of deafness, tinnitus, vertigo, or discharge should be noted. Many children's diseases may affect the auditory nerve, producing various degrees of deafness. Mumps occasionally produce a profound type of deafness without middle ear involvement. Many drugs, especially quinine, salicylates, arsenic, nicotine, mercury, and alcohol, can produce a nerve type of deafness in susceptible people. Interference with the blood supply to the labyrinth as may occur in patients with the various anemias or arteriosclerosis can affect hearing. Eighth cranial nerve deafness in a few cases may be caused by syphilis, especially in the late form. The duration of the deafness, history of onset, and related symptoms are important factors to be recorded, especially if they relate to the chief complaint or correlated symptoms. Vertigo in patients with Ménière's syndrome should not be associated with symptoms of temporomandibular joint dysfunction. Deafness and vertigo have been suggested as symptoms of Costen's syndrome, but these are not acceptable with present concepts. The relationship fo Ménière's disease with periodontal disease or abscessed teeth has not been established. Vertigo and dizziness may be associated with the eighth cranial nerve, brain disease, epilepsy, migraine, severe anemia, or drug reactions.

Nose. Colds must be distinguished from allergic symptoms. Frequent colds give some indication of the resistance of the patient. In children sinusitis may give rise to symptoms that are thought to be caused by frequent colds. Postnasal drip may be a result of an allergic rhinitis, foreign objects, sinusitis, or lesions. Epistaxis may be associated with rheumatic fever, and a history of frequent nosebleeds should lead to questions regarding other symptoms of this disease. Nasal hemorrhage is frequently present in patients with hypertension and various blood dyscrasias, or it may be the result of various chemical irritants such as mercurial and phosphorus poisoning or local conditions such as trauma in the anterior septum where Hassalbach's venous plexus is located. In addition to the function of smell, the nose prepares the air for use by the lungs. It cleans, moistens, and warms inspired air. Breathing through the mouth instead of the nose has an injurious effect on the tissues of the respiratory tract and the oral cavity and is also a factor in maldevelopment of the facial skeleton and malocclusion of the teeth because of the displacement of the normal growth forces. Most individuals have a strong tendency for nasal respiration; however, if the nasal passageways are blocked, the individual will, of necessity, breathe through his mouth.

At this time in the system review, some information relative to the problem of respiration through the mouth instead of the nose should be obtained. During the clinical examination, the effects of mouth breathing as well as whether habitual mouth breathing is occurring can be determined. However, at this time subjective information relative to the altered function is of importance in later direction of the clinical examination and many times determines the necessity for referral to the rhinologist. Habitual mouth breathing may be caused by anatomic malformation such as nasal obstruction, enlarged tonsils, engorged nasal mucosa, and a deviated nasal septum. Probably the size of the airway, plus additional factors such as nasal or pharyngeal obstruction, is the predisposing factor in the mouth breather. Thus a narrow airway coupled with engorgement of the vascular bed or enlargement of the lymphoid masses in the pharyngeal airway may very well result in varying degrees of mouth breathing. Mouth breathing caused by the physiologic hyperplasia of the pharyngeal lymphoid tissue usually occurs between the fourth and twelfth years. Since the lymphoid mass begins to atrophy after the twelfth year, the mouth breathing becomes less frequent because of the decrease in the obstruction to breathing through the nose. However, in many instances mouth breathing is a residual habit even after the nasal obstruction is removed.

Although few patients will admit that they are chronic mouth breathers, a review of some of the factors that predispose to mouth breathing, as well as a review of the precipitating factors, may well bring out the need for examination in this particular area. Allergy, chronic rhinitis, sinusitis, nasal polyps, and a deviated septum are factors that may be important in the etiology. Nasal obstruction is quite common during sleeping hours and is especially prone to occur when the patient is lying on his back. Some children have an open-mouth habit but do not necessarily breathe through their mouths. However, this habit itself may lead to mouth breathing because when the mouth is open it is easier to breathe

through it than to breathe nasally. In mouth breathers or in persons with the open-mouth habit, hyperplastic gingivitis, especially of the anterior portion of the mouth, is likely to occur.

Mouth breathing is a common habit and presents important clinical problems. To treat gingivitis associated with mouth breathing or to intercept certain types of malocclusion associated with mouth breathing, it is necessary to determine the type and character of the mouth breathing. This information will greatly influence the treatment planning. In many instances mouth breathing will be treated by the rhinologist and also by the dentist. Certainly the dentist is in the position to correct habitual mouth breathing when no organic obstruction is noted or after the obstruction, if one is present, has been treated by the rhinologist. In many instances, however, the elimination of a possible organic obstruction should be determined by the rhinologist. Whether there is a necessity for detailed clinical examination for mouth breathing many times is determined during a system review. Testing for nasal and oral breathing that can be done by the dentist and the determination of a rationale for referral to a rhinologist are discussed briefly in Chapter 15 under clinical examination of the patient and indications for referral of patients to specialists. A history of nasal obstruction, allergic rhinitis, and sinusitis, atrophic rhinitis, nasal polyps, or deviated nasal septum coupled with a complaint of difficulty in breathing through the nose, should direct the examiner's attention to a thorough examination of the structures that may be affected by mouth breathing and to a more complete examination of this area than might ordinarily be given. Careful observation of the patient during the history taking offers many clues to the direction one must take for a more thorough evaluation either by a more detailed review of this area or by a more detailed clinical examination. (See references for additional details of the etiology and diagnosis of mouth breathing.)

Throat. A few exploratory questions concerning the throat should be asked even though a patient's complaints are not directed to the throat. The review should cover hoarseness, tonsillitis, and sore throat. Persistent hoarseness should be considered a result of a neoplasm until proved otherwise. Frequent episodes of sore throat and tonsillitis are significant factors in thumb sucking, tongue thrusting, and mouth breathing and are important historically in the evaluation of rheumatic fever. The differential diagnosis of herpetic stomatitis and acute necrotizing gingivitis is facilitated by a positive history of sore throat and dysphagia prior to the onset of oral lesions. Complaints about the throat should direct the examiner to specific areas of consideration during the clinical examination.

Cardiorespiratory system. The symptoms that should be explored that suggest either cardiovascular or pulmonary disease are chest pain, dyspnea, ankle edema, and cough.

The onset of chest pain during exertion or emotional stress may be indicative of angina pectoris. The type of chest pain should be determined as well as its location. A squeezing type of substernal pain that appears with exercise and subsides with rest is typical of myocardial ischemia. Angina of cardiac origin may be first noticed or become more severe during outdoor activity in cold weather. Chest wall pain resulting from spasm of the pectoral or intercostal muscles must be considered when the location of the pain and its relationship to increased cardiac demand are not typical of myocardial origin.

Dyspnea or distress in breathing may be of cardiac, pulmonary, or psychogenic origin. Shortness of breath resulting from mild exercise may be the result of congestive heart failure or impaired pulmonary function. Dyspnea that develops during recumbency or sleep, paroxysmal nocturnal dysp-

nea (PND), is typical of congestive failure, although an asthmatic attack might occur under the same circumstances. Ankle edema accompanying PND is pathognomonic of congestive heart failure. Chronic asthma, pulmonary emphysema, bronchiectasis, and other situations that permanently reduce the efficiency of pulmonary function are accompanied by reduced vital capacity and persistent dyspnea. Dyspnea of psychogenic origin may develop in a patient who is excessively apprehensive about dental treatment prior to or during a dental procedure. The resultant increased rate of respiration produces hyperventilation, which may induce dizziness and mild tetany.

Cough as a symptom may have many origins among which are acute and chronic respiratory infections, chronic pulmonary diseases, congestive heart failure, bronchogenic carcinoma, and chronic irritation from tobacco smoke. The duration of the cough and the type of sputum that is produced are helpful in identifying the origin. The appearance of blood in the sputum is a significant finding but it must be clearly established whether the source of the blood is pulmonary or oral.

Findings suggestive of cardiovascular or pulmonary disease demand that medical evaluation be accomplished before anything but preliminary dental treatment is started. The potential hazards to the patient with untreated cardiovascular and pulmonary disease are several if even certain simple dental procedures are performed.

An interpretative electrocardiographic service is being offered in several communities whereby ECG data from a patient is monitored by a center for computer processing and interpretation. The computer output (Fig. 3-1) is review by a cardiologist prior to transmission of the report. The importance of such a service is obvious in remote areas or where capability for ECG analysis is limited. Although the dentist may not be taking the ECG data, he should have some knowledge of its meaning

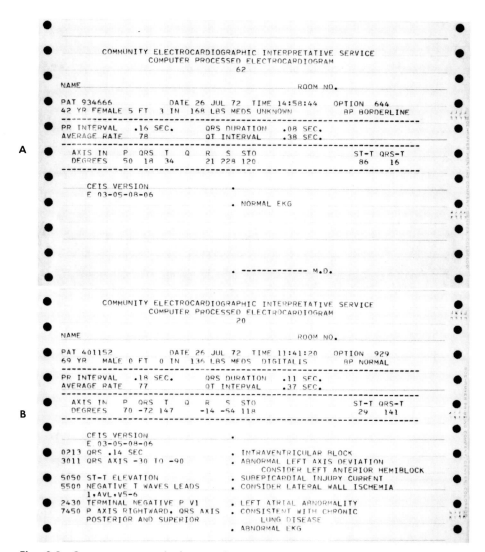

Fig. 3-1. Computer-processed electrocardiogram. Interpretation of ECG data: **A,** Normal. **B,** Abnormal.

to dental treatment, especially in a hospital service.

Gastrointestinal system. A review of the gastrointestinal system serves to systematically recall to the patient's attention any symptoms of disease in this tract, including the mouth, that may have a bearing on his present illness and treatment. The information obtained may be of value because (1)

disease that is manifest in the mouth may be the hallmark of more extensive systemic disease; (2) it is helpful in calling to the examiner's attention the patient's basic desire in seeking dental service, especially if the disturbances of the gastrointestinal tract are considered by the patient to be caused by oral conditions such as poor chewing ability, ill-fitting dentures, or periodontal disease; and (3) the diagnosis of many conditions in the mouth is dependent upon the proper evaluation of the condition of the remainder of the system; that is to say the nutrition, especially of an older debilitated patient, is in many instances dependent upon the proper and comfortable mastication of a proper diet.

More patients have complaints involving the gastrointestinal system than any other system. A complete review of this system should include questions regarding nausea, vomiting, regurgitation, indigestion, anorexia, dysphagia, constipation, diarrhea, hematemesis and melena, jaundice, loss of teeth, toothache, flatulence, excessive thirst, abdominal pain, hemoptysis, bad taste, food impactions between the teeth, salivary changes, difficulty in mastication, pyorrhea, bleeding gums, canker sores, bad breath, loose teeth, pain, pain or sensitivity to heat, cold, or foods, vague feelings of discomfort of the teeth and gums, gumboils, and sharp edges on the teeth.

Although patients frequently tend to underestimate the significance of complaints relative to this system and habitually attribute their discomfort to "something I ate," it is well known that the hallmark of many diseases may be manifest by symptoms in the gastrointestinal system. Such diseases as anemia, allergy, syphilis, vitamin deficiency, leukemia, and acute infections frequently present their chief symptoms in the gastrointestinal tract. A consideration of the symptoms common to the gastrointestinal tract lends itself to their artificial division into three main groups: (1) anorexia, dysphagia, nausea, and vomiting; (2) constipation, diarrhea, and dysentery; and (3) symptoms referable to the oral cavity.

Other than oral complaints, nausea and vomiting are among the most frequent symptoms referable to the gastrointestinal tract. Though the symptoms themselves may appear to point toward a stomach disorder, reflexes that cause nausea and vomiting may rise virtually in any part of the body or nervous system. They may be induced by pain and other sensations and intoxications, by unusual strains and efforts, by emotions and psychic disturbances such as fear, and by other conscious or unconscious mechanisms. Vomiting may be associated with almost any disturbance; unless it is qualified by some other symptom, the act itself may be of little diagnostic importance. The physiologic basis for the symptoms of nausea and vomiting appear to be a diminution in the functional activities of the stomach and alterations in the motility of the duodenum. There are apparently two ways of stimulating the organism to vomit: those that are central in origin and those that are peripheral in origin. Both vomiting stimuli act upon the vomiting center. Nausea and vomiting may be encountered in patients with acute infectious diseases, acute abdominal emergencies, chronic indigestion, diseases of the heart such as chronic heart failure, metabolic disorders such as the crises of thyrotoxicosis, Addison's disease, and disorders of the nervous system. In other instances the effects of drugs and poisons, laryngeal irritation, and psychogenic causes may produce vomiting. In many diseases, such as carcinoma of the stomach in the early stage and chronic indigestion caused by lesions of the stomach, the cause of nausea and vomiting may not be readily apparent.

In a system review, vomiting should be related to the time, volume, contents, relation to food intake, and means of relief. If the volume is small, especially in the morning and after meals, it is often functional; if copious and occurring at night or late in the day, obstruction is suggested. When food content from the day before is seen, obstruction should be suspected. Bile stain indicates an obstruction below the pylorus. Coffee-ground color indicates blood decomposed by acid.

Regurgitating may be differentiated from vomiting. Regurgitation implies an expulsion from the esophagus of undigested food retained because of some obstruction such as occurs with cardiospasm, esophageal varices, or a diverticulum, or an expulsion of gastric contents without preceding nausea. Regurgitation is of dental significance because of the acidity accompanying this type of activity and the decalcification of the teeth.

Indigestion is a term with no specific meaning that is generally used to mean those symptoms occurring after eating such as heartburn, nausea, epigastric fullness, flatulent pains in various combinations, and belching of gas. Nausea and vomiting may also accompany severe cases of so-called indigestion.

Anorexia means lack of appetite and hunger. Clinically, it occurs in so many conditions of ill health, both psychogenic and organic in origin, that its diagnostic significance has little value. However, it may be present in patients with poor oral hygiene, ill-fitting dentures, painful teeth, and periodontal disease. Decreased weight should be associated with this symptom if it occurs in an individual who has just recently had dentures or some other type of dental treatment or in middle-aged or older persons whose appetite previously has been good.

Complaints of persistent indigestion related to a lack of dentures or to new dentures should not be taken lightly. Although the indigestion may be psychogenic in origin as a result of the new dentures, it is also likely that such persistent distress may well be caused by more serious conditions in the gastrointestinal tract. As prevoiusly mentioned, the complaint is the patient's communication in his own terms about his symptoms, but the interpretation of the complaint is the responsibility of the dentist. In many instances the patient already had a complaint of indigestion prior to the time the dentist was consulted. Not knowing the true significance of his complaint, the patient may well have considered that his difficulty was caused by ill-fitting den-

tures and that new ones would take care of his complaint of indigestion.

There are symptoms so universally associated with unimportant illnesses that scant attention is given to them, with the result that serious disease is sometimes neglected. For example, a hoarse voice resulting from carcinoma of the larynx may be permitted to go untreated for a considerable length of time under the misapprehension that it is caused by laryngitis. In the same manner a patient may seek out a dentist for treatment of ill-fitting dentures under the mistaken idea that his indigestion is caused by the ill-fitting dentures.

Dysphagia, which means difficulty in swallowing, is a symptom that is usually of special significance to the dentist because of its relation to his field of interest. It may be caused by mechanical obstruction in the esophagus, to lesions of the mouth, pharynx, or larynx, or to disturbances of the neuromuscular components used in swallowing. The most common cause of dysphagia is mechanical obstruction of the esophagus, and by far the most common obstruction of the esophagus is carcinoma. Thus the first and most important symptom of carcinoma of the esophagus is difficulty in swallowing. Dysphagia from carcinoma usually has a gradual onset but may suddenly become progressively increased until even liquids are unable to pass through the esophagus. Regurgitation and pain are usually inconspicuous or absent. It can be readily understood that the dentist is in a prime position to evaluate changes in the swallowing ability of his patients. Dysphagia may also result from disturbance in neuromuscular mechanisms. The Plummer-Vinson syndrome is generally considered in this category since the difficulty of swallowing in this condition resembles that caused by a neuromuscular disorder; the actual cause of dysphagia is not clear. Patients with this syndrome are usually middle-aged women who present the characteristics of a chronic idiopathic microcytic anemia in conjunction with signs of vitamin B complex deficiency. Thus dysphagia, anemia, and atrophy of the mucosa of the upper gastrointestinal tract are symptoms of this syndrome. These patients also usually have relative degree of acrodynia and sore mouths. Spoon-shaped fingernails are not uncommon findings. In some instances hyperkeratotic white plaques may be found on the buccal mucosa and throughout the mouth. These lesions apparently have a tendency to regress to carcinoma. Symptoms of dysphagia considered in the system review should include a reference to the time of onset and its relationship to hoarseness, coughing, and eating.

Constipation is an undue delay in the evacuation of feces. Diarrhea is the elimination of watery feces with excessive speed. Constipation is the most common of all symptoms referable to the gastrointestinal tract. Even though some investigators do not consider constipation, per se, to be physiologic, much attention has been placed on changes of bowel movements in an attempt to increase the awareness of the public to the possibility of cancer of the gastrointestinal tract. Though it is popularly believed that at least one satisfactory bowel movement a day is sufficient and that less than this constitutes constipation, such factors are quite variable and some healthy persons will form a stool of normal consistency that is passed only every 2 or 3 days. These individuals are not constipated, for the stool has not been excessively dehydrated in its passage through the distal colon and has not been unduly delayed in evacuation. Constipation and diarrhea may be central, reflex or mechanical in origin. The emphasis placed on constipation as a symptom is probably unwarranted. However, when constipation is recent and progressive, a serious psychogenic or organic cause must be suspected. The onset of constipation after middle life should raise a suspicion of organic disease of the bowels, especially if the disorder is progressive.

Diarrhea is as difficult to define as constipation. There are disturbances that by any standard can be called diarrhea. These are more likely to be termed dysentery than diarrhea. The concept of diarrhea varies with the training, education, culture, and habits of the patient. Recurrent or chronic diarrhea may occur after acute infectious dysentery. These are diarrheas caused by neoplasms, protozoa, bacterial molds, drugs, worms, allergies, radiation, vitamin deficiencies, and other specific agents. Diarrhea of brief duration is commonly caused by dietary indiscretion, food intolerance, or infections by organisms of the salmonella group. Prolonged diarrhea suggests some type of infection, and it may result from bacillary dysentery, tuberculosis, enteritis, dietary deficiency, or such intractable disorders as idiopathic ulcerative colitis or regional enteritis. The latter are usually severe enough to force a patient to see a physician, and the dentist is only indirectly concerned with these diseases.

A positive history of hematemesis (vomiting of gross blood) and melena (passing of tarrish stools) are, with rare exceptions, manifestations of hemorrhage in the upper digestive tract. Peptic ulcers are the most common cause of hematemesis. Carcinoma of the stomach and portal hypertension are less frequent causes. Although hematemesis and melena may be caused by a large number of disorders, one must keep in mind that about 90 percent of all cases result from primary intragastric diseases.

Jaundice is a term that refers to a discoloration of the skin with bile pigments. The scleras, skin, and to some extent the mucous membranes assume a greenish yellow hue; however, the intensity of the jaundice color varies greatly. The bile pigments causing the discoloration are derived from the red corpuscles. The term yellow jaundice often means more to the patient than to the dentist. However, the dentist should always check misinterpretation of the sallow complexion of general ill health by asking the patient about the urine and stool color and the doctor's statement at the time of the discoloration. Jaundice may be separated clinically into primary obstructive, hemolytic, and hepatocellular types. *Obstructive jaundice* may be caused by lesions within the lumens of the bile ducts, lesions in the wall of the bile ducts, or lesions causing compression of the bile ducts. *Hemolytic jaundice* is caused by excessive breakdown of erythrocytes and a rapid production of bilirubin. The causes include pernicious anemia, sickle cell anemia, malaria, certain drug sensitivities (for example, sulfanilamides, chemical agents such as acetanilid, lead, and bile salts), erythroblastosis fetalis, and Cooley's anemia. *Toxic* or *infective jaundice* is associated with portal cirrhosis, allergy (such as arsphenamine, sulfanilamide, mercury, and so on), hepatitis, amebiasis, leptospirosis, and yellow fever. Thus jaundice is a *symptom* of an underlying disturbance located in the liver, bile ducts, gallbladder, or a combination thereof.

It is important to know historically when teeth have been lost, reasons for loss, sequence of eruption, presence or absence of disease in formative periods, presence or absence of toothaches, location, and presence of drainage in the mouth. In periodontal therapy it is significant to determine whether or not teeth were lost because of dental caries or because of periodontal disease. It is important to know how long the disease has existed and if the loss of teeth is associated in any way with an acute disease process in the past. The presence of many periodontal abscesses with sudden loss of tissue tone suggests the possibility of uncontrolled diabetes mellitus.

A statement that a toothache is without apparent cause usually results from the observer's inability to make a diagnosis. Such conditions as sinusitis, anemia, cardiac failure, very slight trauma, pregnancy, menses, angina pectoris, mumps, neuroses, changes in altitude, and trigeminal neuralgia may many times produce toothaches without the presence of obvious disease in the tooth.

In some instances there is a direct time correlation between the occurrence of gastrointestinal disturbances and the insertion of a new partial or complete denture or the extraction of several teeth. Gastrointestinal disturbances associated with the insertion of dentures may be psychogenic in origin as a result of increased salivation or may be coincidental with more serious disorders not attributable to oral changes. Sensitivity reactions to denture material are not common and are exceedingly difficult to demonstrate because of the common occurrence of denture-sore mouth from ill-fitting dentures. Poor patient preparation without attention to what the patient expects from new dentures might well be the basis for some of the so-called "poor-denture" patients and untoward reactions.

Cacogeusia (bad taste in the mouth) may be caused by blood, pus, stagnant food, debris, or metals. The presence of a metallic taste should lead to investigation of metal intoxication with a consideration of occupational hazards. Pus from periodontal packets and periodontal abscesses gives a particularly disagreeable taste, although many degrees of appreciation of these factors are present from one individual to the next. The establishment of an appreciation of what a clean mouth feels like is one phase of dental education and home care. Food impaction is a common cause of the feeling of bad taste. A history of food sticking between the teeth is suggestive of functional inadequacy in the area of impaction. Since the olfactory sense accounts for much of a person's ability to taste, the history of bad taste should lead to questions concerning conditions of the nasal passage. An associated productive cough may well mean that there is some pulmonary disease such as bronchiectasis or tuberculosis. Malfunction of the cardia with the regurgitation of food particles is not a too frequent cause of bad taste. In making an evaluation of bad taste in the mouth, one needs to determine the duration and association of other factors such as coughing, vomiting, gastric disturbances, sinusitis, and cold. The quality of the taste (sweet, sour, salty, or metallic) should be determined and evaluated.

Increased flow of saliva may be associated with metal intoxication, mercurial therapy, wearing of dentures, Vincent's infection, herpetic stomatitis, and other functional disorders. Decreased salivation (xerostomia or dry mouth) is seen occurring after irradiation, in old age, and with functional disorders. Decreased salivation and dry mouth may, in some degree, be caused by obstruction of the salivary gland ducts by inspissated material or calcareous deposits. Dry mouth and drooling are terms used by patients to describe the symptoms of a change in the quantity of the flow of saliva. A history of endemic parotitis may at times aid in making a differential diagnosis, since it is unlikely that a patient who has had bilateral mumps is suffering from this disease when presenting with an enlargement of the parotid glands.

When a patient has previously been fitted with a prosthetic appliance but now keeps it in a drawer and never uses it or just uses it on special occasions, questions should be asked regarding the complaints associated with the appliance. A review of the conditions in the past allows a better understanding of the problems to be encountered by the practitioner as well as a chance for patient education. The same is true of patients who, when told of periodontal diseases, are troubled because previous treatment was supposed to have cured the condition. An adequate history of previous diseases of the oral structures in relation to further treatment is necessary not only to bring out objective dissatisfaction, but also to learn of personality problems that have to be considered for successful treatment of the patient.

A patient who expresses difficulty in masticating food may do so because of painful teeth, malocclusion, periodontal disease, insufficient occlusal surfaces, temporomandibular joint disease, oral lesions, muscular dysfunction, or lack of training after long disuse. The most frequent cause of such difficulty is loss of posterior teeth without replacement. In some instances, tipping and extrusion of posterior teeth, especially third molars, may lead to trauma of the temporomandibular joint through occlusal disharmony. Very frequently the patient may trace his difficulty to the loss of teeth, placement of restorations, or eruption of third molars.

A history of orthodontic treatment should include the reason for the treatment and the apparent results in terms of the patient's satisfaction.

Genitourinary system. The principal historic manifestations of disorders in the urinary system are dysuria, polyuria, hematuria, and edema. In a review of this system, positive statements regarding a history of these manifestations of disease, as well as venereal disease, should be made. A history or the presence of disorders is of importance to the dentist because of the relationship between oral health and the general health of the patient. The value of the information obtained may be found in the following relationships: (1) Manifestations of serious metabolic disorders such as diabetes mellitus are frequently suspected because of disorders of urinary function, namely, polyuria. Though this symptom may be transient, it may also be of primary consideration in directing the examiner's attention to other contributory symptoms of diabetes mellitus. (2) Edema that is generalized or limited to areas particularly susceptible to accumulations of a transudate because of dependency or laxness of the skin is of dental significance because of the frequent association with cardiac insufficiency. This factor, as well as other diseases of renal and nutritional disorders, is of primary concern to the oral surgeon contemplating surgical procedures. (3) A history or presence of venereal disease is of importance because of its possible relation to disease of the mouth, such as syphilitic glossitis, Hutchinson's incisors, and mulberry molars, and because of possible contraction of the disease by the dentist. Rarely gonorrhea may lead to acute pyogenic arthritis of the temporomandibular joint.

Questions regarding venereal disease require tactful inquiry by name and symptom: for example, gonorrhea, "clap," penile discharge in the male; vaginal discharge with low abdominal pain and dysmenorrhea or a disease diagnosed as "inflammation of the tubes" in the female; and syphilis, "bad blood," "haircut," chancre, or prolonged "needle treatments for bad blood." Tests of food handlers and premarital tests usually suffice to obtain valuable information concerning serology; patients should be questioned about previous tests when venereal disease is suspected.

Catamenia. The menstrual history is of importance as an index to a woman's health and as a means of detecting an early sign of genitourinary cancer and a bleeding tendency. Odontalgia, mucosal ulceration, salivary gland swelling, and gingival hemorrhage are associated with menstruation in some women. Pregnancy complicates dental care in several aspects; increased carbohydrate intake in patients with so-called morning sickness may contribute to an increase in the rate of dental caries. Dental appointments may necessarily be avoided in the morning when "morning sickness" is a factor.

So-called pregnancy gingivitis, gingival "tumors," and the tendency for an increase in the severity of an existing gingivitis may be seen in pregnant women. The apparent increase in gingivitis may be caused by several factors, including less inclination on the part of women to maintain good oral hygiene because of an "ill feeling" and because of hormonal imbalance and vascular changes during this period.

The climacteric should be evaluated in the female patient because of the changes occurring in the mucous membranes and because of the psychic factors involved. The main symptom of the menopause is the so-called hot flash, which is often accompanied or followed by sweats. Such flushes may occur for no apparent reason or may occur in association with a temporary psychic unrest—dental procedures involving discomfort, and so on. They usually affect only the upper portion of the body and produce a sensation of warmth over the chest, head, and neck. The skin may flush and turn red, and there may be a sensation of choking and suffocation. Flushes are likely to appear during the night as well as during the day. Other symptoms, such as tinnitus, palpitations of the heart, loss of appetite, bitter taste in the mouth, flatulence, nausea, vomiting, abdominal cramps, diarrhea, or constipation (or both) may be produced. The patient may have headaches ranging from an occasional dull ache to an intense ache that lasts for days and weeks. The hot flushes may cause the hands and the whole body to tremble. Vague pains such as backaches, numbness, and tingling sensations may also be present. Induced menopause may result in the same symptoms. The development of symptoms of anxiety, depression, tension, or hysteria in the premenstrual period is a well-recognized and accepted feature of the menstrual cycle in the female.

In the menopause there is a decrease in ovarian function and sufficient hormonal imbalance in some patients to produce noticeable symptoms. Along with the shift in hormonal balance, in many patients there appears to be a pronounced shift in stability of the autonomous nervous system. As a result there are frequent discharges of sympathetic activity that result in the symptom called hot flushes and in nervousness. The other symptoms that appear during and after the onset of the menopause are caused by the gradual decrease of estrogen. This decrease makes itself manifest by a gradual decrease in the thickness of skin and mucous membrane and in the size and tone of muscles, the appearance of atrophy of the vagina, the endometrium, and the breasts, and a relative decrease in the formation of bone matrix. This latter condition results in senile osteoporosis because of the relative failure of osteoblastic activity to provide an abundant organic matrix for the deposition of calcium. This is more noticeable in some patients than in others. Such senile osteoporosis is evident by radiographic examination in many patients, especially in the mandible. In some instances these areas of radiolucency have been mistakenly described as pathologic conditions.

Although men may suffer from symptoms of the climacteric, this is very uncommon and should not be emphasized since it is probably of no clinical significance. In women, osteoarthritis may first become symptomatic at the time of menopause. when complaints of osteoarthritis are already present, symptoms may be sharply accentuated with the onset of the menopause. One must remember that age, wear and tear, trauma, abnormal occupational stresses, congenital and developmental defects, infection, and neuromuscular disease are all considered to be causes of osteoarthritis, and thus it may be difficult to assess the importance of the menopause in the etiology of osteoarthritis of the temporomandibular joint. Clinically, osteoarthritis of the temporomandibular joint is asymptomatic even in the presence of extensive articular damage.

Premenstrual tension and dysmenorrhea are often accompanied by menstrual irregularity and premenstrual pain. Premature occurrence of amenorrhea after less than the average span or normal menstrual cycles is called early menopause. The onset of female climacteric before the age of 45 years is definitely abnormal and is probably related to an early depletion of primordial follicles. Thus it is possible for an individual in the early menopause to show the characteristic menopausal symptoms, including osteoporosis of the mandible and atrophic gingival changes.

Between the ages of 45 and 50 years is progressive irregularity in frequency, duration, and amount of menstrual flow until only an occasional period or spotting occurs; complete amenorrhea then occurs. A recurrence of bleeding after a period of amenorrhea in patients over the age of 45 years must be considered to be caused by ovarian or uterine neoplasms until proved otherwise. Hyperhidrosis, rapid gain in weight, atrophic arthritis, and osteoporosis are not uncommon findings after the menopause.

It is obvious how the symptoms of the climateric may present problems in diagnosis and treatment of dental conditions. In patients with gynecologic disorders occurring after menopause it is not uncommon to find sore and tender mouths and certain forms of gingivitis. Patients in the menopause commonly complain of dryness or a burning sensation in the mouth. Lesions of the buccal mucosa consisting of irregular grayish white areas that are expressions of atrophic changes are not infrequently mistaken for leukoplakia or lichen planus.

The dentist should not overlook the psychic factor in his evaluation of any dental problem in the patient in the menopause, since the "human equation" may be of considerably more imporance than technical perfection. For example, dentures may be technically perfect, yet some patients, because of emotional imbalance during the menopause, may not be able to adjust and train themselves in their use.

Neuromuscular system. A complete review of the neuromuscular system should contain at least sufficient questions to assure an adequate coverage of any history of syncope, convulsions, anesthesias, paresthesias, paralysis, mental confusion, memory loss, sudden changes in temperament, bruxism, neuralgias, neuroses, trismus, and myositis. The extent of the review will depend in part upon the type of information to be obtained and in part upon the emphasis that may be directed toward this system, especially from the *chief complaint* and *present illness.* Of primary interest to the dentist are the relation of syncope to dental procedures, paresthesias and anesthesias related to dental extractions or traumatic injury, major and minor neuralgias of the mouth and face, bruxism associated with occlusal dysfunction, and oral, systemic, and psychic changes associated with convulsions, mental confusion, and cerebral damage.

Syncope or fainting may result from psychic stimuli, emotional upsets, hypodermic injections, pressure on the carotid sinus, postural hypotension, myocardial infarction, hyperventilation, hypoglycemia, hysteria, and occasionally from heart disease. When there is a positive history of frequent syncope, the patient should be questioned regarding the time of onset, position of patient at onset, duration of a syncope, and any alleviating circumstances. Orthostatic syncope associated with rigid attention and lack of muscle movements is of much less significance than recumbent syncope. A past history of syncope is very likely to be related to emotional upsets or apprehension; however, a complete history should cover the possibility of other factors that may have been responsible.

Syncope should not be confused with the transient blackouts of petit mal (epilepsy) because posture and activities may be little affected during the blackouts. Unconsciousness, arising from circulatory disorders that cause cerebral ischemia, varies from momentary fainting (postural syncope) to prolonged unconsciousness (apoplexy). A history of convulsions should be described as to the presence or absence of self-injury from falling, tongue biting, and cheek biting since these factors rarely accompany hysteria.

Anesthesias and paresthesias should be described as to location, duration, mode of onset, and associated symptoms. Transient perioral numbness or paresthesia of both hands is a common symptom of hyperventilation. It is not uncommon for a patient to complain of anesthesia and paresthesia of the side of the face and lips after extraction of a difficult third molar. These symptoms usually subside, but occasionally they may persist. Not infrequently, when damage to the mandibular nerve is great, traumatic neurofibromas may develop and the patient may be troubled with varying degrees of discomfort.

Inquiry into a history of paralysis of the mouth and face should include questions concerning transient or developing muscular weakness and the development of speech defects not related to dentures. In tertiary syphilis (paresis) the gait is often shuffling, and the patient may not be able to keep his eyes off his feet while walking. An ataxic gait, though somewhat characteristic in itself, may occur in many conditions and diseases besides tertiary syphilis. In general, an individual who has been seriously debilitated will initially have difficulty in walking in addition to other manifestations of weakness. Cerebrovascular accidents may cause a patient to be paralyzed in any portion of the body. It is not uncommon for a patient who has experienced a cerebrovascular accident to have a complete or partial paralysis of the muscles of facial expression and mastication on one side of the face. Such a patient has difficult problems in oral hygiene as well as problems in restorative dentistry. Those with severe paralysis affecting an arm may find it difficult to place or to remove partial dentures.

A history of bruxism may be difficult to obtain at the first interview since many patients are unaware of this condition. It may be necessary to ask the patient to determine its presence for himself. He may be completely unaware of any clenching or grinding habits even though there may be clinical signs of their presence. Other members of the family may be aware of this condition, especially when the bruxism occurs when the patient is asleep. Bruxism is of extreme importance in the etiology of traumatic occlusion and its basis must be determined, whether it be psychogenic or occlusal in origin.

A complaint and history of odontalgias and referred pain require careful questioning about the time of onset, duration, type of pain, extent, spread, and factors such as heat, cold, and eating that may be the precipitating agent.

Bones and joints. A review of the bones and joints may contain questions directed toward previous trauma, pain, swelling, heat, limitation of motion, duration of symptoms, mode of onset, mode of relief, association of complaint with the use of the bone or joint, previous history of infantile scurvy, rickets, fractures, osteomyelitis, poliomyelitis, cerebral palsy, muscular atrophy, and hemophilia. When a chief complaint and related symptoms are located within this system, a detailed account much more extensive than that just indicated may be necessary before an adequate coverage of the system can be considered to have been accomplished. Although the primary concern to the dentist is the review of the bones and joints of the masticatory system, diseases of the bones and joints outside this area may be of significant importance to the formulation and treatment of oral disease.

Certainly no dentist would consider the evaluation of the temporomandibular joints complete without a consideration of the other joints of the body, since the same disease may also be present in the other joints. In some instances the diagnosis of temporomandibular joint disease may be dependent upon the presence or history of disease elsewhere in the body. The question of whether the historian should cover the bone and joint system more extensively will depend upon the type of examination and the presence of disease in the bones and joints of the masticatory system.

When a history of joint disturbances is suspected, questions should be asked relating to trauma, muscular imbalance, degenerative diseases, neuropathic joint disease, specific infectious arthritis, acute rheumatic fever, rheumatoid arthritis, and the effects of movement. When the attention of the examiner is directed toward the temporomandibular joint, a more complete review of the symptoms of disease of this joint must be carried out.

It must be remembered that the temporomandibular joint is only a part of the masticatory system and that, as a functional part of this system, diseases and other components may reflect to the temporomandibular joint. Thus the symptoms of temporomandibular joint abnormality may be associated with injuries to the jaws, occlusal disharmony, oral habits, faulty dental therapy, lack of replacement of lost teeth, and bruxism. It is not uncommon for a patient with arthritis of the joint to complain of painful sensations in the ear or around the temporomandibular joint that have no organic origin within the temporomandibular joint or ear. In these instances the patient may consult a otolaryngologist first and be told that he has no ear disease. With such a history the examiner should make a detailed inquiry for symptoms of dysfunction not only of the temporomandibular joint, but also of other components of the masticatory system.

The most important symptoms of disturbances of the temporomandibular joint are related to various degrees of trauma. Complaints associated with acute symptoms can usually be related to a known traumatic injury. After the injury there is a painful restriction of mandibular movements and in some instances pain of a continuous nature. Chronic trauma related to chronic subluxation of the temporomandibular joint and occlusal disharmony are the most frequent causes of disturbances of the joint. These symptoms include clicking or snapping noises upon moving the mandible, unilateral mastication with restriction of mandibular movements, and referred pain to the ear, occipital and temporal regions, and in some instances the neck, tongue, jaws or sinuses. The patient will often have have remissions of the symptoms but occasionally will have acute exacerbations.

Symptoms involving the temporomandibular joint may also arise from disease of the joint itself. Rheumatoid arthritis, degenerative joint disease, infective arthritis, rheumatic fever, bursitis, and nonarticular rheumatism may produce symptoms of pain and limit the jaw movements. Systemic symptoms may be present with infective arthritis, namely, fever, chills, sweats, malaise, and anorexia.

Atypical facial neuralgias, Ménière's disease, headaches, and psychogenic complaints may be difficult for the examiner to evaluate in a differential diagnosis of temporomandibular joint disturbances. Thus, when a complaint involves the temporomandibular joint, it is important that the examiner be aware of the other factors that may produce complaints referable to the joint. A diagnosis of temporomandibular joint dysfunction should be based on the examination of the joint and on obtaining and evaluating a history of the patient's complaints. Though the physical examination of the joint is a necessary procedure, initially it is probably not as important as proper collection of the facts concerning the patient's complaint. Because of the common relation of occlusal dysfunction to temporomandibular joint dysfunction, examination of the occlusion is of primary importance. However, a careful analysis of the complaint and associated symptoms should be made to rule out other causative agents.

There may not be a characteristic or prodromic illness prior to the onset of inflammation of the joints in rheumatoid arthritis; on rare occasions it may involve the temporomandibular joint first. The nature and intermittent character of complaints with remissions and exacerbations associated with swelling and stiffness of joints suggests rheumatoid arthritis. The proximal interphalangeal joints almost always are involved ultimately. Almost all disorders of joint function are characterized by the association of two or more related symptoms. An investigation of these symptoms would generally lead to an understanding of the related complaints and of the underlying basic disturbance. For example, in a complaint of chronic joint pain it is significant to know that recently a third molar was extracted and that prior to this there was frequent subluxation of the mandible. Although it is possible for the extraction itself to be responsible for the complaint, the prior chronic subluxation must be evaluated before treatment can be instituted. Although a patient is primarily interested in alleviation of the pain in the temporomandibular joint, treatment of symptoms, such as injections of cortisone or hyaluronidase into the joint space or immobilization of the jaws, will probably not give permanent relief. However, a complete review of the masticatory system will serve to direct the examiner in his examination to the underlying basis for the disturbed function of the joint and provide a rational basis for therapy. It is to be expected in the example given that the examiner will find evidence of disturbed occlusal harmony and that a permanent therapy must include an occlusal adjustment. The third molar may well be responsible for the occlusal disharmony, but in view of the persistent complaint the clinical examination will probably show additional occlusal disharmony. Thus the chronology of the complaints and a clinical examination of the occlusion are both necessary before adequate therapy can be undertaken. Moreover, an adequate history and examination will serve to rule out other possible causative agents.

In some instances an examiner may elicit the symptoms of temporomandibular joint disturbance and also occlusal disharmony but fail to discover significant symptoms of emotional disturbances. This often results in poor treatment planning and ineffective therapy since no therapy for the adjustment of the occlusion and palliation of the temporomandibular joint symptoms can be adequate in the presence of perpetuating emotional disturbance. Thus the examiner must be adept in collecting the facts, have a basic knowledge of the disease processes responsible for the symptoms collected, and be able to synthesize these two components in the formulation of a diagnosis.

REFERENCES

Alexander, H. L.: Reactions with drug therapy, Philadelphia, 1955, W. B. Saunders Co.

Bacterial endocarditis, J.A.D.A. **85:**1177, Dec. 1972.

Bottomley, W. K.: How the dentist can protect his patients from bacterial endocarditis, Mich. Dent. A. J. **51:**149-151, 1969.

Carr, E. A.: Drug allergy, Pharmacol. Rev. **6:**365-424, 1954.

Comroe, B. I., Collins, L. H., and Crane, M. P.: Internal medicine in dental practice, ed. 3, Philadelphia, 1949, Lea & Febiger.

Cuttita, J. A., et al.: Self histories; an adjunct to history taking, J. Periodont. **35:**489-494, Nov.-Dec., 1964.

Dingman, R. O., and Hayward, J. R.: The value of writing case histories, J. Oral Surg. **5:**123, 1947.

Donaldson, K. I.: Pain; the chief complaint, Austral. Dent. J. **12:**9-11, Feb., 1967.

Emslie, R. D., Massler, M., and Zwemer, J. D.: Mouth breathing, J.A.D.A. **44:**506-521, 1952.

Fulton, M., and Levine, S. A.: Subacute bacterial endocarditis with special reference to valvular lesions and previous history, Amer. J. Med. Sci. **183:**60-77, 1932.

Gilman, S.: The treatment of dangerous reactions to novocain, New Eng. J. Med. **219:**841, 1938.

Herrmann, G. R.: Clinical case taking, St. Louis 1945, The C. V. Mosby Co.

Horder, T. J.: Infective endocarditis, Quart. J. Med. **2:**289-329, 1909.

Hughes, F. W.: New psychotherapeutic drugs, J. Indiana Med. Ass. **50:**293, 1957.

Landa, J. S.: The dynamics of psychosomatic dentistry, Brooklyn, 1953, Dental Items of Interest Publishing Co., Inc.

Massler, M., and Zwemer, J. D.: Mouth breathing; diagnosis and treatment, J.A.D.A. **46:**658-671, 1953.

McCarthy, F. M.: Emergencies in dental practice, Philadelphia, 1967, W. B. Saunders Co.

Meakins, J. C.: Symptoms in diagnosis, ed. 2, Boston, 1949, Little, Brown & Co.

Millard, H. D., and Tupper, C. J.: Subacute bacterial endocarditis: a clinical study, J. Oral Surg. **18:**224-229, 1960.

Modell, W.: The relief of symptoms, Philadelphia, 1955, W. B. Saunders Co.

Nyquist, G.: A study of denture sore mouth, Acta Odont. Scand. (supp. 9) **10:**1-154, 1952.

Prevention of bacterial endocarditis, J.A.D.A. **85:**1377-1379, Dec. 1972.

Rostenberg, A., Jr.: Eczematous sensitization, Arch. Dermatol. **56:**222-232, 1947.

Seabury, J. H.: Subacute bacterial endocarditis, Arch. Intern. Med. **79:**1-21, 1947.

Walton, C. H., and Bottomley, H. W.: Allergy to aspirin, Canad. Med. Ass. J. **64:**187-190, 1951.

4

Significance of drugs in oral diagnosis

The practice of medicine and dentistry is highly complicated by the use of a large number of drugs that produce extensive alteration in the physiologic reactions of patients to whom they are administered. Durgs given for specific effect on one system for the treatment of a specific disease may alter considerably the functions and reactions of the entire organism. The effects of many drugs may be potentiated by the administration of other drugs for an entirely different disease. A patient receiving a specific drug for the treatment of a systemic disease may be given a drug for his oral disease that will be incompatible with the drug already being used. The side effects produced by the initial drug may be intensified by the administration of a second drug. The interaction of the two drugs may intensify the initial disease. It may increase the side effects of the initial drug, or it may initiate another disease state. Some interactions or synergistic effects may cause a new disease state or intensify the original disease to such a degree that it causes death of the individual. Because of these possibilities, it is important that the dentist know what types of drugs are given for specific disease states. Conversely, it is important to know that when a patient is receiving a particular drug this indicates a specific disease state. It is also important to know which classes of drugs are incompatible and what side effects are produced by various drugs. It is important in arriving at a diagnosis and dictating a treatment plan to give consideration to these various interrelationships of drugs and disease states.

As a brief guide, the various classes of drugs used for management of specific disease states are listed and the significance of each group of drugs as they relate to dental diagnosis and treatment planning is indicated.

Adrenocorticosteroids and corticotropin. Drugs of anti-inflammatory nature are used to treat a wide range of diseases, and the patient taking corticosteroids must be questioned about the type of disease for which they are being treated. The adverse reactions to steroids are as numerous as the diseases treated so that patients taking these drugs should be carefully evaluated before treatment procedures are begun. It is important that one using these drugs in therapy have a thorough knowledge of the pharmacology of this class of drugs.

Analgesics. This class of drugs is divided into those of mild and strong action. The mild analgesic drugs are codeine, ethoheptazine (Zactane), dextropropoxyphene HCl (Darvon), aspirin, and aminopyrine. These drugs produce only limited side effects unless given in large quantities, with the exception of aminopyrine, which causes agranulocytosis in a significant number of individuals. The continuous use of these drugs usually indicates some musculoskeletal disease for which relief of pain and anti-inflammatory reaction is desirable. Large doses of aspirin may affect hemostasis. The strong analgesics are morphine and its derivatives. Synthetic drugs in this class are meperidine HCl (Demerol) and methadone. The chief side effect of this class of drugs is respiratory depression that can be potentiated by alcohol, barbiturates, and antipsychotic agents. These drugs are usually given for the control of severe pain, and therefore the patients who are using such drugs and presenting in the dental office may be addicted to the drug. It is important to know whether patients are drug addicts before prescribing other forms of drugs.

Antianemic compounds. A large number of women are given these drugs to correct a reduction in hemoglobin or red blood cell count and are used in the treatment of pernicious anemia. Patients with mild to severe anemia may complain of a burning tongue and atrophy of papillae along with chronic fatigue, weakness, and tingling of extremities.

The types of drugs used as antianemic drugs are iron compounds, vitamin B_{12}, folic acid, and liver extract. The iron compounds may produce pigmentation of the teeth if given in liquid form. The solutions are usually acid in reaction and may enhance caries activity. Gastric intestinal disturbances also frequently occur from iron therapy.

Vitamin B_{12} and folates are nontoxic, and there are almost no complications related to their administration. The use of vitamin B_{12} or folic acid may indicate treatment of pernicious anemia, which is often accompanied by neurologic symptoms that may complicate the diagnosis of oral symptoms.

Antianginal drugs. Such drugs as nitroglycerin and amyl nitrite are used for the relief of anginal pain produced by coronary ischemia and other pain associated with cardiac disease. Patients who have angina pectoris may have symptoms initiated or potentiated by the injection or administration of vasoconstrictor drugs. Therefore the use of local anesthetic containing epinephrine and its derivatives is contraindicated for patients with angina pectoris.

Antianxiety drugs (ataractics). The use of meprobamate (Miltown, Equanil), chlordiazepoxide (Librium), chlorpromazine

(Thorazine), and diazepam (Valium) usually indicates that the patient has emotional problems and anxiety. This type of drug is frequently taken by patients before dental appointments, and it would be desirable to know this before other similar drugs are prescribed. A variety of actions and reactions are produced by this group of drugs. The drugs act as depressants of the central nervous system. Side reactions are dizziness, drowsiness, headache, and moderate xerostomia. Patients taking these drugs develop dependence to the same extent as barbiturates and have similar withdrawal symptoms. Physical coordination, judgment, and mental alertness are all reduced by these drugs. These drugs also provide muscle relaxation and may be prescribed for that purpose.

Antiarrhythmic drugs. Frequently antiarrhythmic drugs are given to help establish normal heart rhythm when the individual has either bradycardia or tachycardia. The drugs most often used that indicate the patient has cardiac arrhythmia are digitalis and quinidine. Anxiety, local anesthetic, or any cardiac stimulant, such as caffeine in APC, may initiate the arrhythmia and should be used with caution. Quinidine in some individuals is responsible for thrombocytopenia so that gingival bleeding in a patient using this drug might result from the drug.

Antibiotics (tetracyclines, penicillins, erythromycins, and chloramphenicol). Antibiotics are used for the treatment of a variety of disease processes produced by microorganisms. Some of the antibiotics, especially chloramphenicol, produce bone marrow depression in some patients on large doses. The depression may be manifest as either agranulocytosis or purpura. Also patients who take antibiotics for prolonged periods may, because of altered symbiosis, develop an overwhelming increase in fungal organisms. This is especially true of *Candida (Monilia) albicans,* and the patient develops thrush as a complication. One should consider this situation when evaluating patients with a history of prolonged antibiotic therapy or if prolonged use of antibiotic therapy is prescribed. Steroid and immunosuppressant drugs given with antibiotics enhances the development of fungal disease.

Anticoagulants (heparin and coumarin derivatives). Anticoagulants are given to patients who have thromboembolic states such as cardiovascular disorders, peripheral vascular disease, cerebrovascular disease, various surgical procedures, and pulmonary embolism. The effect produced by the anticoagulant drugs is a prevention of blood clotting. Individuals taking this class of drugs should be continually monitored by prothrombin tests to determine when there is a tendency for hemorrhage. Careful supervision of a patient on anticoagulation therapy, using the one-stage prothrombin time test, is mandatory when the patient receives other medication. The prothrombin time should also be evaluated previous to any elective surgical procedure. Deep subgingival curettage, gingivectomy, and extraction may result in severe hemorrhage if the level of anticoagulant is too high.

Anticonvulsants. Anticonvulsant drugs are used primarily for the treatment of petit or grand mal seizures (epilepsy). Phenobarbital is also commonly used for the treatment of convulsive disorders (see the discussion on barbiturates). The chief anticonvulsant drug other than phenobarbital is diphenylhydantoin (Dilantin). The prolonged use of these drugs especially in childhood produces hyperplastic gingivitis of considerable severity. These drugs have sedating effects. Nearly any type of allergic reaction can result from the use of hydantoin drugs. The most severe reaction is bone marrow depression with the development of agranulocytosis and bleeding states.

Antidepressants. This class of drugs includes the amphetamines (Benzedrine, Dexedrine) used to treat patients with central nervous system depression, but they may be used without need by many individuals. Side effects produced by these drugs are dry mouth, nervousness, collapse, and syncope. These drugs also potentiate the effect of procaine, barbiturates, alcohol, and many of the analgesic type of drugs. It is therefore important to know whether patients are using these drugs before other drugs are prescribed for sedation or pain control.

Antigout drugs. Those agents most often used to treat gout are colchicine, corticotropin, indomethacin (Indocin), phenylbutazone (Butazolidin), and probenecid (Benemid). The drugs used for the treatment of gout are a widely differing group, but there is some common ground for consideration of adverse reactions. All produce gastrointestinal disturbances and activate existing peptic ulcers. All may produce skin reactions or mucous membrane lesions. The action of antigout drugs such as probenecid (Benemid) may be negated by aspirin.

Antihistamines. The list of antihistamines available is extensive. They may be purchased over the counter or by prescription. They are taken routinely as antiallergic drugs and irregulary as treatment for upper respiratory infections. A history of patients taking antihistamines is essential if the drugs are to be prescribed as a part of dental treatment.

Antineoplastics. Patients taking antineoplastic drugs (cyclophosphamide [Cytoxan], fluorouracil, methotrexate, mercaptopurine) frequently develop oral ulcerations of a type seen in agranulocytosis. In fact, some patients with prolonged heavy dosage of antineoplastic drugs develop agranulocytosis from depression of hemopoietic tissue. Surgical procedures should not be carried out for patients on antineoplastic drugs because of the delay in healing and the possibility of initiating a septicemia or hemorrhage. Patients on antineoplastic drugs should not be given drugs that might produce bone marrow depression. When patients are taking antineoplastic drugs, the situation usually indicates that the individual has an advanced and probably incurable neoplasm and thus a short life expectancy, which would dictate the accomplishment of palliative rather than extensive definitive treatment.

Antispasmodics. Patients with hyperactive smooth muscle of the gastrointestinal tract and peptic ulcer are treated with antispasmodic drugs, such as belladonna, atropine, hyoscyamine, methantheline (Banthine), and propantheline (Pro-Banthine). One of the common side effects of this class of drugs is the extreme dryness of the mouth often accompanied by burning and difficulty in swallowing. Uninformed patients may associate the problem with oral or salivary gland disease and seek dental advice. The xerostomia enhances the carious activity of the patient.

Antituberculosis agents. Patients who have tuberculosis are treated with a variety of drugs (aminosalicylate, cycloserene, ethionamide, and streptomycin). When these drugs are used individually, drug-resistant forms of *Mycobacterium tuberculosis* develop so that a treated patient may still be infectious. Although the patient is symptom free, he may have active drug-resistant organisms present, which could be transmitted to one in close contact with the patient. Personal protection with a mask is advisable when the patient gives a history of being treated with any of the antituberculosis drugs. The prolonged use of these drugs produces neurotoxic effects involving hearing and vision. The neurotoxic reactions may result in confusion with symptoms of oral disease.

Bronchial dilators. The bronchial dilators are used for the treatment of bronchial asthma and emphysema. Those most often used are adrenergic agents (epinephrine [Adrenalin], ephedrine), isoproterenol, theophylline, and corticosteroids. The chief side effects produced by these drugs involve the cardiovascular and central nervous system. Tachycardia associated with the use of bronchial dilators may be intensified by the administration of local anesthetics. Central nervous system stimulation may also be enhanced by the use of local anesthetics. It is also important to realize that asthmatic attacks may be initiated by the anxiety of dental treatment and by drugs used for treatment.

Diuretics. There are several types of drugs used to eliminate excess fluid by increasing urinary output. Some of these same drugs are used as antihypertensive drugs. Drugs in this category are aminophylline, chlorothiazide (Diuril), and others such as ammonium chloride. Prolonged use of these drugs results in loss of potassium with alteration of electrolyte balance. These drugs also produce xerostomia.

Estrogens, progestogens, oral contraceptives, and ovulatory agents. Large numbers of postmenopausal females receive estrogen therapy without any appreciable side effects. Many postmenopausal women have mucosal atrophy and "burning mouth," which is on a hormonal basis. Before these drugs are prescribed for this condition, one should determine whether the patient is already receiving estrogen therapy. Gingival disease has been attributed to oral contraceptive drugs, but positive association except in rare cases has not been demonstrated.

Hypotensive drugs. Hypertension is treated with (1) oral diuretics (thiazides), (2) sympathetic nervous system inhibitors (rauwolfia, reserpine, methyldopa), or (3) a drug acting directly on smooth muscle (hydralazine [Apresoline]). These drugs may cause weakness, mental depression, dizziness, and dryness of the mouth. Patients on any form of diuretic may develop xerostomia with pronounced increase in dental caries as a secondary result.

Sedatives and hypnotics. The drugs used as sedatives and hypnotics are classified as barbiturates and nonbarbiturates. The barbiturates produce respiratory depression, which is intensified by alcohol. These drugs are habituating and patients develop psychic dependence so that they should not be prescribed in therapeutic doses for long periods. These drugs reduce mental alertness, judgment, and physical coordination; so patients should be warned of this when the drugs are prescribed.

DRUG-INDUCED DISEASES

Certain disease states are produced by the reaction of an individual to a specific drug. Some of the type reactions that may be caused by a variety of drugs are mentioned.

Agranulocytosis is produced by such drugs as aminopyrine, anticonvulsants, chloramphenicol, phenylbutazone (Butazolidin), thiazides, antihistamines, and ataractics. *Anemias* may be produced by any of the drugs that depress bone marrow or affect the absorption of iron. In addition to the above, indomethacin, phenacetin, aspirin, and tetracyclines should be added to the list of drugs that produce anemia. *Anginal pain* may be induced by epinephrine and isoproterenol. These same drugs may produce arrhythmia. *Drug dependence* may result by the prolonged use of amphetamines, narcotic analgesics, codeine, meprobamate, pentazocine lactate (Talwin),

oxycodone (Percodan), ataractics, and opiates. *Syncope* may be produced by injection of local anesthetics, aminophylline, amphetamine, chlordiazepoxide (Librium), meperidine (Demerol), penicillin, and quinidine. *Tardive dyskinesia,* rhythmical involuntary movements of the tongue, face, mouth, or jaw, may appear in some patients on long-term use of phenothiazines and certain other antipsychotic medications. *Thrombocytopenia* (allergic purpura) is produced as a reaction to many drugs in those who have an allergy or hypersensitivity to the drugs. Some of the drugs that should be considered are quinidine, anticonvulsants, aminosalicylates, antineoplastic agents, chloramphenicol, heparin, indomethacin, and phenylbutazone.

REFERENCES

Accepted dental therapeutics, 1972-73, ed. 35, Chicago, American Dental Association.
AMA drug evaluations, Chicago, 1971, American Medical Association.
Evaluations of drug interactions, Washington, D. C., 1973, American Pharmaceutical Association.
Grollman, A., and Grollman, E. F.: Pharmacology and therapeutics, ed. 7, Philadelphia, 1970, Lea & Febiger.
Millard, H. D.: Failures in medication, Dent. Clin. N. Amer. **16:**201, 1972.

SECTION II
THE CLINICAL EXAMINATION

The clinical examination of a patient should be based on a discipline that will enable an examiner to identify the cause of disease for which a patient seeks help and to detect disease that is unknown to an apparently well patient. The principles should be the same for the complete, screening, or emergency type of examination. The clinical examination, regardless of its purpose, is not a diagnosis but a step toward diagnosis, and the discipline by which it is carried out is the same irrespective of the omission of some of the elements of the complete type of examination. Therefore, the fundamentals necessary to carry out a complete and thorough examination should be the basis of knowledge for all practitioners who seek to satisfy the principles of an adequate clinical examination. The practitioner who is well grounded in the methods of a thorough and complete examination is generally in a position to know what elements can be omitted without interfering with the formulations of a complete diagnosis even though it is necessary to utilize the screening or emergency type of examination.

The omission of some of the elements of a complete examination for the purpose of screening patients is justifiable only when the limitations of the omission are well understood. The justification for an incomplete or emergency type of examination is based upon the relative efficiency of such an examination in the recognition of obvious disease and the relief of symptoms. This use, even when its limitations are known, does not justify teaching it in a course of oral diagnosis to the exclusion of a complete discipline that is so necessary for the development of competence in oral diagnosis. Once all the elements of a complete examination are mastered, the type of examination or its contents may be easily modified to meet the circumstances. Therefore, all the procedures necessary to carry out a complete examination are given here.

After a general survey of the patient's health, the examiner should carry out a detailed and systematic examination of the mouth. The order begins with the lips and traverses the buccal mucosa and contiguous structures, the hard and soft palates, the tonsillar region, the floor of the mouth, the tongue, the gingivae, and the teeth. The examination should be carried out systematically and routinely in this manner so that no portion will be missed.

The plan to be followed here is based on the concept that the examiner should learn how to examine the mouth, know what to expect in the normal mouth, and know what variations of the normal to consider. It is only logical to assume that he will not be able to detect the abnormal unless he is aware of the normal and its variations. It is suggested that the student should make a record of his examination findings regardless of the presence or absence of pathologic conditions. After he has acquired skill in the procedures of the examination and has developed an appreciation for the normal findings, he may eliminate the inclusion of such negative findings except in those instances in which the absence of pathologic conditions is of significance.

Thus it may be necessary to make a positive statement regarding the absence of certain features of a disease in order to provide the negative and positive correlative data necessary for a diagnosis. It is best not to write "negative" in recording the absence of disease; it is better to remove any doubts about the area having been examined by a positive statement as to the regions covered. When no disease is present, the student examiner should give a description of the normal. If diagnosis is to be complete and if obscure lesions are to be noted, the technic of oral examination must be careful and exacting and should include more than a "checkup" of the teeth.

OUTLINE FOR CLINICAL EXAMINATION

PRINCIPLES OF THE CLINICAL EXAMINATION

Inspection
Palpation
Percussion
Auscultation

CLINICAL EXAMINATION—GENERAL

General appraisal (including temperature, pulse rate, and blood pressure when indicated)

Head

Skull—facies, facial form, symmetry
Eyes—scleras, pupils, eyelids, conjunctival lesions
Nose—deformity, obstructions, mouth breathing

Skin

Pigmentation, hair, texture, scars, lesions
Fingernails—biting, disease

Neck

Lymph nodes, scars, lesions, swelling, tenderness, pulsations, deviation of the midline

Jaws

Symmetry, anteroposterior relationship, closure pattern, lateral and protrusive movements

Temporomandibular joints — clicking, snapping, swelling, tenderness

CLINICAL EXAMINATION—ORAL

Soft tissues

Lips

Inspection and palpation of the physiologic and anatomic features of the lips in health and disease —form, position, function, color, texture

Labial and buccal mucosa

Inspection and palpation of the physiologic and anatomic features of the labial and buccal mucosa in health and disease—color, texture, glands, ductal orifices, attachments of the frenula

Palate

Inspection and palpation of the physiologic and anatomic features of the hard and soft palates in health and disease—color, texture, glands, ductal orifices, density, rugae, function

Oropharynx

Inspection of the physiologic and anatomic features of the tonsils and throat in health and disease—color, size, form

Floor of the mouth

Inspection and palpation of the physiologic and anatomic features of the floor of the mouth in health and disease—sublingual and submaxillary glands and ductal orifices, lymph nodes, sublingual sulcus, lingual aspects of the mandible

Tongue

Inspection and palpation of the physiologic and anatomic features of the tongue in health and disease—color, papillae, lymphoid tissue, glands, attachment, position, function, size, texture

Periodontium

Inspection of the physiologic and anatomic features of normal and healthy gingiva—color, form, density, level of epithelial attachment, depth of gingival crevice

Findings in disease—alteration of normal color, form, density, and attachment

Examination procedures

Charting—free gingival margin, depth of gingival crevice, level of epithelial attachment, mobility of teeth

Teeth

Inspection, exploration, and percussion of the physiologic and anatomic features of the teeth in health and disease—color, size, form, structure, number, erosion, abrasion, fractures, functional contours, carious lesions, contact relationship of the teeth, marginal bit of restorations

Charting—caries, decalcification, vitality, missing teeth, restorations

Occlusion

Inspection, palpation, and analysis of the physiologic and anatomic features of the dentofacial structures in health and disease—facial form analysis, primary dentition analysis, mixed dentition analysis, adult occlusion analysis, functional analysis of the masticatory system

Edentulous and partially edentulous mouths

5

Principles of the clinical examination

The clinical examination is based on the principles of inspection, palpation, percussion, and auscultation. In general, these technics are applicable to the examination of the entire mouth and adjacent structures. All too often the examiner uses only the procedure of inspection. This is a mistake since palpation, percussion, and auscultation may be of considerable value in the examination of many areas and conditions.

Inspection. Inspection is the systematic visual assessment of the patient under examination. By inspection, assessment may be made of the color of the skin and mucosa; surface contours and proportions of the body and its parts; functional movement; and various bodily states that reflect in part the physiology and psychologic constitution of the individual. Thus, the examiner uses inspection every moment he is looking at his patient, noting anatomic, physiologic, and psychologic landmarks. Surface contours are influenced by the state of development of the musculature and the amount of fat in the superficial tissues. The prominences produced by underlying structures and easily seen in a thin person may be obscured in a fat one. In a thin individual, muscles of mastication such as the temporalis and masseter may be easily seen either when they are at rest or during function, whereas in a fat person the form and size are usually obscured even during function. Tumescence from a pathologic state such as enlargement of any of the glands of the neck may be obscured in an obese individual, whereas in a thin one a surface contour may be considerably changed and easily seen. Despite the fundamental similarity of structure in all patients, individual variations do occur. Almost everyone is familiar with the differences in musculature and other anatomic features of the various races. Thus certain peculiarities of external form are characteristic of certain people. A slight asymmetry affects both the proportions and the movements of the body and its parts.

Palpation. Palpation is a procedure whereby the examiner feels or presses upon the structures or portions of the body. An examiner skilled in the palpation of the normal body structures and their variations will find this procedure of significant value in discovering conditions outside the range of normal. The method of palpation depends upon the area to be examined. In some areas, such as the floor of the mouth, bimanual palpation is the method of choice (Fig. 5-1, *A*). Bidigital palpation is the method of choice for the lips (Fig. 5-1, *B*). With these methods, the intervening tissue is pressed and gently rolled between the two hands or fingers. The use of two hands or fingers allows for greater depth of coverage and movement of the tissues than is possible with the use of only one hand or finger. Also, with two hands more support can be given to those tissues that are freely movable than is possible when only one hand is used against unsupported tissue. At other times two hands are used to inspect the same structures on each side of the body; this is bilateral palpation (Fig. 5-1, *C*). This method gives the examiner some basis of comparison provided that both

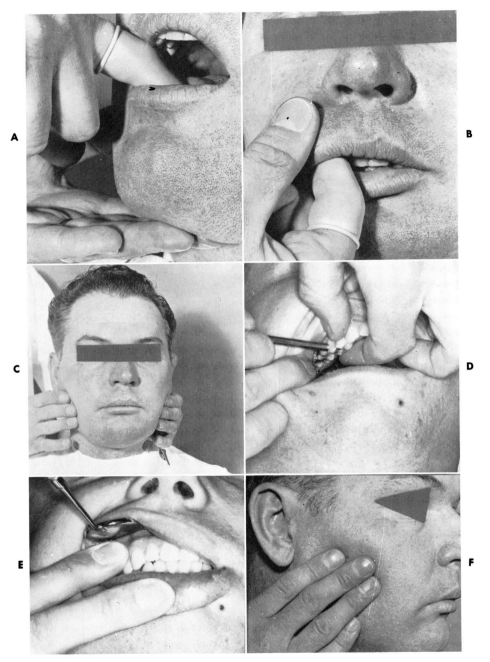

Fig. 5-1. *Palpation.* **A,** Bimanual palpation. **B,** Bidigital palpation. **C,** Bilateral palpation. **D,** Palpation of the teeth for mobility. **E,** Direct palpation to determine movement of a tooth during function. **F,** Palpation by compression; note fingers are held together to determine texture of underlying tissue.

sides are not abnormal. In addition to the comparison of bilateral structures for abnormalities, the examiner must keep in mind what should be normal in the average individual. Adequate palpation does not require undue pressure on the tissues with resulting discomfort to the patient; the procedure should be such that it causes very little discomfort.

By palpation the competent examiner is able to tell much about the tissue he is evaluating. It is necessary that he have an adequate knowledge of the anatomic and physiologic states of the tissue he is to consider. Only by practice will he learn to differentiate muscle tissue, glandular tissue, tendinous tissue, and osseous tissue in their normal anatomic and functional relationship. In the palpation of a salivary gland, the examiner should determine its boundaries, density, attachments, anatomy of its surface, and its relationship to other structures. Where possible, palpation and expression of saliva is desirable to allow inspection of the saliva and its freedom of flow. The palpation of muscle should reveal its boundaries, attachments, consistency, size, changes during function, and the presence or absence of tenderness. Palpation of bones should be done to reveal normal bony landmarks such as fossae, joints, tubercles, and muscle attachments; normal bones should be nontender and nonyielding except in areas of contiguous cartilage. Bones should be tested also for continuity, at rest and during function. Bilateral palpation for alterations in size and form is a desirable procedure.

Where possible, the potential spaces should be examined for the presence of density changes; accumulations of pus may fill the spaces and give the area a hard boardlike density. Palpation of the surface of the mucous membrane and skin is also an especially desirable procedure; texture, density, and resilience are significant factors in the examination of these tissues. Palpation of the teeth should consist of manual movement of the teeth by the examiner (Fig. 5-1, *D*), feeling for excessive movement of the teeth during functional movements of the jaws while chewing, and feeling for excessive movements of the teeth when the teeth are in contact and various excursions of the mandible are being performed (Fig. 5-1, *E*). In palpation of the skin, its texture, resilience, density, and lubrication should be considered. Depending upon the location, as much of the surface of the hand or fingers as possible should be brought to bear on the part to be inspected. Thus, where circumstances permit, the fingers should be held together and the hand should remain flat (Fig. 5-1, *F*).

Percussion. Percussion is the technic of striking the tissues with the fingers or an instrument so that the examiner may listen for the resulting sounds. The response of the patient to the procedure is also noted. Percussion is valuable for the evaluation and localization of inflammation of the periodontal membrane and secondary pulpitis. In many instances tenderness of the teeth may be localized to a single tooth because of the response of the patient to the technic of percussion. Changes in the character and density of the supporting tissues and the amount of alveolar bone surrounding a tooth may be evaluated to a certain extent by the sounds elicited by percussion. The difference in the sound produced may be easily appreciated by comparing percussion notes of the teeth on one side of the mouth with their counterparts on the opposite side. In general, a tooth with normal support will give rise to a rather high-pitched sound, whereas one with less support or less dense support will give rise to one of lower pitch. A difference in the percussion note of a given tooth and that of its counterpart on the opposite side of the arch does not necessarily indicate the presence of an abnormality of the supporting structures. In any case variations of the normal, as well as the presence or absence of other contributory signs and symptoms of disease, must be taken into consideration.

The composite sound of percussion, which is produced by the patient tapping his teeth together in centric relation or in acquired centric occlusion, is of value in making a general appraisal of the degree and localization of premature contacts. A light tapping of the teeth together from the rest position of the mandible may serve to elicit or to demonstrate hypertonicity and spasticity of the muscles of mastication. Tapping of the muscles themselves may also produce the same effect. Percussion of the teeth is best carried out with the handle of an explorer (Fig. 5-2, *A*). It should be directed at right angles to the incisal, occlusal, lingual, buccal, or labial surfaces. Very light tapping is all that is necessary, and it goes without saying that pounding is

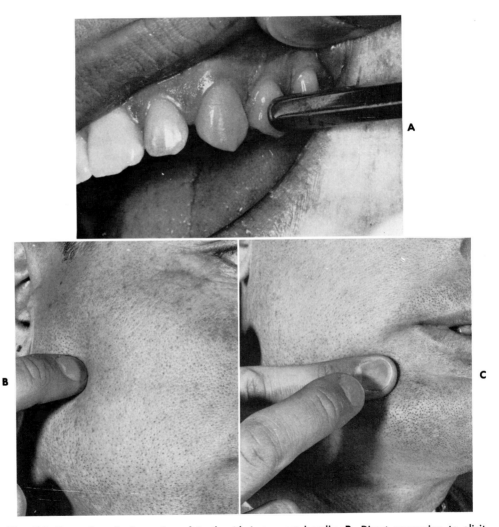

Fig. 5-2. *Percussion.* **A,** Percussion of teeth with instrument handle. **B,** Direct percussion to elicit nerve response. **C,** Indirect percussion; note that pleximeter finger is percussed immediately over point of contact.

entirely unnecessary. A pain response or an abnormal percussion note may be elicited when the percussing instrument is directed in any or all directions.

The technic of percussion of muscle and bone consists of sharply tapping the area to be tested with the tips of two or three fingers. An area is tapped twice and the sound or response compared with that produced in its like area on the other side of the face. The fingers should be flexed to a right angle at the first interphalangeal joint (Fig. 5-2, *B*). This method of percussion is of value in observing muscle-reflex mechanisms of the mandible, muscle tenderness, hypertonicity of the muscles of mastication as evidenced by localized contraction at the site, and a demonstration of Chvostek's sign (in latent tetany, tapping over the facial nerve in front of the ear causes twitching or spasm of the facial muscles).

Percussion applied by tapping bone with the fingertips may be useful in locating tender areas in the mandible or maxilla. Percussion to determine the density of structures such as bone is best carried out by placing a finger of one hand on the area to be evaluated and striking it a blow with the tip of one of the fingers of the other hand (Fig. 5-2, *C*). The middle finger of one hand (pleximeter finger) is held firmly but not uncomfortably against the bony structure to be percussed. The middle finger of the other hand (plexor finger), flexed at a right angle at the first interphalangeal joint, is used to strike the pleximeter finger two quick sharp blows. The action is done entirely by the wrist, and the plexor finger is removed quickly from pleximeter finger to prevent dampening of the sound. Differences in the density of the bone and underlying structures may be clearly differentiated where they exist. As in palpation and inspection, like areas on two sides of the face must always be compared.

Auscultation. Auscultation is the act of listening for sounds produced within the body. The development of a sense of hearing for the various sounds of interest to a dentist is one of the least appreciated facets of the clinical examination. Unless the examiner's attention is receptive to the sounds of abnormal breathing, clicking and snapping of the temporomandibular joints, vocal fremitus, and other abnormal sounds, it is quite likely that a complete appraisal and diagnosis of a patient's abnormality may be overlooked in many instances. Though it seems unlikely that any dentist would undertake therapy in an asthmatic or dyspneic individual with abnormal breathing sounds without further systemic evaluation, it does happen, for it is not uncommon to completely overlook this phase of auscultation. This may be further emphasized by pointing out the failure of many clinicians to recognize snapping and clicking of the temporomandibular joint as a symptom of disturbance of this joint. Another use of auscultation that appears to be overlooked by many is the determination of the relationship of oral structures to the production of normal speech. The loss of teeth, placement of artificial teeth, cleft palate, and muscle paralysis can give rise to serious impairment of speech. Another abnormal sound of considerable significance to a patient wearing full dentures is constant clicking of the teeth during speaking and mastication.

Occasionally a patient will complain of a peculiar "squeak" that may be elicited by clenching of the teeth. The cause of such an abnormal sound may be difficult to locate and may necessitate special procedures. However, it is usually caused by the abnormal movement of teeth whose approximating surfaces have been restored with improperly finished amalgam. The sound is not unlike that of the "tinner's cry" of fresh amalgam being squeezed. The placement of flat wax dental floss between the contact areas of the suspected teeth may serve to localize the offending restorations.

6

Clinical examination—general

The clinical or physical examination of the patient should include the exposed parts of the body and the structures of the mouth. A logical and orderly scheme of examination should be practiced. Even though the physical examination may consist of only an examination of the affected part as determined by the chief complaint, only a thorough and complete examination can be expected to produce a high yield of unsuspected disease or even the "obvious" disease.

General survey

The clinical examination should begin with a general appraisal or survey of the patient's well-being; it begins when the patient is first observed. This part of the examination will allow the dentist to make an overall evaluation of gross alteration of body habitus, state of nutrition, body build, constitution, intellectual achievement, personality, speech, mental alertness, psyche, and general hygiene. When indicated, the examiner should record body temperature, pulse rate, blood pressure, weight, and respiration.

The examination of the exposed parts of the body is not to be considered a medical examination but rather a review of parts immediately related in health and disease to the mouth and to dental treatment; this review is within the scope of the responsibility of the dentist in rendering a health service. In the general survey an attempt should be made to evaluate the individual in relation to this disease, including his psychologic adjustment to his disorder. Obser-

vations should be included that relate to the natural course of the disease and alterations caused by therapy.

The general survey does not take the place of a routine systematic clinical examination; however, it does serve to facilitate the examination by directing the examiner's attention to certain areas or systems for a more detailed consideration than might be otherwise considered routinely. The general appearance of a patient may suggest such entities as pernicious anemia, thyrotoxicosis, tic douloureux, tabes dorsalis, or an endocrine disturbance, yet the true nature of the disease remains to be substantiated by further detailed examination. Therefore, early in the clinical examination, the findings from the general appraisal will serve as a guide for the rest of the examination.

Constitution and stature of an individual represent not only characteristics of inheritance, but also the influence of the endocrine system. Inasmuch as diseases of the endocrine system may affect the characteristics of stature and body build, variations from the range of normal may characterize a particular disturbance of the endocrine system.

Examination of a child should begin with a general appraisal of the status of general growth and development. The examiner may use anthropometric charts showing so-called norms of growth and development at various age levels, provided that he keeps in mind that each child has his own pattern of growth and development. It is more significant to know that a child is consistently within the same percentiles for weight and height than it is to know whether he is tall or short, overweight or underweight. One must keep in mind that there may be no sharp line of differentiation between the normal and abnormal child in respect to the features of body build or growth such as size or rate of growth. However, it is well to know how growth and development can be influenced by such factors as genetics, disease, malnutrition, and endocrine disturbances. This phase of the examination is of considerable importance in the interception of malocclusion, diagnosis of malocclusion, and the formulation of an orthodontic treatment plan.

It is not the purpose of this book to point out and describe all the findings in disease that may relate to abnormalities of body build, growth, and development. Although great variations of body build do exist in the range of normal, and the body habitus of all individuals may not be characteristic enough to fit into a clear-cut category, it is to be expected that the student and practitioner will have a sufficient knowledge of the range of normal to detect abnormal body proportions and qualitative abnormalities of secondary sexual characteristics. It is most important that they develop an appreciation for variations from the normal in growth and development of children and for variations of body build and stature in adults. Descriptions of the normal constitution and body habitus and the effects of disease upon growth and development can be found elsewhere. The primary consideration of the dentist in his clinical examination of the patient is to recognize that abnormalities of constitution and body habitus may play an important part in the diagnosis and treatment of oral disease.

It is not unusual for the experienced examiner to sum up the appraisal of the patient's weight and nutrition by the phrase "well developed and well nourished." This does not simply imply well-developed musculature or an abundance of avoirdupois.

The phrase "well developed" should be used to mean normal body proportions consistent with the size, age, and sex of the individual. The phrase "well nourished" should be used to mean the absence of any evidence of disease caused by malnourishment. Weight is only one feature in the nutritional state of an individual. Probably the most common disorder in this country is obesity. Thus the term "well nourished" means the absence of evidence of avitaminosis, hypoproteinemia, iron deficiency, mineral deficiency, and excessive variation in the person's ideal weight.

A partial survey of the neurologic and musculoskeletal systems can be made from an observation of an individual's gait. There is considerable variation in normal gait; however, systemic and local disease, especially of the feet and the hip joints, may considerably influence gait. Diseases involving pyramidal and extrapyramidal tracts, cerebellar disease, and other diseases involving posture columns may produce rather characteristic abnormalities of gait; for example, ataxic patients may keep their eyes fixed on the floor while walking with a shuffling gait and a patient with hemiplegia associated with apoplexy (cerebral vascular accident) usually walks with a circumduction of the hip with plantar flexion and inversion of the foot and with the flexed arm of the afflicted side held rigid. Thus the presence of an abnormal gait may be somewhat diagnostic and also introduce the examiner to the possibility of paralysis in other area such as the facial muscles and those of mastication. It goes without saying that the examiner must attempt to identify the areas that are involved since dental treatment many times will be dictated by the extent and location of the paralysis.

The patient's body temperature should be recorded if the presenting complaint involves constitutional symptoms that include fever. In taking oral temperatures, the thermometer should be left in place for at least 3 minutes. The bulb should be placed under the tongue and the mouth should be kept closed. The use of hot or cold fluid just prior to taking the temperature may lead to erroneous results. Fever is a reaction of the body to physical or somatic disturbances. The degree of elevation of body temperature depends on many factors; the two most important are the type and severity of the pathologic process and the individual reaction of the patient to the disease. Increased pulse rate, increased respiratory rate, and increased basal metabolic rate usually accompany fever. The most common cause of fever is the response to local or systemic infectious agents such as bacteria and viruses. Another cause is malignant neoplasms. This is especially true in the lymphomatous diseases, including the leukemias. Injuries may cause a rise in body temperature. Thus fever may be related to specific injury to the central nervous system or to dead or dying tissue. The most common causes of fever in patients seen by the dentist are abscessed teeth, acute necrotizing gingivitis, and herpetic gingivostomatitis. The severity, type, character of onset, and time relationship of the fever to tissue lesions are significant factors in the differential diagnosis of herpetic gingivostomatitis and acute necrotizing gingivitis.

When a patient's history is being taken, his speech should be evaluated because of its frequent importance as a diagnostic clue. Disorders of speech may be of no diagnostic importance or may be associated with neurologic lesions, inability to enunciate, disturbances of the larynx, harelip, cleft palate, nasal obstruction, or other serious diseases. For example, an anxious and tense individual is likely to speak rapidly and at a high pitch; however, these same speech mannerisms are likely to be present in the thyrotoxic patient. A chronic alcoholic or an individual with general paresis may have difficulty in speaking and in enunciating; such difficulties should alert the examiner to the possibility of the presence of disease.

Though hoarseness may be associated with a cold or an upper respiratory tract infection and is usually of a transitory nature, persistent hoarseness may suggest the presence of a tumor or paralysis of the vocal cords. Of special interest to the dentist are lisping associated with tonguetie, inability to pronounce labials associated with harelip or cleft palate, and difficulties of enunciation related to loss of teeth, encroachment on the tongue space, ill-fitting dentures, and macroglossia.

Respiration should be noted for rate and rhythm if surgery is to be performed and there is a past history of heart disease, lung disease, or asthma. In the patient with asthma, orthopnea may or may not be present and wheezing may be present on expiration and inspiration. With asthma, the accessory chest and neck muscles labor to push the air in and out of the lungs. In left ventricular failure, which the dentist is not likely to see except as an associated complaint, expiration takes little effort, and orthopnea is usually present. Observation of respiration is done only to recognize signs of respiratory embarrassment. The presence of respiratory embarrassment, however slight, should be evaluated. It is under these circumstances that precautionary measures should be taken and in some instances a medical referral made.

The pulse should be taken whenever heart disease is suspected or has appeared in the patient's history. Although the stethoscope reveals more than the pulse rate, the average practicing dentist is not equipped or trained to auscultate sounds of the heart. However, it is possible for him to palpate one of the larger peripheral arteries rather easily and to discover the presence of cardiac disease. The radial artery is most often used. In addition to noting any thickening of the arterial wall (quite common with advancing age), the course of the artery, its compressibility and fullness, and its rate and rhythm should be evaluated. In general, tortuosity is indicative of arteriosclerosis; a palpable cordlike structure in both diastole and systole is seen in patients with hypertension; a full, or bounding pulse is found with increased cardiac output, after exercise, and in persons with hyperthyroidism and similar conditions; a rapid and "thready" pulse may occur when there is an insufficient quantity of blood and weakened ventricular systole; a pulse with a sharp rise and fall with a sharp summit and wide pulse pressure (Corrigan's or water-hammer pulse) is typically present in patients with aortic regurgitation and may be found to a certain degree in those with anemia and hyperthyroidism.

Tachycardia and bradycardia should be noted and correlated with the patient's history of cardiovascular disease. Without auscultation of the heart, it is impossible to actually evaluate either of these two signs. Tachycardia, bradycardia, and heart irregularities may be normal findings, but in the presence of a history of cardiac disease such findings give basis for medical referral.

Palpitations of the heart may be considered as an awareness of the pounding, rapidity, or irregularity of heart action. Although some forms of palpitation may be extremely serious, the phenomenon usually causes distress beyond its significance. The dentist is usually confronted with immediate concern when a patient complains of an awareness of pounding of the heart. Occasionally the symptoms include tachycardia and paroxysmal arrhythmias. These symptoms may produce fright, weakness, vasomotor disturbances, or collapse. It is not uncommon for the disturbances in rhythm to cause this type of distress and yet cause no interference with cardiac efficiency. These symptoms may arise in any normal individual exposed to dental procedures, especially when treatment tends to cause anxiety. Occasionally the use of drugs or anesthetic will cause tachycardias or cardiac arrhythmias. Thus disturbances in rhythm of the heart occur not only in normal individuals under unusual circumstances but also in patients who have heart disease. A history of cardiac arrhythmias prior to dental operation or oral surgery may serve to direct the treatment of the patient by the dentist in case such conditions arise while he is treating the patient. If there is a history of heart disease, the onset of tachycardia may be a threat to the patient. If a patient is known to have auricular fibrillation and is using a drug to slow the ventricular rate, it is well to know that he has taken such medicine prior to dental procedures.

Other findings of significance in the evaluation of a patient with heart disease are malar flush, clubbing of the fingers, and distention of the neck veins. A malar flush may indicate hypertension, fever, or mitral stenosis. Cyanosis and clubbed fingers may be related to pulmonary disease or heart disease. Pronounced substernal pulse may be caused by aortic insufficiency, hypertension, or an aneurysm. If a patient who is seated in a dental chair and breathing normally has significant distention of the neck veins, heart disease or mediastinal obstruction should be suspected.

When oral surgery is considered and symptoms suggest the presence of cardiac disease, a determination of blood pressure should be made. In most dental offices this procedure is not routine; its use is limited to emergency situations. In those instances where the other examination procedures indicate the presence of cardiovascular disease, the recording of the patient's blood pressure hardly seems necessary. However, in instances of transient or recurrent hypertension, it would appear wise to record the blood pressure prior to surgical procedures.

The brief evaluation of the patient's cardiac status should not be considered as exhaustive or final. Whatever precautions the dentist may take for the safety of his patient are taken for the purpose of referring the patient, when necessary, for more adequate evaluation. Thus the emphasis on the cardiac evaluation is not upon the discovery and diagnosis of cardiac disease itself but upon the discovery of signs of cardiac disease that might be of significance in dental treatment.

In most instances it might appear to the casual observer that a general appraisal of the patient is not warranted since the yield of information appears to be small. Fortunately most clinicians make a gross appraisal of a patient's health without being really aware of it. Actually it takes but little more concerted effort to broaden the scope of the practitioner's awareness of his patient's general appearance. It is the development of a systematic awareness that enables the good diagnostician to detect all the significant deviations from normal health. Obvious signs of disease may be entirely lacking in the oral region, yet the examiner's considered general appraisal of the patient may dictate to him the necessity for a medical referral for the patient's good. Even the simplest considerations of the patient's health and well-being are obvious signs to the patient of the dental practitioner's interest in him as a whole individual. All too often the criticism of "playing doctor" is leveled at the conscientious dental practitioner showing any interest in his patient other than to search for dental caries. This criticism cannot be justified except in rare instances in which a dentist enters into those areas that are unrelated to his responsibility and for which he is not qualified by training.

Head

The examination of the head should include a brief review of the skull (including facies, facial form, symmetry), eyes, and nose. The objectives of this part of the examination are to evaluate briefly those abnormalities of the head that may be related to the patient's general well-being and to evaluate those abnormalities that may be directly or indirectly related to the diagnosis and treatment of disease within the province of the dentist. The primary consideration is the recognition of abnormalities. The next procedure is the interpretation and evaluation of the results of the examination. How the examiner handles the facts that he has collected will depend to a large extent upon his ability to determine which findings are contributory, which are related to predisposing and exciting causes, and which are related to the signs and symptoms of oral disease. Thus the prerequisites to formulation of a diagnosis are the collection of the facts and a descriptive knowledge of those diseases responsible for the observed abnormalities.

Once it is recognized that an abnormality exists, it is possible for the examiner to make an evaluation of it in terms of disease processes. The recognition of the abnormality will be considered here; the relationships of these abnormalities to disease will be found more aptly in those textbooks concerned with descriptions of disease. The primary purpose of the examination of the head is not to make a diagnosis of disease but to recognize the presence of an abnormality that can, with proper knowledge of the signs and symptoms of disease, be related to oral disease. Therefore, the examiner's attention should be initially concerned with the discovery of those features of the head that are outside the range of normal. To be concerned primarily with the diagnosis of an abnormality generally precludes the recognition of any disease other than that of which the examiner has a descriptive knowledge. This is especially true in the examination of the head since many clinicians are familiar with only the most important abnormalities of the head and are unaware of the relationship or importance of abnormalities of the skull, eyes, and nose to diseases of the oral structures.

Skull. The external features of the cranium may give some clue as to congenital deformity, growth and development, asymmetry, general effects of disease, and endocrine disturbances. Deformities of the skull can be more readily determined by an examiner who has acquired an appreciation for the normal through systematic observation. The contour and size of the skull varies considerably within the normal limits, and even extreme deviations from normal may not indicate any disturbance. However, mild degrees of altered contour and size, which may be difficult to detect, may result from a pathologic disturbance. This should not imply futility but rather the need for considered observation.

The presence of signs of disease, injury, and operations may play a significant role in the evaluation and differential diagnosis of disease of the mouth and adjacent structures. Textbooks on pathology and oral medicine are usually replete with descriptions of abnormal findings of contour and size of the skull. Pictorial descriptions of an abnormally large head related to hydro-

cephalus, osteitis deformans (Fig. 6-1), leontiasis ossea, and acromegaly are well known. The "square head," which appears abnormally large (though actually it is not), is frequently attributed to prominent "bosses" of the frontal bones and may occur in the healing of the bone lesion of either rickets or congenital syphilis. Less well known is the importance of the signs of injuries and operations of the head. The scar of an operation for tic douloureux, intracranial tumor, or gunshot wound may be the basis for dysfunction of the oral structures.

The term "facies" refers to the appearance of the patient's face as a whole. The appearance may be suggestive or characteristic of certain disease conditions. Of special interest to the orthodontist is the adenoid facies seen in children. It is characterized

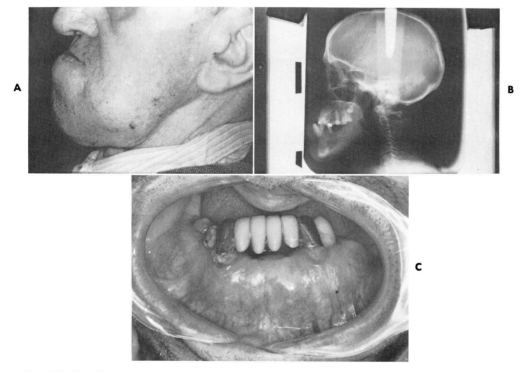

Fig. 6-1. *Paget's disease.* **A,** Apparent enlargement of mandible with prognathism and lateral enlargement. **B,** Radiograph showing prognathic enlarged mandible of patient shown in **A. C,** Enlarged and expanded mandible of patient shown in **A.**

by a thin face, pinched nose, high arched palate, mouth breathing, and, frequently, a languid expression. Other rather characteristic facies include those of acromegaly (Fig. 6-2), cherubism (Fig. 6-3), goiter (Fig. 6-23, *C*), mongolism (Fig. 6-4, *A* and *B*), cretinism (Fig. 6-4, *C*), achondroplasia, myxedema, and Cushing's disease (Fig. 6-5). The facial appearance may show evidence of dehydration—dry wrinkled skin with sunken cheeks and hollow eyes. The face may also show evidence of edema—pale and puffy; this may be especially prominent beneath the eyes. The facies of the chronically ill and the psychiatric patient may also be of diagnostic significance.

Examination of the profile facies may reveal much about the positions of the teeth and jaws. The "Andy Gump" type and the "Hapsburg" jaw are fairly characteristic signs of malocclusion, malfunction, or maldevelopment (Fig. 6-6). The facial profile should be evaluated not only in terms of osseous structures, but also in terms of the muscles supplied by the fifth and seventh cranial nerves. Extreme malpositions of the teeth are seldom seen without accompanying muscle strains and unilateral contractions of the facial muscles.

Symmetry must also be considered. Normally the skull and face are fairly symmetrical; however, perfect symmetry is not usually found, and the two halves of the face and skull will invariably differ somewhat. A demonstration of this fact may be shown by producing two faces from a photograph whose negative is cut vertically in the center and using each half to make a complete print. It is necessary that the examiner develop an appreciation for asymmetry of the face in order to recognize skeletal defects that may have an important bearing on growth and development of the jaws, to properly evaluate past injury, and to recognize the presence of disease whose beginning may be manifest only in slight facial asymmetry. The most common asymmetries encountered by the dentist are seen in association with alveolar abscesses, abscesses of the soft tissues, paralysis of the facial nerve (Bell's palsy, Fig. 6-7), functional and organic malpositions of the jaws, tumors, diseases of the parotid glands, and post-traumatic swelling (Fig. 6-8).

The obvious signs of gross enlargement which give the face and jaws asymmetry

Text continued on p. 96.

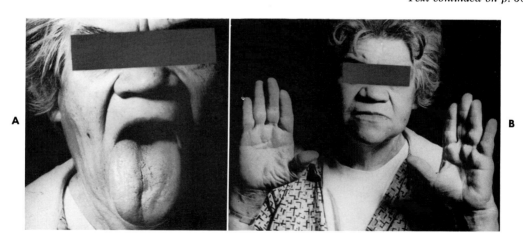

Fig. 6-2. *Acromegaly.* **A,** Apparent enlargement of tongue. **B,** Thickening of skin has resulted in thick lips and lids, broad nose, coarse features, and enlargement of hands with thick blunt fingers and heavy palmar pads. (Courtesy Dr. S. Fajans.)

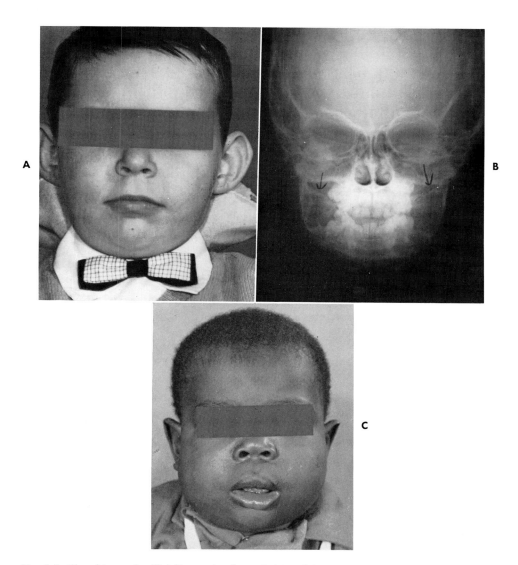

Fig. 6-3. *Cherubism or familial fibrous dysplasia.* **A,** Note fullness of lower face providing a round or square face. **B,** Bilateral involvement of angle and body of mandible with destructive lesions, which produce bulging of buccal plate. **C,** More severe example of cherubism; note symmetrical enlargement of lower face. (**A** and **B,** Courtesy Dr. W. G. Shafer; **C,** courtesy Dr. C. Witkop.)

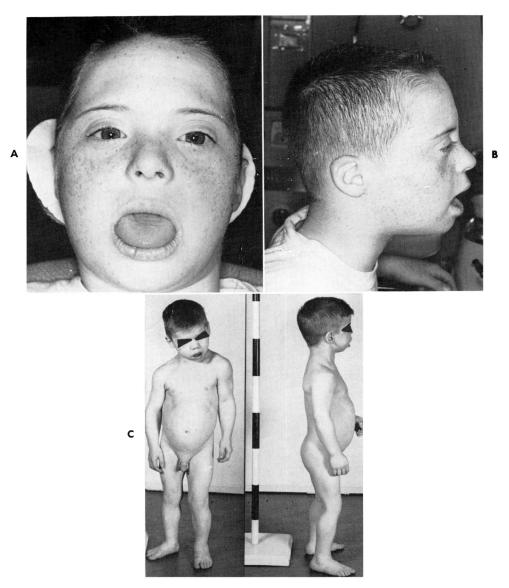

Fig. 6-4. *Characteristic facies in mongolism and cretinism.* **A,** Mongolism; note transvere grooves on tongue and characteristic mongoloid facies. **B,** Profile of typical mongoloid facies. **C,** Typical facies and habitus in cretinism. (**A** and **B,** Courtesy Dr. J. Hartsook; **C,** courtesy Dr. W. Beierwaltes.)

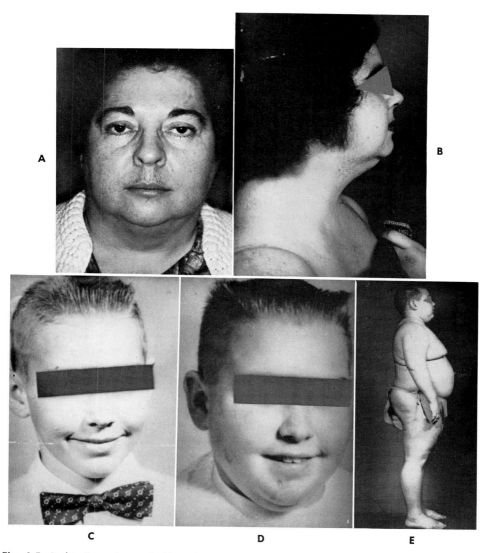

Fig. 6-5. *Cushing's syndrome.* **A,** Moon face, eruptions, and hirsutism secondary to steroid therapy. **B,** Enlargement of fat pad of upper back ("buffalo hump") secondary to steroid therapy. **C,** Early development, 9 years of age. **D,** Progress of disease with development of round facies, 14 years of age. **E,** Further progress of disease with greater change in face and development of typical habitus. (Courtesy Dr. S. Fajans.)

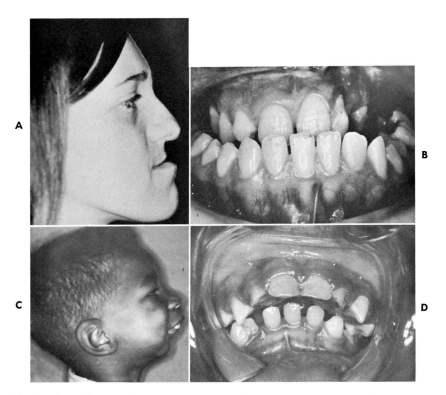

Fig. 6-6. *Facial profile.* **A** and **B,** Prognathism, Angle's class III malocclusion. **C** and **D,** Micrognathia and resultant malocclusion.

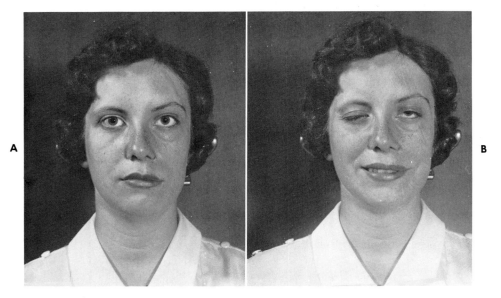

Fig. 6-7. *Facial asymmetry.* **A,** Note droop of left angle of mouth and wide opening of left eye at rest. **B,** Note inability to retract left angle of mouth and to close left eye.

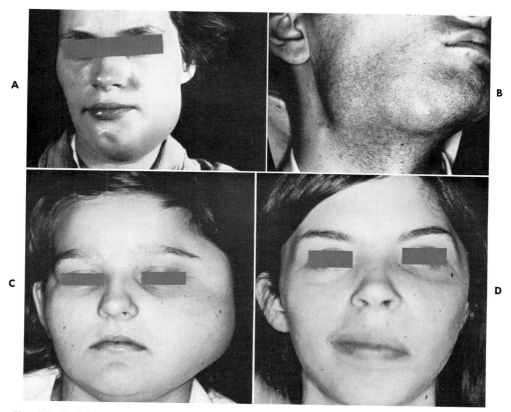

Fig. 6-8. *Facial asymmetry.* **A,** Swelling caused by extension of periapical infection. **B,** Nodular lateral swelling produced by actinomycosis. **C,** Facial asymmetry caused by a fibrosarcoma. **D,** Enlargement of left mandible and maxilla caused by fibrous dysplasia.

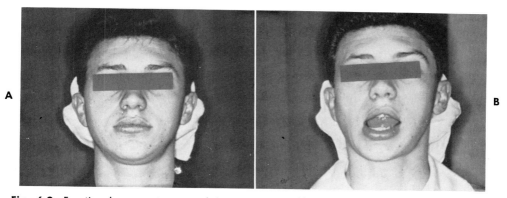

Fig. 6-9. *Functional asymmetry caused by temporomandibular joint ankylosis.* **A,** Closure. **B,** Opening; note shift of mandible to the right.

are important; however, even more important are the slight degrees of asymmetry that herald the onset of disease. Thus the emphasis is upon the slight degree of asymmetry and its recognition rather than simply upon gross deformities. This does not mean that gross deformities are unimportant; it does suggest that most examiners will see the obvious signs of asymmetry but will fail to recognize equally significant signs of slight asymmetry. The cause of jaw and facial asymmetry may be skeletal, muscular, glandular, occlusal, or soft tissue in origin. Asymmetry may be manifested only when the mandible is opened (Fig. 6-9). Functional deviation of the mandible may be caused by a disturbance of the temporomandibular joints, muscle disturbances, and disturbances of neurogenic origin. Deviation of the mandible when the teeth are occluded may be skeletal or occlusal in origin. On occasion disharmony between centric relation and acquired centric occlusion will result in a midline deviation of the mandible. This deviation may be grossly apparent or observed by comparison of the midline of the maxilla and mandible. Deviation of the midline may also be caused by malposition of the teeth; therefore, the mandible must be placed in centric relation to determine whether the deviation is a result of occlusal disharmony and premature contacts or of malposition of the teeth.

The analysis of facial form is of considerable importance in the evaluation and diagnosis of malocclusion. Its relation to the development of occlusion will be found in Chapter 10.

Eyes and adnexa. The eye is more commonly affected by constitutional disease than any other organ or system. The information gained from the history and from a brief clinical examination may indicate the true nature of oral disease and the necessity for additional investigation by an ophthalmologist. The dentist must limit his examination to subjective findings derived from the patient's statements and from a general inspection of the eye and adnexa for gross departures from the normal. Although the ocular manifestations of systemic disease not infrequently herald widespread or distant disorders, the dentist cannot recognize many of them because of their location in the eye beyond his examination. However, many diseases may be manifest in a location that he may observe by simple inspection. The objective signs of disease that may be seen by the dentist include Argyll Robertson pupil, exophthalmos, conjunctival petechiae, nystagmus, pigmented pingueculae, interstitial keratitis, corneal ulcerations, lid lag, widening of palpebral fissures, icterus, ptosis of the eyelid, miosis, and exudation.

Ptosis is drooping of an eyelid caused by paralysis of the levator palpebrae superiosis resulting from dysfunction of the third cranial nerve. The cause may be congenital in origin or may be caused by any condition such as tabes dorsalis, multiple sclerosis, and neoplastic or inflammatory disease. In Bell's palsy, there is inability to close the lid, and the constant irritation causes excessive lacrimation (Fig 6-7). Exophthalmos (Fig. 6-10) is a protrusion of the eyeball and is a characteristic finding in Graves' disease. Lid lag may be demonstrable in patients with thyroid disease. As the eye is rotated downward, the lid fails to follow synchronously. Corneal ulcerations, infre-

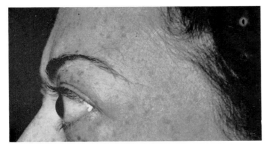

Fig. 6-10. *Exophthalmos.* Graves' disease with characteristic protrusion of the eyes. (Courtesy Dr. W. Beierwaltes.)

quent blinking, and widening of the palpebral fissures are also likely to be present in the patient with hyperthyroidism and exophthalmos.

The sclera is normally bluish white, and variation in this color may be readily appreciated by simple inspection. Icterus may be seen in the sclera. Of dental significance is the relationship of blue scleras to osteogenesis imperfecta and odontogenesis imperfecta. The conjunctiva may give valuable signs of vitamin A deficiency (Bitot's spots) and jaundice and may contain petechiae associated with subacute bacterial endocarditis and purpuras. Interstitial keratitis may give the cornea a grayish ground-glass appearance. This, as well as the other elements of Hutchinson's triad (notched incisors and middle ear deafness), is seen in congenital syphilis. Vitamin A deficiency may be manifest in the cornea by keratotic changes. Riboflavin deficiency may also produce changes, although these are difficult to see with the naked eye. The corneal reflex may be lost with sensory disturbances of the trigeminal nerve.

The change in the pupil most significant to the dentist is miosis associated with tabes dorsalis (Argyll Robertson pupil) and the pinpoint pupil of the narcotic addict. Pupils of unequal diameter may be of congenital origin or may be related to disease of the nervous system. Some ocular-oral syndromes of dental significance include Behçet's syndrome, consisting of a recurrent iritis, aphthae in the oral cavity, and ulcerations on the genitals; Stevens-Johnson syndrome, consisting of a severe conjunctivitis in association with an eruptive fever and stomatitis (the lesions are of an erythema multiforme character); and Sjögren's syndrome, consisting of conjunctivitis caused by dryness and stomatitis caused by diminished secretions of the mouth and pharynx.

Nose. An examination of the nose should include observations of gross deformity (saddle nose of syphilis [Fig. 6-11], achondroplasia, fracture, lesions), inflammation of the turbinates with possible relation to toothaches not otherwise placed as to origin, the presence of discharge and its relation to postnasal drip, allergy, lesions, epistaxis, and nasal obstruction, and the ability of the patient to breathe through his nose. Obstruction of the nasal cavity may be caused by polyps, foreign objects, large turbinates, tissue hypertrophy, and habit. The relationship of nasal breathing to mouth breathing is of primary consideration to periodontal and orthodontic therapy (Fig. 6-12).

Chronic mouth breathing may result from

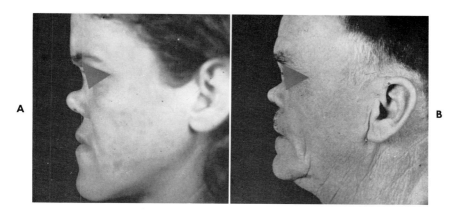

Fig. 6-11. *Saddle nose.* **A** and **B,** Congenital syphilis; note disproportionate development of maxilla and mandible in patient shown in **A.**

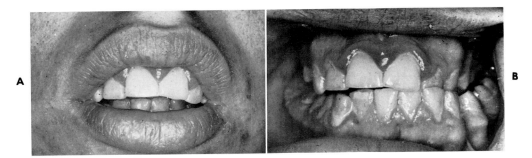

Fig. 6-12. *Mouth breather.* **A,** Note short upper lip and exposure of gingiva. **B,** Note outline of gingival hyperplasia.

habit or from obstruction to nasal breathing. The habit may be secondary to the obstruction in nasal breathing. This habit is not infrequently established from an inability to breathe through the nose because of enlarged adenoids, deviated septum, allergic rhinitis, frequent colds, polyps, or nocturnal and recumbent engorgement of the vessels of the nasal mucous membranes. All chronic mouth breathers should be evaluated by an otolaryngologist for possible nasal obstruction. Dental appliances for breaking the habit will not be of value unless the underlying cause is removed. The chronic gingivitis seen so frequently in the mouth breather cannot be treated effectively unless the mouth breathing is eliminated first.

Skin

The skin should be examined for abnormal texture (Fig. 6-13), color, pigmentation, scars, eruptions (Fig. 6-14), lesions (Fig. 6-15), and indications of local and systemic disease such as pallor, cyanosis, suborbital edema, and jaundice. It must be given careful consideration not only because it frequently reflects manifestations of systemic disease and the health of the individual, but also because it may be of considerable importance in the differential diagnosis of dermatologic lesions that ap-

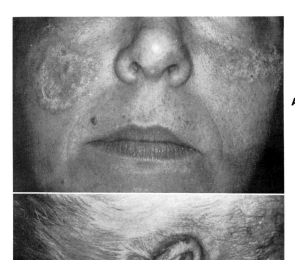

Fig. 6-13. A, Bilateral patches that are slightly elevated with violaceous center and scaly appearance at periphery and are typical both in character and location of chronic discoid lupus erythematosus. **B,** Senile keratosis and other changes typical of those occurring in skin of elderly people, especially those who have had constant exposure to sunlight. Note crustlike keratotic lesions on upper border of helix, pigmented areas of hair of temple, and atrophic changes in skin of face.

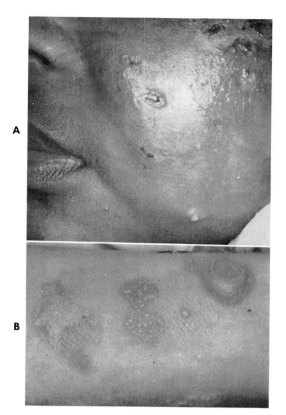

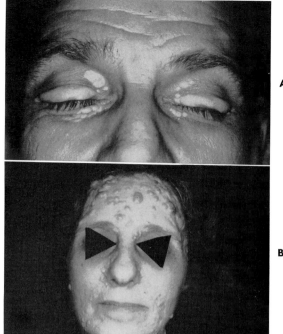

Fig. 6-15. A, Xanthoma palpebrarum caused by deposit of cholesterol in and about eyelids. Margin of upper lid is noticeably thickened. Small nodules surround inner canthus. **B,** Numerous varying-sized nodules covering face are adenomas of sebaceous gland origin.

Fig. 6-14. A, Swelling of entire lateral aspect of face with multiple draining sinuses typical of actinomycosis. Sinus in lower right shows drop of pus at opening. Most of the other sinuses are closed at this time. **B,** Large bullae, some of which are intact and filled with fluid; others have ruptured and collapsed, leaving a wrinkled membrane over surface. These lesions are typical of those seen in epidermolysis bullosa.

pear only in the oral cavity or simultaneously on the skin and in the oral cavity (Figs. 6-16 to 6-18). The texture of the skin of a normal healthy young individual has a certain degree of elasticity and thickness that causes it to quickly return to normal after it has been picked up in a fold between the thumb and index finger. In the older individual, as the skin loses some of its elasticity, there is some delay in the resumption of its former contour, when it is picked up and released. The elasticity generally decreases rapidly after the menopause, and in the senile person the skin is usually inelastic, thin, atrophic, and parchment-like. Such diseases as hypothyroidism, myxedema, and hyperthyroidism produce various changes in the texture of the skin. In hyperthyroidism the skin feels smooth and silky and is generally moist and elastic. In hypothyroidism and myxedema, dryness and inelasticity are generally found. These changes may not be sufficiently clear cut to be diagnostic, but such skin changes are highly suggestive of systemic diseases.

Color of the skin of the face may be compared with that of other areas of the body. However, since the dentist will be examining only the face and neck and exposed parts of the body, he must keep in mind that alterations of the color and texture may be physiologic in origin, for example, the changes of suntan associated with constant exposure to the sun versus the lack of tanning or a sallow skin associated with an indoor life. The color of the skin is derived chiefly from its vascular bed and from the amount and distribution of its pigment. It may vary because of age, regional distribution of pigments, sex differences, and climatic differences.

In abnormal states the skin may be yellow, olive green, lemon-yellow tinted, red, bluish red, light brown, or dark brown. Many factors control pigmentation, and one of the principles of the anterior pituitary gland appears to have considerable im-

portance in the alteration of skin color, especially for protective purposes. In general, the underlying basis for alteration of skin color may be related to changes in the vascular bed, blood and bile pigments, metallic pigments, and melanin pigments. Thus any physiologic and pathologic changes that may affect these various factors may give rise to alterations.

Paleness or pallor cannot be considered as especially indicative of the presence of an anemia; however, it is sometimes suggestive enough to warrant this consideration. Pallor may be related to factors other than anemia such as vasomotor phenomena. It must be differentiated from the sallow color of chronic illnesses or the lack of exposure

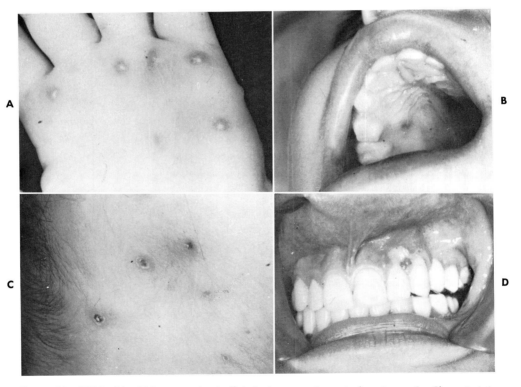

Fig. 6-16. *Child with chicken pox (varicella).* Lesions are in vesicular stage. **A,** Characteristic vesicular lesions on palms. **B,** One of several palatal lesions. Other areas of oral mucosa also are affected. **C,** Resolving lesions of varicella in an adult showing the pitlike character. **D,** Chronic lesion of same duration as those shown in **C** involving marginal gingiva between maxillary left lateral incisor and cuspid.

to sunlight. Pallor of the skin or mucous membrane may be caused by a decreased flow of blood to these structures or to an actual loss of hemoglobin. The color of an anemic patient varies with the factors responsible for the diminution of the hemoglobin; thus a combination of pallor and jaundice may be produced in hemolytic anemia. If pallor is to be used as a sign of anemia or as a sign of changes in the hemo-globin content of the blood, then the areas to be observed should be those that are less well melanized and nonkeratinized and that contain a minimal stratum corneum, such as the lips, palpebral conjunctivae, and mucous membranes (the fingernail beds are also useful because of the translucency of the nails). Pallor or paleness, per se, is difficult to detect and, when it is believed to be present, the examiner should evaluate

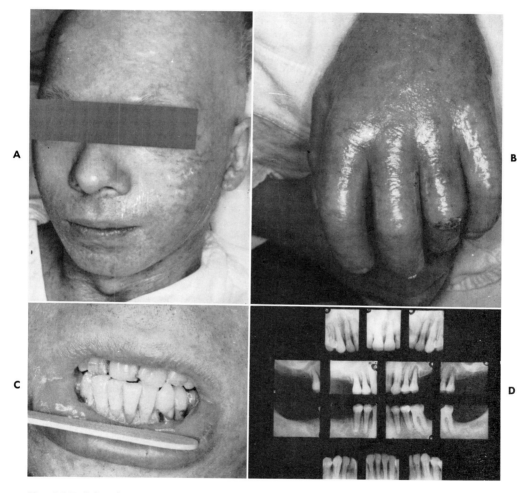

Fig. 6-17. *Scleroderma.* **A,** Loss of natural wrinkles, providing masklike appearance. Note also telangiectasia and reddish-purple blotches. **B,** Tense atrophic shiny skin, with ulceration over the knuckle of ring finger. **C,** Atrophy of mucosa and loss of elasticity of skin resulting in limited oral opening. **D,** Changes in supporting tissues demonstrated radiographically by widening of periodontal space, finely trabeculated bone, and horizontal bone loss.

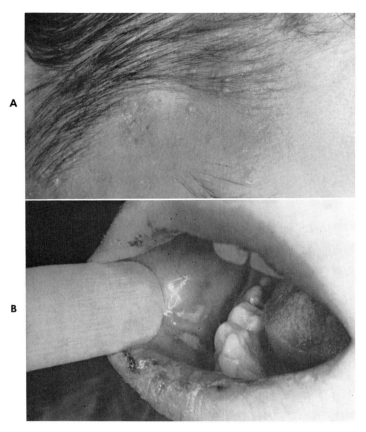

Fig. 6-18. *Herpes zoster.* **A,** Note vesicular lesions between eyebrow and hairline and beneath hair. **B,** Numerous crusted lesions on lip and ruptured lesions covered with fibrinous membrane on buccal mucosa.

the possibility of its cause. It may result from a decrease of hemoglobin pigment, a diminished flow of blood to the tissues, the presence of edema, or a decrease in melanin pigments. One must remember that melanin pigment can effectively screen out much of the color or lack of color caused by altered hemoglobin or vascular changes. The detection of erythema, cyanosis, and pallor should be observed in those areas of the body that have a minimal or absent melanization.

An increased redness of the skin may be caused by capillary dilatation, or associated with blushing, fever, burns, exposure to sunlight, and telangiectasia resulting from x-ray therapy (Fig. 6-19). In rare instances generalized redness may be caused by polycythemia vera. The tissues may be quite red in inflammatory changes. Areas of ulceration that allow the color of the underlying vessels to be readily seen may show an intensive red color. Where there is an increased desquamation of the skin or mucous membranes, such as may occur in the red beefy tongue of deficiency glossitis and desquamative gingivitis, the more superficial position of the capillary vessels may show more easily the color resulting from oxyhemoglobin. Vascular nevi give the skin involved a port-wine color; the gingivae may also be affected (Fig. 6-20).

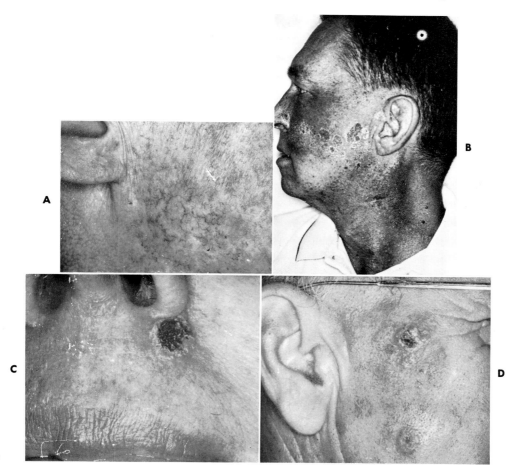

Fig. 6-19. *Changes in skin associated with irradiation.* **A,** Note atrophy, epilation, and telangiectasia. **B,** Acute irradiation effects manifest as hyperpigmentation and crusting. **C,** Squamous cell carcinoma appearing as slightly elevated, ulcerated lesions covered by black crust and having rolled border with some desquamation. Changes in skin are caused by irradiation. **D,** Multiple lesions on side of face. Uppermost is an elevated, crusted, indurated lesion—an advanced carcinoma of the skin. Lower lesion is an elevated, indurated, slightly hyperkeratotic process—senile keratotic plaque. Two pigmented areas can be seen just below and anterior to the ear. The four lesions demonstrated by this patient are all reactions to exposure.

Cyanosis is a term used to designate the predominance of reduced hemoglobin in the blood. It results when the absolute reduced hemoglobin in the blood reaches 5 gm. The color of the tissues as a result of cyanosis varies considerably, depending upon the modifying factors. In general, it varies from a deep purplish blue to heliotrope. Thus, the color produced by an alteration of the hemoglobin pigments may vary from the purplish blue of cyanosis to the generalized redness of polycythemia vera.

Changes in the color of the skin or mucous membranes caused by altered melanin pigmentation may be related to local changes such as prolonged irritation or to diseases of systemic origin such as Addison's disease. Most cases of altered skin color not resulting from hemoglobin, melanin, or metallic pigmentation are caused by bile pigments that produce a yellow color. The most common cause of a yellow skin color is bilirubin pigment and is associated with prehepatic, hepatic, or obstructive jaundice. The skin may not be simply yellow in character but may also appear to be pale since, for example, in hemolytic anemia the combination of pallor and a yellow tint give the skin a lemon-yellow appearance. In other types of jaundice bile pigments may impart a fairly yellow tint to the skin and to all the other tissues except the teeth. As the disease or obstruction increases in severity, the yellow color may become quite pronounced and may become greenish yellow or darker. Jaundice associated with these disorders may be present generally throughout the skin areas and the scleras and the mucous membranes. Hyperpigmentation caused by carotene such as

may be seen in myxedema and carotenemia is more characteristically localized in the palms, soles, and face. Yellow pigmentation may also be caused by drugs, chemicals or chronic uremia. Thus mere discoloration of the skin must be differentiated from the yellow discoloration of the skin caused by exposure to certain chemicals such as quinacrine (Atabrine) and carotene.

Melanin pigmentation is a normal component of the skin structure, and normally the degree of melanization varies from one individual to the next, depending upon their complexion, exposure to sunlight, or racial group. Alterations in the content of pigment are usually only of significance when the change is of recent origin. Melanosis or increased melanin pigmentation may result from external causes such as sunlight, mechanical irritation, wind, and heat. Systemic diseases, as well as many skin disorders, may produce melanosis.

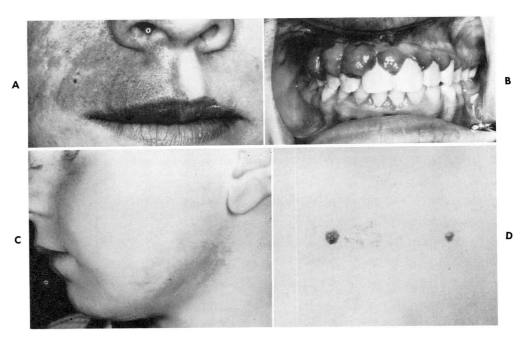

Fig. 6-20. *Discoloration resulting from hemangioma.* **A,** Port-wine stain of upper right lip, cheek, and nose. **B,** Gingival involvement in same patient. **C,** Very light red to pink, smooth, nonelevated discoloration of skin, over posterior lateral border and angle of mandible. **D,** Vascular nevi on neck.

Melanosis may be seen in nutritional deficiency states such as pellagra or may be the result of hormone imbalance. Representative examples of the latter are pigmentation of the face in pregnancy (chloasma gravidarum) and the accentuation of the areas of primary melanization such as the nipples and areolae. Not infrequently in Addison's disease there is an increased melanin pigmentation of the buccal mucosa. The nature of the mechanism of melanosis in Addison's disease is not clear; however, it is well established that primary adrenocortical insufficiency does cause melanosis, whereas adrenocortical insufficiency secondary to hypopituitarism does so only rarely. In general, there is no characteristic pattern of melanosis aside from that produced from an increased number of melanoblasts. Melanosis is usually not uniform in character but is predisposed to certain areas of the body. Thus, it may occur in those areas of the body that are exposed to sunlight, in the so-called primary zones of melanization, and in association with localized external causes.

Although many diseases do not produce an unequivocal clinical picture of melanosis

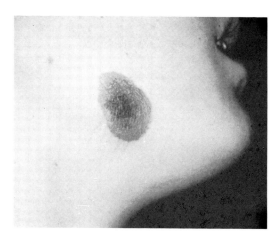

Fig. 6-21. Pigmented nevus over labial aspect of face bearing oval, dark brown, smooth patch with elevated black center. Black hairs originate from dark center.

that will allow a diagnosis on the basis of this picture alone, a few diseases show a melanotic skin picture that is suggestive of basic systemic diseases. The objective of the dentist is not to diagnose these diseases but to recognize that there is an alteration of the basic pattern of pigmentation. Inasmuch as the dentist sees his patients fairly frequently, he is in a position to notice changes or alterations in their normal pigmentation (Fig. 6-21).

Melanin pigmentation in the mouth is not usually seen in white persons of light complexion but is quite frequently observed in Negroes and in Caucasians with natural deposition of pigments. Melanin areas in the mouth are termed "melanoplakia" and are of diagnostic significance when seen in a person of light complexion or if known to be of recent origin. It is not known to what extent melanoblasts in the oral mucosa react to local physical factors such as irritation, heat, and chemical agents. In Negroes melanosis is detected more easily on the tongue than on the buccal mucosa. Of special interest to dentists is the increase in pigmented spots around the oral cavity, lips, and mouth associated with intestinal polyposis.

Exogenous metallic pigments may be responsible for changes in the skin color; the patient's occupation should be considered because of the possibility of metals and paints, insecticides, beverages, wallpaper, and electrotyping solutions being the causative factors. Though most metallic pigments are exogenous in origin, an important exception to this hemosiderin, an iron-containing pigment resulting from the destruction of blood or from a defect in iron metabolism.

The texture of the hair, as well as the amount present, may be suggestive of endocrine disturbances. In hyperpituitary disturbances the hair may be silky, of the lanugo type, and profuse on the cheeks. In hirsutism the distribution of hairs is universal in extent, with the tendency for a masculine distribution; the hair is coarse and black and appears abundantly on the chin and upper lip (Fig. 6-5). This is especially noticeable in the female. In hypothyroidism there may be a diffuse loss of hair and what hair is present is harsh, dry, and brittle. Also, the skin is dry, and the nails are brittle. The reverse is true in hyperthyroidism. These findings should not be confused with the increase in growth and change in color of hair that may be seen in women after removal of the ovaries or after menopause. Loss of the outer one-third of the eyebrows is seen at times as the result of hypothyroidism or syphilis.

A general survey of the patient should include a brief examination of the nails. This can be accomplished easily by a brief glance at the nails for obvious signs of disease; additional careful inspection may be made if indicated. The fingernails are important because they may show the presence of systemic disease. When disease is present in the nails of both the hands and feet, the disease is likely to be systemic in origin rather than local.

Onychophagia is of importance in dentistry because of its association with malocclusion, trauma to teeth, and gingivitis (Fig. 6-22, *A*). In the presence of diseases of the nails such as onychomycosis and mycotic paronychia, nail biting may spread the causative agent of the nail disease to the mouth. Nail changes caused by roentgen rays include longitudinal ridging, slow growth, and brittleness. Koilonychia, or spoon nails, may be seen in association with anemia and is a part of the Plummer-Vinson syndrome. Chronic paronychia should be differentiated from the change of the nail base angle seen in clubbing of the fingers associated with hypertrophic osteoarthropathy (Fig. 6-22, *B*), which may be idiopathic in origin or result from atelectasis, bronchiectasis, heart failure, or other pulmonary disease. Excessive tobacco stain on the fingers is some indication of mental unrest and is partially a quantitative estimate of the amount of smoking that the patient does. This may be related, if necessary, to cough, gingivitis, stomatitis, and so on. Personal care of the fingernails gives some indication of what to expect in the way of care of the mouth. Although not all patients who take care of their fingernails also take care of their mouth, they are more likely to do so than those who have no time for manicures and for other aspects of their personal hygiene.

It is not to be expected that the dentist should be able to make a diagnosis of diseases of the fingernails in general; however, he should have sufficient knowledge of changes to recognize a deviation from normal and in some instances to relate changes in the nails to systemic disorders and to disorders of the mouth. For example, he should correlate chronic nail biting with

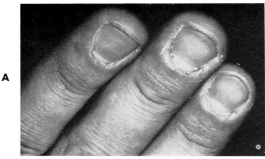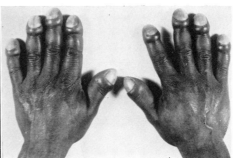

A **B**

Fig. 6-22. *Fingernails.* **A,** Nail biting. **B,** Hypertrophic osteoarthropathy.

small fractures of the incisal edges of the anterior teeth and with gingivitis associated with the trauma from continual nail biting. It is necessary that the nail biting habit be eliminated before satisfactory periodontal therapy or restorative therapy can be undertaken. Furthermore, in some instances nail biting reflects psychologic unrest and this in itself may call for specialized therapy by a psychiatrist. It is not altogether easy at times to differentiate between a habit and a compulsion to satisfy some psychic tension. Not infrequently the patient with bruxism, fingernail biting, excessive smoking, or other oral habits is emotionally disturbed to the extent that proper dental therapy cannot be accomplished.

Neck

An examination of the neck should be made for lesions, scars, lymph node enlargement, glandular enlargement (Fig. 6-23, A), deviations of the trachea, and the presence of developmental defects within the lateral aspects and the midline. Palpation should be done by comparison of both sides alternately or at the same time. Enlargement of lymph nodes may result from local inflammation, neoplastic metastasis, or systemic disease. Examination should include palpa-

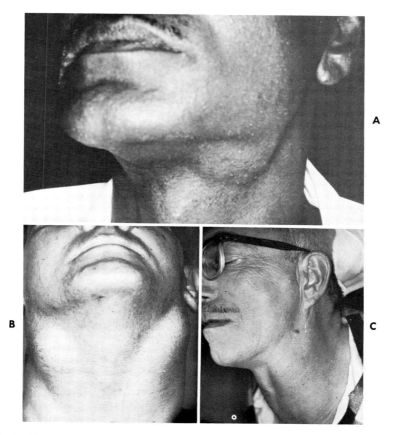

Fig. 6-23. *Swellings of neck.* **A,** Unilateral swelling beneath angle of mandible caused by chronic obstructive sialadenitis. **B,** Bilateral enlargement of cervical lymph nodes typical of Hodgkin's disease. **C,** Note bilateral fullness of lower neck caused by colloid goiter.

tion of the posterior auricular, submental, and anterior and posterior cervical nodes and, when indicated, the supraclavicular, infraclavicular, epitrochlear, and axillary nodes. A differential diagnosis of swelling in the neck region makes necessary the differentiation of glandular elements, lymph nodes, fascial spaces, bones, and muscles.

Of special significance in the examination of the neck are the lymph nodes. In the normal individual very few lymph nodes are palpable even on careful clinical examination; however, their strategic location along the lymph channels makes them likely to be involved in a variety of infections and in various types of malignancies. Enlargement may be confined to small areas or may be widespread in nature and may be characterized by the cardinal signs of inflammation. Sequelae of involvement may be necrosis, rupture of the nodules, and the formation of a sinus. It is possible, however, for considerable enlargement to take place in the absence of any signs of inflammation. If the examiner discovers an enlargement or a mass in the usual location of lymph nodes, he should determine whether it is a solitary nodule or multiple masses. By bilateral palpation he should determine whether the process is unilateral or bilateral, whether the masses are discrete or matted together, and whether or not there is any tenderness present. The consistency must be noted to determine if the mass is hard, firm, or fluctuant. Palpation must be carried farther to determine the presence of fixation to an underlying structure such as the mandible. The first evidence of lymph node enlargement may be pressure associated with the enlargement or signs of systemic involvement if the condition is inflammatory in character.

The most common causes of lymph node enlargement are acute and chronic infections of regional or systemic origin, so-called primary lymph node disease, such as Hodgkin's disease (Fig. 6-23, *B*), reticulum cell sarcoma, and lymphosarcoma, and the enlargement associated with leukemia and metastases from malignant disease. Lymphadenopathy associated with pulpal disease is most commonly found by the dentist. Tuberculosis (Fig. 6-23, *C*) and syphilis were formerly the most common causes of lymphadenopathy from specific infections.

The regional lymph nodes associated with the primary lesion of syphilis are characterized by a firm, painless swelling; in the secondary phase of syphilis, there is a generalized distribution of firm, shotty, nontender nodes. Enlargement resulting from metastasis of neoplastic lesions is characterized by being distinctly localized and very hard. The location of the lymphadenopathy may suggest the site of the origin of the disease since certain anatomic areas are drained by known groups of regional lymph nodes. The sequelae of any inflammation may leave the lymph node enlarged, firm, and easily palpable. Thus a differential diagnosis of enlargement must consider the possibility that previous injury or infection may be responsible for the enlargement that is felt at a later time. For example, in palpating enlargements in the neck such as a single mass in the midline just below the tip of the chin, the history and the physical characteristics of tumefaction, shape, size, consistency, attachment, and location must be determined. In this instance the physical characteristics are best defined by pressing the enlargement or node against the jawbone or toward the floor of the mouth. If the enlargement is tender, has been present for only a short period of time, and is associated with a reactive lesion of the lower lip, the tip of the tongue, or the floor of the mouth, the diagnosis of metastatic carcinoma must be suspected. Lymphadenopathy in association with a metastatic carcinoma does not invariably mean that the lymph node enlargement is caused by metastasis; enlargement secondary to ulcerating carcinoma may be the cause. When many of the lymph nodes of the neck are involved or multiple masses appear bilaterally in the neck rather suddenly in association with fever and malaise, the disease is usually of a general infectious nature.

In acute infectious diseases, the nodes may increase rapidly in size and become tender; they are usually discrete and firm but not hard and can be moved freely in their bed. When enlargement of the lymph glands of the neck begins insidiously in one area and spreads to other regions with a progressive increase in the size of the nodes, a chronic disease of the lymph nodes is usually present. In general, the glands are freely movable and are not tender. These are not characteristic findings of any specific chronic inflammatory process but may be seen in the specific infective granulomas, leukemias, Hodgkin's disease, lymphosarcoma, or malignant metastases.

Cervical lymphadenopathy may occur in Vincent's infection and in herpetic gingivostomatitis. Occasionally these two conditions may present diagnostic problems to the dentist, and a history of the time of onset of the lymphadenopathy is of importance in making the differential diagnosis. In herpetic gingivostomatitis the regional lymphadenopathy occurs prior to the lesions in the mouth, whereas in Vincent's disease the cervical adenopathy occurs after the lesions in the mouth. In acute infectious adenopathy the swelling usually subsides as soon as the primary lesions have healed; however, there may occasionally be suppuration with abscess formation. Infrequently the infection may break through the capsules of the gland and involve the surrounding glands. Where considerable scar tissue results, the lymph nodes may be palpable for many weeks and even months.

Lymphoid hyperplasia associated with many diseases is common in childhood, and adenopathy without any specific causative factor is also common. In the middle-aged or older individual the presence of localized and hard lymph nodes without obvious cause should direct the examiner's attention to the possibility of malignant metastasis. Lymph node enlargement from metastases may involve a single node or, in most instances, more than one node. At first the nodes involved are freely movable and do not exhibit tenderness when palpated. But as the disease progresses, they become matted together and fixed to the surrounding structures; at this time they exhibit their characteristic hardness. Whenever such adenopathy is found in the neck region, especially in the submaxillary or superior deep cervical chains, carcinoma within the mouth, nasal pharynx, or nose should be suspected, and a diligent search should be made for a primary lesion in these regions. Occasionally malignant tumors may metastasize from distant parts of the body to the neck. Lesions involving the midline may involve the lymph chains on both sides. In the absence of sialolithiasis or a history of contact wtih epidemic parotitis or of a surgical procedure that might suggest operative parotitis, the examiner should direct his attention to the possibility of a neoplasm of the parotid gland. Although radiographs with radiopaque fluid serve to assist in determining the extent and character of neoplasms of the parotid gland, it remains for the pathologist to make the precise diagnosis by studying a section of tissue from the gland.

An examination of the neck should include inspection of the veins of the neck. The position of the patient in the dental chair is such that congestion and pulsation of the jugular veins may sometimes be noticed in association with vascular hypertension, severe thyrotoxicosis, and congestive heart failure. Thus, in general, engorgement of the veins of the neck is suggestive of right-sided congestive heart failure or of some obstructive process that prevents the return of blood flow. When it is bilateral, the pathologic process may be of mediastinal or cardiac origin.

Swellings in the lateral aspect of the neck

may be developmental, inflammatory, or neoplastic in origin. Branchial cleft cysts may be found along the anterior border of the sternocleidomastoid muscle, and Warthin's tumors may be found at the angle of the jaw. As in other masses found in this area, it may be necessary to perform a biopsy to determine the exact nature of the lesion. An adequate history and a complete examination of the mass are important in order to determine the true nature of the lesion. It is the history and the clinical examination that will determine whether a biopsy is to be performed.

The presence of a smooth, firm, solitary swelling along the anterior border of the sternocleidomastoid muscle that has been present since childhood and has not changed its characteristics is highly suggestive of a branchial cleft cyst. However, because of the presence of teratoma-like tumors in the area that have a tendency to become malignant in the fourth or fifth decade, a positive diagnosis of the swelling should be made (Fig. 6-24).

The examination of a patient with an enlargement or a mass in the neck should include an examination of the oral cavity for possible associated lesions. In the presence of a vague history and the absence of a contributing lesion in the oral cavity, the patient should be referred to a physician for consultation. When a lesion exists in the mouth, its exact nature should be determined.

In summary, an examination of the neck should be made for the presence of lesions, scars (Fig. 6-25), lymph node enlargement, enlargement of the salivary glands, deviation of the trachea, and developmental defects in both the lateral aspects and the midline. A mass in the neck should be regarded as neoplastic until proved otherwise. When a swelling in the neck exists and is attributed to a pathologic process in the jaws such as an abscessed tooth, the following should be determined: whether there is involvement of the fascial planes and potential spaces, whether the enlargement is firm or fluctuant, whether the overlying skin is red and fixed, whether the center of the mass is soft, and whether the patient has constitutional symptoms of malaise and fever. Localization of the suppu-

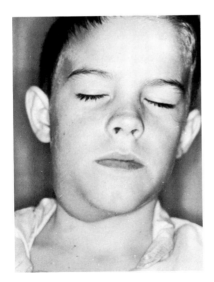

Fig. 6-24. Unilateral swelling of upper lateral neck caused by branchial cyst.

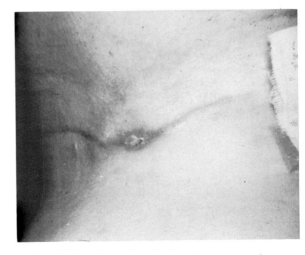

Fig. 6-25. *Lesion of neck.* Scar from surgical removal of thyroglossal duct cyst.

ration and abscess formation is necessary so that precise surgical intervention may be accomplished.

The parotid glands should be palpated for enlargements; this may be done at the time that the neck is examined. It is difficult to palpate all of the parotid gland because of its extensive nature. One should remember that it extends posteriorly and upward to the lobe of the ear as well as below it and anteriorly to the anterior border of the masseter muscle. The dense fascia that surrounds the parotid glands does not permit any great amount of swelling to occur as a result of an inflammatory process without severe pain. The external features of the gland are palpated during the examination of the neck; however, the examination of the ducts and orifices is best accomplished by bimanual extraoral and intraoral palpation during the examination of the mouth. The external features may be altered by inflammatory processes, obstruction of the ducts, and neoplasms.

It should be pointed out again that the objective of this book is not to give a detailed descriptive review of all the diseases that produce swelling in these areas but to present to the examiner a systematic approach for the detection of enlargements or masses in these areas. It is hoped that this will alert him to the cause of the enlargements so that he will more effectively utilize reference books containing a descriptive review of the lesions.

The technic of examination of the neck is based upon a knowledge of the location of anatomic structures most frequently involved by pathologic processes and a division of the structures into areas that are more easily covered by a systematic examination. In order for the examiner to carry out a thorough examination of the neck or lymphadenopathy, he must be aware of the anatomic location of the glands and the areas that they drain.

The *submental lymph glands* are located in the midline of the jaw just below the chin and between the attachments of the anterior digastric muscles. They drain the central portion of the lower lip, the tip of the tongue, and the anterior portion of the floor of the mouth. The *submaxillary lymph glands* are located below the midportion of the mandible about the submaxillary gland. This location can be best palpated by beginning at the anterior quarter of the masseter muscle and moving toward the midline. These glands drain the sides of the nose, the upper lip and lateral portions of the lower lip, the buccal mucosa and cheek, the midportions of the eyelids, and the anterolateral margins of the tongue. The *superficial cervical lymph glands* are located about the external jugular vein. They drain the external ear and the parotid gland and can be best palpated by manipulation of the tissues anterior to the sternocleidomastoid muscle. The deep superior and inferior cervical lymph glands are found along the course of the carotid artery and the internal jugular vein. These glands lie behind the sternocleidomastoid muscle and are especially numerous at the bifurcation of the common carotid artery. The deep superior cervical glands drain the back of the neck, the occipital region of the scalp, portions of the external ear, and the posterior and central portions of the tongue, palate, nasopharynx, nose, larynx, and upper part of the esophagus. The deep inferior cervical glands drain the back of the neck and the lower portion of the occipital scalp and superior anterior chest wall.

The examination of the neck and adjacent structures is one of the most important elements of the clinical examination of structures outside the mouth. This anatomic region is not only important to disease of the mouth and contiguous tissues, but also is often related to disease distant from the neck, especially disease of the chest. As previously mentioned, cardiac and pulmonary diseases are prime examples.

Examination procedure. Of initial importance is the correct seating of the patient in a relaxed unstrained position in the dental chair, preferably without head support. The examiner should be able to move the patient's head freely to relax muscle tension so as to facilitate palpation (Fig. 6-26). Depending upon the site to be examined, palpation is bilateral or unilateral. The position of the examiner depends upon the particular procedure used. Bilateral palpation is usually best accomplished with the examiner standing behind the patient, whereas unilateral palpation can usually be best accomplished with the examiner standing in front of the patient.

The first step in the examination is inspection of the neck for changes in contour and symmetry, changes in color and texture of the skin, scars, and dilatation and pulsation of the neck veins. The inspection should be systematic, and like areas should be compared. Inspection should follow a definite procedure beginning with the parotid gland area. It should then proceed to the areas at the angles of the mandible, the borders and base of the mandible, the sub-

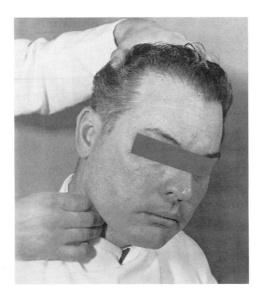

Fig. 6-26. *Palpation of neck. Note head position to facilitate relaxation of muscles.*

mandibular areas, the submental region, the midline of the neck, the anterior triangles of the neck, and along the borders of the sternocleidomastoid muscles. After inspection of these areas and while the patient is still facing the examiner, an inspection of general contours should be made while the patient moves his head slowly from side to side. This procedure may serve to bring out masses or demonstrate a lack of mobility.

Palpation of the neck and contiguous structures should be carried out with a definite procedure in mind. After the initial inspection, the examiner should start the palpation procedure standing behind the patient. The muscles should be completely relaxed. The examiner should begin by placing the flat surfaces of the fingertips at the same position on both sides of the neck and bilaterally palpating the parotid region and the tissue between the ascending ramus of the mandible and the sternocleidomastoid muscle. The head should be moved from side to side sufficiently to allow free access to the structures beneath the areas.

The examiner then should palpate bilaterally down the angles of the jaw, along the bases of the mandible, and below the mandible to the midline (Fig. 6-27). In the midline, the tissues and nodes in the submental region should be palpated by pressing them upward against the symphysis of the jaw. Later, during the examination of the floor of the mouth, bimanual palpation serves to retest some of the structures present in this area. Any deviation of contour that is abnormal in itself or different from the other side of the jaw should be noted. The midline of the neck should be examined, and the hyoid bone and thyroid cartilage should be palpated while the patient is at rest and while he is swallowing. The thyroid gland is attached to the larynx and trachea and will ascend during the swallowing act. Unless a pathologic process associated with the thyroid gland has caused

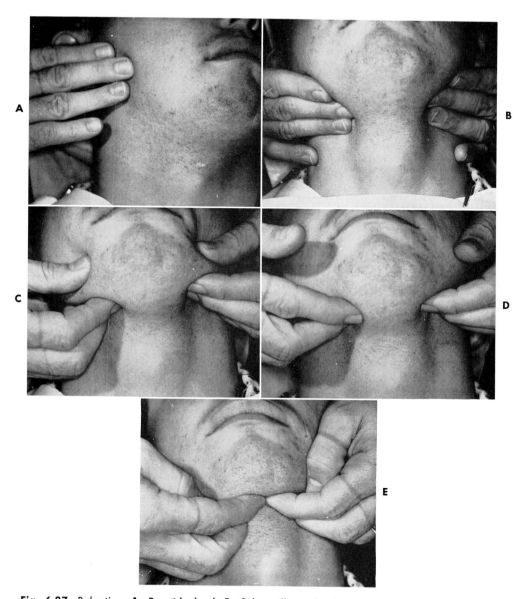

Fig. 6-27. *Palpation.* **A,** Parotid gland. **B,** Submaxillary gland. **C** and **D,** Submaxillary lymph nodes. **E,** Submental lymph nodes.

fixation of the surrounding structures, any such lesion will ascend with the thyroid gland when the patient swallows (Fig. 6-28). The examiner should extend the palpation to the lateral areas of the neck by passing the closed fingers along the anterior and posterior borders of the sternocleidomastoid muscles while the patient is in a forward position and during rotation and lateral bending of the neck. The palpation should extend the length of the sternocleidomastoid muscles and upward to behind the ears (Fig. 6-29).

During the examination the examiner should be alert to rigidity of muscles, tenderness, induration, and solitary or multiple masses. In many instances the history will serve to enhance the physical examination procedure. The possible relationship to disease in the oral region or elsewhere must be recognized.

A brief review of the lesions found in the several areas of the neck seems in order at this time. Single masses that appear in the midline may be related to lymphadenopathy, thyroid disease, developmental disturbances such as thyroglossal duct anomalies, and cellulitis. Single masses in the submaxillary region may be cellulitis, sialolithiasis

of Wharton's duct, neoplasms of the submaxillary and sublingual glands, and regional lymphadenopathy associated with inflammatory lesions of the oral cavity. Palpation of this area is overlapped by intraoral and extraoral palpation of the floor of the mouth. Single masses in the lateral aspects of the neck may be developmental anomalies such as branchial cleft cysts and hygroma colli cysticum, regional lymphadenopathy, and neoplastic disease. Multiple masses in the neck are most usually the result of lymph node involvement. This may result from hyperplasia associated with infectious disease, secondary inflammatory hyperplasia associated with acute or chronic oral lesions, or neoplasia.

Jaws

In the examination of the jaws, the functional movement of the mandible and the temporomandibular joints with the jaws separated, the anteroposterior relationship of the mandible and maxilla, the symmetry of the jaws, the presence of "clicking" and "snapping" of the joints, and the presence of swelling and tenderness of the jaws and joints should be considered. Further evaluation of the temporomandibular joints in

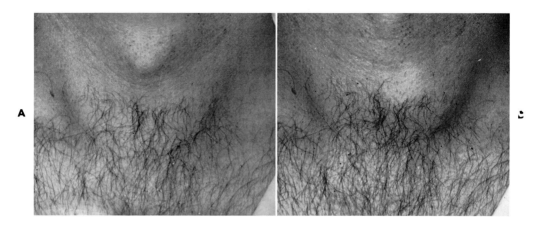

Fig. 6-28. *Thyroid adenoma.* **A,** Note apparent absence of lesion in area of suprasternal notch prior to swallowing. **B,** Enlargement caused by adenoma may be seen as patient swallows.

relation to occlusion should be carried out in the analysis of the occlusion and masticatory system.

The examination should be routinely carried out for the sake of thoroughness and is a necessity whenever the chief complaint and related symptoms are referred to this area. All of the principles of the physical examination may be used.

Inspection should be carried out with the examiner standing directly in front of the patient. The symmetry of size and functional lateral movements of the jaws (with the teeth apart) should be noted. The pa-

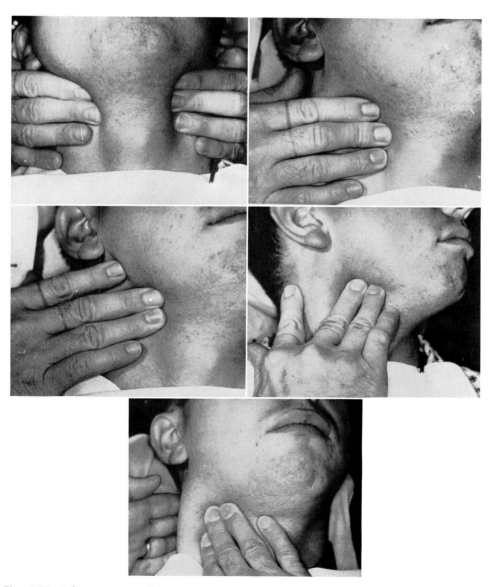

Fig. 6-29. *Palpation.* Cervical lymph nodes. Note position of head and displacement of muscle to facilitate palpation.

tient should be able to move the mandible equally well from side to side. The joints and muscles attached to the mandible should be observed during movement. The movements should be carried out easily without muscle spasms or undue strains of the facial muscles. The patient should be instructed to carry out protrusive movements of the mandible with the teeth sep-

arated. The examiner should pay special attention to deviation of the jaw from the midline and to jerky movements. The presence of abnormal, nonsymmetrical, and jerky movements suggest the possibility of joint or muscle disorders. Traumatic injury of the joints, infections of the joints, muscle hypertonicity or hypotonicity, and fractures of the jaw are common causes of ab-

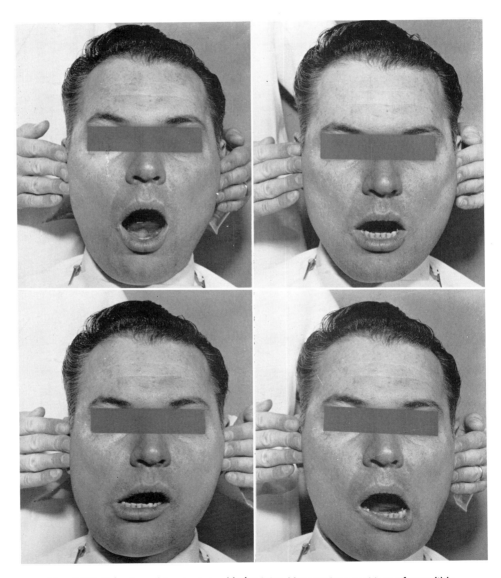

Fig. 6-30. *Palpation of temporomandibular joint.* Note various positions of mandible.

normal jaw movements. Abnormal movements may also be related to neuromuscular disease.

Palpation of the muscles and joints is best accomplished with the examiner standing behind the patient. Bilateral palpation is the method of choice since movements of the joints demand contralateral action of the joints and muscles (Fig. 6-30). The examiner should feel for smoothness in the function of the joints. With the closed fingers of both hands placed on the temporomandibular joint areas, the examiner should ask the patient to make opening movements from rest position, right and left lateral movements with the teeth apart and then together, protrusive movements with the teeth together and then apart, and closing movements from rest position to initial contact of the teeth and maximum occlusal contact. The movements of the joints should be smooth and free from jerky and abnormal action. In lateral movements there is a slight lateral shift or movement of the joint on the side toward which the movement is being made. The opposite joint will move forward and somewhat medially. The possibility of conditioning and training the patient's muscles should be considered before the examiner unequivocally states that abnormal function exists or that there is loss of function. Even so, conditioned movements are important findings since they have important relationships to the muscles, joints, and occlusion. Occasionally ankylosis of the joint may produce abnormal findings on palpation of the joints. Occlusal interferences will also produce jerky and abnormal movements of the joints. This is discussed in greater detail in Chapter 10. The joints should also be palpated for swelling and tenderness.

The muscles responsible for movement of the mandible should be palpated for signs of tenderness, enlargement, muscle spasm, and tonicity. This should be done while movements of the type just described are carried out. Those muscles that are suitably located for palpation are the anterior, middle, and posterior portions of the temporalis and masseter muscles. The digastric muscles are less effectively palpated, and the external and internal pterygoid muscles are less easily palpated. The known functions of the pterygoid muscles allow their action to be grossly evaluated.

Auscultation of the joints can be accomplished simply by listening for any abnormal sounds of "snapping," "grating," or "clicking" that may occur during the movements just described. A stethoscope has limited use but may be of value to one trained in its use for the temporomandibular joint sounds.

Percussion of the jaws may be of value when cavities, fractures, or reflex movements of the mandible are to be evaluated. Percussion should be indirect when percussing for cavities and fractures of the bone and direct when testing for reflex action of the mandible.

REFERENCES

Draper, G., Dupertuis, C. W., and Caughey, J. L.: Human constitution in clinical medicine, New York, 1944, McGraw-Hill Book Co.

Jeghers, H.: Pigmentation of the skin, New Eng. J. Med. 231:88-100, 122-136, 181-189, 1944.

Kampmeier, R. H.: Physical examination in health and disease, Philadelphia, 1954, F. A. Davis Co.

MacBryde, C. M. (editor): Signs and symptoms. Applied pathologic physiology and clinical interpretation, ed. 3, Philadelphia, 1957, J. B. Lippincott Co.

Monash, S.: Normal pigmentation of the oral mucosa, Arch. Dermatol. 26:139, 1932.

Moorrees, C. F., et al.: Principles of orthodontic diagnosis, Angle Orthodont. 6:25-62, July, 1966.

Pullen, R. L. (editor): Medical diagnosis. Applied physical diagnosis, ed. 2, Philadelphia, 1950, W. B. Saunders Co.

Zegarelli, E. V., Kutschen, A. H., and Hyman, G. A.: Diagnosis of diseases of the mouth and jaws, Philadelphia, 1969, Lea & Febiger, pp. 583, xxiii.

7

Examination of soft tissues

General appraisal

The clinical examination of the mouth should begin with a general appraisal of the patient's oral health. The appraisal should include a brief survey of the patient's oral hygiene, state of the teeth, presence of lesions of the soft tissues, presence of acute or chronic distress, presence or absence of prosthetic appliances, presence of edentulous areas, presence of calculus, presence of stains on the teeth, and presence of halitosis. Thus the general survey may be recorded in the following manner: "This is a partially edentulous patient wearing a maxillary full and a mandibular partial denture that appear to be functioning adequately and not causing the patient any distress; the teeth are in good alignment and the color is normal for the patient's age; the oral hygiene is good and there is no evidence of halitosis; there are no lesions of the soft tissues or obvious signs of gross dental decay." In another instance the summary might be as follows: "This is a patient with multiple edentulous spaces without restoration; the remaining teeth show rampant decay, excessive attrition, and a lack of adequate dental care; the oral hygiene is poor and the breath presents an offensive odor; there is evidence of periodontal disease and extensive ulceration of the gingiva that is causing the patient acute distress."

A general appraisal of a patient's mouth serves to inform the examiner how extensive the examination will be and how much time will be required to perform it. It may also indicate what instruments will be needed for the examination and may suggest the necessity for special examination aids. It may also serve to establish a general outline of the areas that should be given special consideration. This part of the examination may be done prior to the rest and thus allow the examiner to make another appointment with the patient at a time when the complete examination can be given more time. It may serve to point out immediately the necessity for referral and consultation.

Obvious signs of rampant dental decay, especially in young patients, should alert the examiner to the necessity for caries control as well as restoration of the teeth. The possibility of control and prevention of decay can be best accomplished through the use and evaluation of carious activity tests. The examiner may elect to carry out these tests at the time of the general appraisal and have their results at hand for the remainder of the examination and for the diagnosis, prognosis, and treatment plan.

The examiner may also wish to have the radiographs taken at this time, including any special radiographs that might be considered necessary. Thus he may elect to carry out the history, the general examination of the patient, and the general appraisal of the patient's mouth and then schedule an appointment for a time after the radiographs are ready to be read.

It is not unusual nor does it lack rationale for an examiner to make a general appraisal of the mouth before any history is obtained or the examination procedure carried out. The procedure has merit when used correctly and does not exclude a more thorough examination. It is usually only justifiable for screening purposes or for evaluating emergency complaints. The latter purpose serves to orient the examiner as to the parts of the history and examination that may be ommited temporarily until relief of acute symptoms can be accomplished.

Under ordinary circumstances the breath of a patient with a normal healthy mouth does not attract the attention of the examiner. The odor of garlic, onions, alcohol, and tobacco may be readily recognized on the breath. Disagreeable odors that are sometimes considered to be somewhat characteristic may be found in association with poor oral hygiene, periodontal disease, rhinitis, sinusitis, tonsillitis, and necrotizing gingivitis. Vincent's or necrotizing gingivitis is considered to have a characteristic fetid odor. Foul breath may also accompany bronchiectasis, lung abscesses, and gastrointestinal upset. Occasionally the fruity odor of acetone can be recognized on the breath of an individual with diabetes mellitus. It is not necessarily, however, a constant finding and may be found only when the patient is in diabetic coma. The appraisal of breath odors may remind the examiner that certain features of the patient's general health history have been over looked. It is not unusual for a patient to be concerned with halitosis; its evaluation at this time in the examination will generally help to remind the examiner of the necessity for a detail examination for its cause.

The general appraisal helps to establish rapport and reminds the patient that his complaints will not become lost in the intricacies of the examination procedures. Many patients are impatient to learn of the evaluation of their oral health before an adequate examination can be accomplished. A brief review and discussion of their oral problems will aid in establishing the need for more extended examination procedures.

Thus, in many instances, it may be rational and even a necessity to make the general appraisal before any history is taken or any other examination procedure carried out. After the initial survey the examiner may then continue with the detailed examination of the mouth, using all the necessary principles of the physical examination —inspection, palpation, percussion, and auscultation. Once again it must be stated that the patient must be made aware of the necessity for a complete examination even though the examination procedure does not appear at times to concern immediately those areas he considers important. It is probably a god practice to enlighten the patient along these lines before beginning the detailed clinical examination.

The instruments and materials necessary for the examination need not be extensive; the following are suggested as basic requirements (Fig. 7-1):

Mouth mirrors No. 5, No. 7
Explorers No. 3, No. 6, No. 17
Periodontal pocket measuring probe, U. Mich. No. 0
Cotton pliers
Cotton
Sponges—2 by 2 inches
Finger cots

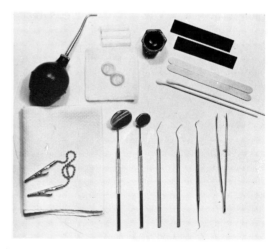

Fig. 7-1. *Examination.* Instruments and their arrangement for the examination.

Dental floss—silk or nylon
Chip syringe or air-jet
Water syringe
Articulating paper
Disclosing solution
Tongue depressor

Good illumination is a primary prerequisite for a thorough examination of the teeth. The patient should be seated properly and comfortably for proper instrumentation and access to all areas of the mouth.

Lips

The lips should be inspected and palpated for variations of the normal and for evidence of disease. Inspection is directed toward changes in color, form, texture, and

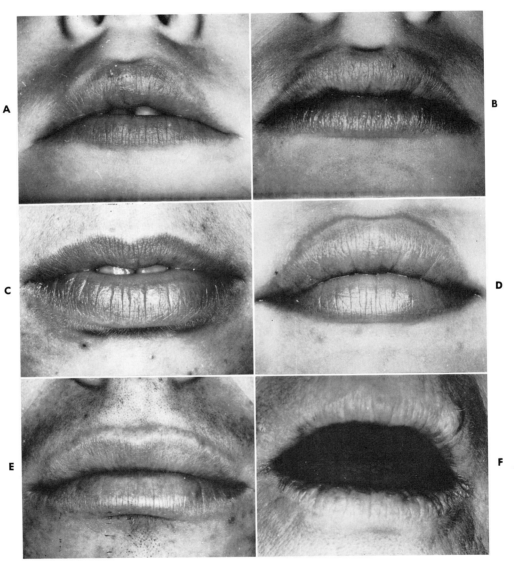

Fig. 7-2. *Lips.* **A** and **B**, Children. **C** and **D**, Adolescents. **E**, Young adult. **F**, Senile person. Note relation of the teeth to the position of lips.

obvious lesions. Palpation is carried out bidigitally to determine the texture, pliability, and firmness of the underlying and surface tissues. Induration, hyperkeratosis, and glandular involvement can be determined by this procedure.

The actual examination of the mouth begins with an inspection of the lips with the mouth unopened. Inspection of the lips is performed first because these are the first structures to attract attention in approaching the examination of the mouth. Normally they are smooth and pink in color, and in the younger individual fissuring is minimal (Fig. 7-2). With advancing age a curl develops in the corner of the mouth medial to the lower end of the mesiolabial sulcus. This is known as the labiomarginal sulcus. It becomes more prominent as the individual becomes older because of the loss of tissue tone and the decrease of fat in the tissues (Fig. 7-3). Various patterns of facial expression and loss of teeth tend to accentuate these grooves.

The patient should be requested to open his lips just slightly, and the line represented by the lower edge of the upper lip should be noted for its relationship to the teeth. The line that the lower border of the upper lip makes with the teeth may vary normally from an approximation to the incisal edges of the lower teeth to the cervical one-third of the maxillary teeth. The patient should also be asked to smile or to show his teeth so that the examiner can note what portion of the teeth may be seen readily; this may be an important consideration in dental restorations. The portion of the tooth structure and gingiva that can be observed when the subject speaks varies normally from a complete exposure of the mandibular incisors and cuspids to a complete blocking of the maxillary teeth by the upper lip. In others it may vary from a complete blocking of the lower incisors by the lower lip to a complete exposure of the maxillary teeth and gingiva.

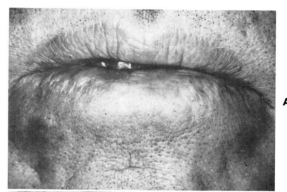

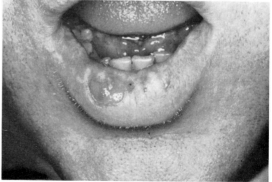

Fig. 7-4. *Lips.* **A,** Senile cheilitis; atrophy and hyperkeratosis associated with age and exposure to weather. **B,** Loss of all normal fissures of lower lip caused by atrophy. Clean, shallow ulcer with very thin border suggests delayed healing and is typical of ulcers that result from acute exposure of lip showing solar cheilitis.

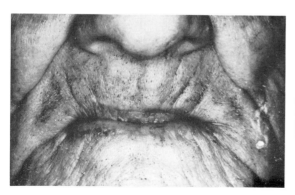

Fig. 7-3. *Lips.* Changes associated with age and loss of teeth; note development of prominent lateral labial sulcus.

The integrity of the seventh cranial nerve can be tested by instructing the patient to show his teeth or to smile (Fig. 6-7). Normally these movements will show a symmetrical position of the lips and the angles of the mouth. The posture of the upper and lower lips is related to the anatomic contours of the jaws and teeth, tonicity of the muscles, and the size of the lips. When the mandible is in the tonus rest position, the lips should just be in approximation without undue strain on the lip muscles.

Usually the color of the upper and lower lips is the same, except in individuals exposed to sunlight and wind. In these instances the color of the lower lip may be masked by some scaling and desquamation. Prolonged exposure to the elements, as occurs in farmers, cowboys, and sailors, may cause permanent changes in the lips (Fig. 7-4). Though these changes are variations of the normal and are not the result of disease, they are of considerable importance in the etiology of leukoplakia and carcinoma. In prolonged exposure to the elements the mucous membrane becomes thickened and is of a bluish to purplish color. A histologic section of the lip of an individual exposed to wind and sun may show scarring and chronic inflammation as a result of the effects of ultraviolet rays and dehydration. In these instances the capillary routes become prominent and are seen clinically as red dots over the lips.

When the individual is a mouth breather, the lower lip may be chapped and dry. This, too, will alter the coloration, since the flaking and desquamation of the epithelium tend to mask the underlying red color of the lips. Therefore, when the upper and lower lips are compared, the upper one appears to be brighter in color. Children, and sometimes adults, have a peculiar habit of sucking or chewing on their upper or lower lip (Fig. 7-5). This causes excessive desquamation of the epithelium and increased circulation of that particular lip. In these instances the lip that is being manipulated is more red in color than the other lip.

The color of the lips is often more significant than the color of other areas because of their thin epithelial covering and their capillary supply. Any disease that affects the number of red blood cells, the amount of reduced hemoglobin, or the oxygen-carrying capacity of the blood may cause various changes in the normal color of the lips. In cardiac failure the lips may have a bluish tint, and in congenital shunts the color may be almost purple. Emphysema, increased blood volume, increased viscosity of the blood, and disturbances of the hemoglobin molecule may produce varying degrees of the blue color of cyanosis.

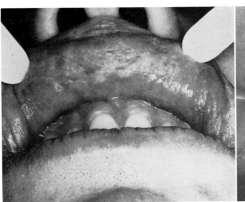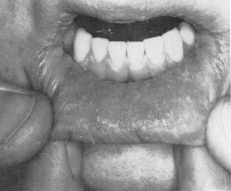

Fig. 7-5. *Lips.* Roughness and hyperkeratinization associated with chewing of lips.

Palpation of the lips may be done at this time or during the inspection of the labial mucosa. The presence of external lesions suggests the earlier time. The lips should be palpated between the index finger and the thumb while the muscles are relaxed and then while they are pursed. When the lips are relaxed, they are soft and resilient throughout the outer surfaces, and the bands of the orbicularis oris muscle can be felt in the body of the lips. When the lips are pursed or tensed, occasionally a secondary fold of soft tissue may be felt just inside the lip and has frequently been called a second lip (Fig. 7-6). Though this is a fairly common occurrence, it may be extensive enough to present anesthetic problem. This is especially true when the individuals are public speakers or singers. Ectopic sebaceous glands are seen so frequently on the vermilion border of the upper lip that they may be considered to be a variation of normal. They are of little significance except in those instances in which they are very extensive and cause esthetic problems. Changes in the lip caused by habits or exposure to wind and sunlight are not in themselves pathologic conditions, but they may be of significance in the diagnosis of orthodontic and periodontal problems. Thus the posture, color, form, texture, tonus, and activity of the lips may relate to mouth breathing or undue pressure on the teeth; these are of significance often in the diagnosis of malocclusion and gingivitis (Fig. 7-7).

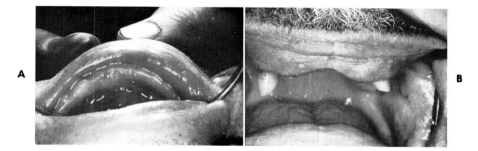

Fig. 7-6. *Lips.* **A,** Double lower lip produced by accessory vestibular fold. **B,** Double upper lip caused by developmental overgrowth.

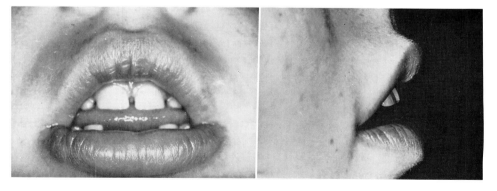

Fig. 7-7. *Lips.* Mouth breathing; note the difference in shade, texture, form, and position of the lips and the position of the tongue.

Findings in disease. The size and form of the lips should be examined for evidence of disease. Large lips may be an expression of a variation of normal or may be caused by angioedema or neoplasms. The lips are frequently thickened in cretinism, and they appear to be protruded in acromegaly. Swelling of the lips is most commonly a result of edema associated with injury or exposure to an offending allergen. In the latter instance a history of reaction to dental agents such as oil of cloves and other dental drugs, systemic therapeutic agents, and cosmetic agents will provide the clue to the cause of the edema. In these instances the response to elimination of the suspected agent and to the use of antihistamines should be noted. (Remember that an individual may be sensitive to antihistamines, too.) Generally, sudden enlargement of the lips suggests an allergic etiologic agent (Fig. 7-8). The size and form as well as texture and tonicity of the lip vary within normal limits with age, sex, race, and exposure to the weather.

Obvious signs of disease such as primary and secondary lesions can best be evaluated on the basis of the type of lesion present and the history of the lesion (Figs. 7-9 to 7-12). The first step in the diagnosis of any lesion of the lip is to determine whether the history and the signs and symptoms presented are suggestive of a developmental, dermatologic, traumatic, metabolic, allergic, or neoplastic disease. In general the history and location of the lesion will be the primary evidence for the diagnosis of a developmental disease. Traumatic lesions can best be related to their history of occurrence; however, occasionally a biopsy may be necessary to make a differential diagnosis from neoplastic disease.

Fissuring at the corners of the mouth (Fig. 7-13) should direct the examiner's attention to vitamin deficiencies or, in elderly patients (in whom the labiomarginal sulcus is deep and excessive salivation or xerostomia is present), toward ulceration of the sulcus and infections with yeast or bacteria. The contiguousness produced by the accentuation of the labiomarginal sulcus results in an extension of the commissures of the upper and lower lips into skin areas that are not suited to continuous wetting or drying; these areas are then prone to cheilitis. Fissuring may also occur from extensive stretching of the mouth; this may be seen in association with dental procedures. The secondary ulcerative lesions of herpes simplex are also seen frequently at the commissures after dental procedures. Longitudinal fissuring of the lower lip should direct the examiner's attention toward the possibility of actinic cheilitis, dehydration, and mouth breathing. Fissures that have been present for a long period of time have a tendency to bleed, and if indurated should be evaluated for neoplastic disease. Ulceration characterized by chronicity, failure to heal, induration, and lymphadenopathy suggests neoplastic disease (Fig. 7-12). Hyperpigmentation of rather recent onset accompanied by other signs and symptoms of a systemic nature should suggest the possibility of metabolic disorders such as Addison's disease.

The foregoing discussion is not meant to be an extensive categorization of all the diseases that may affect the lips. When a more descriptive account of lesions of the lip is

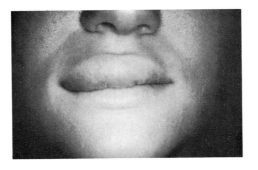

Fig. 7-8. *Lips.* Pronounced and sudden swelling of one or both lips, especially accompanied by swelling of the eyelids, is indicative of angioneurotic edema. This is usually an allergic response.

needed for a final diagnosis, the examiner is referred to textbooks of oral pathology or dental medicine.

Labial and buccal mucosa

The examination of the mucosa should begin with reflection of the upper and lower lips and inspection of the color and texture of the labial surfaces (Fig. 7-14). The lips should be palpated in a systematic manner, and this should be a routine part of the examination. The presence of unsuspected mucous retention cysts is not an uncommon finding when the routine practice

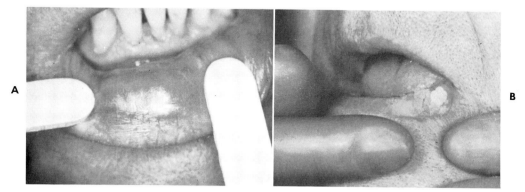

Fig. 7-9. *Lips.* **A,** White, thin plaque of vermilion mucosa called "smoker's patch." This is an example of focal hyperkeratosis produced by mechanical, chemical, and thermal injury. **B,** Typical picture of "smoker's cancer." Left lateral one-third of vermilion is covered by thin, opaque, keratinized plaque. The most lateral zone has recently become thicker, whiter, and more firm, and there is slight rolling of the most lateral border.

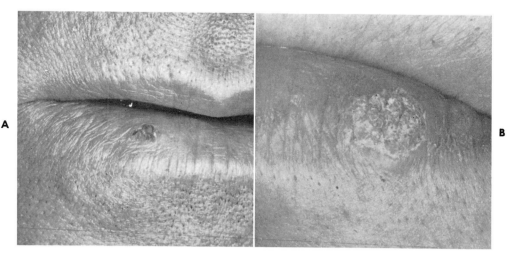

Fig. 7-10. *Lips.* **A,** Small, elevated, crusted lesion on vermilion border of lip—early squamous cell carcinoma. **B,** Crusted, verruca-appearing, 1 cm. lesion, slightly elevated above the surface, on the middle, one-third of the left vermilion. The lesion is indurated. This type of squamous cell carcinoma is frequently mistaken for a "cold sore."

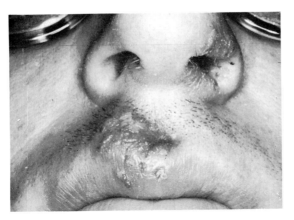

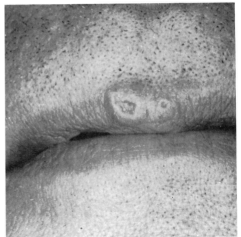

A

Fig. 7-11. *Lips.* Two vesicular, crusted lesions, one involving upper lip and one involving left nares; note the well-demonstrated conglomerate character so typical of herpetic lesions.

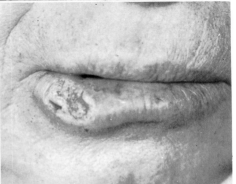

B

Fig. 7-12. *Lips.* **A,** Lesion involving mucocutaneous junction in midline of upper lip, with elevated border about depressed center. Rolled border is feature of neoplasia; the lesion is a basal cell carcinoma. **B,** Some deformity of lip produced by slightly craterous ulcer of vermilion with rolled, white border—moderately advanced squamous cell carcinoma.

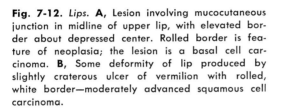

A

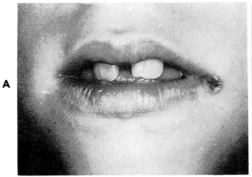

B

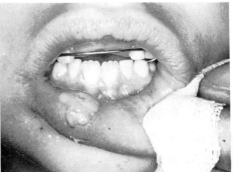

Fig. 7-13. *Lips.* **A,** Angular fissure, traumatic in origin; note change in shape of lower lip associated with lip biting. **B,** Vermilion of lip and vestibular mucosa demonstrating irregularly contoured, elevated, yellowish adherent, soft membrane. This yellowish membrane is composed of fibrin that has exuded from area of traumatized mucosa.

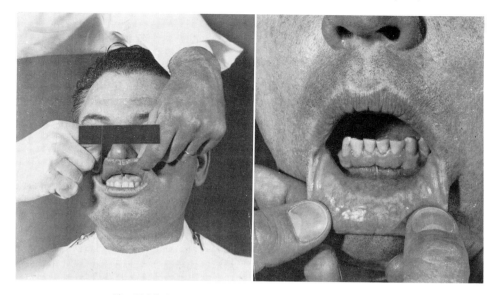

Fig. 7-14. *Lips.* Inspection of lips and vestibular mucosa.

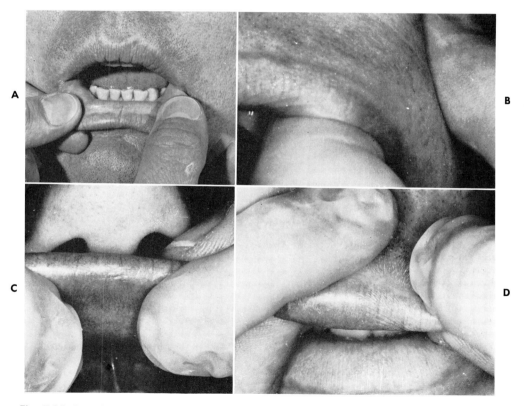

Fig. 7-15. *Lips.* **A,** Inspection. **B,** Bidigital palpation. **C** and **D,** Bilateral and bidigital palpation.

of bidigital palaption is carried out. Palpation should start with the outer edge of the lip and proceed to the vestibule. It may be bilateral as well as bidigital (Fig. 7-15).

Inspection and palpation of the labial surfaces of the lip will show varying degrees of nodularity associated with numerous mucous glands that are situated in the submucous tissue (Fig. 7-16). These glands have a granular feeling somewhat analogous to cooked tapioca. The degree of nodularity may be increased by chronic irritation, especially the use of tobacco.

Several folds of tissue, called frena or frenula, traverse the vestibular fornix (Fig. 7-17). In the midline, sagittal folds connect the alveolar process with the upper and lower lips. In children, before the eruption of the teeth, the superior labial frenulum is attached to the crest of the alveolar process and forms a raphe that may reach to the palatal papilla. With the eruption of the teeth and vertical growth of the alveolar process, the attachment migrates superiorly and can be found normally on the attached gingiva or may be restricted to the aleovlar mucosa of the vestibule. Most frequently in the adult it is found at the junction of the attached gingiva and alveolar mucosa. The inferior labial frenulum is found most often attached at the junction of the alveolar mucosa and the attached gingiva. However, it may extend for some distance onto the attached gingiva. The position of the attachment is related to the eruption of the teeth and vertical growth of the alveolar process. The lateral frenula are present in the area of the cuspids and bicuspids. They are usually more prominent in the lower arch than in the upper. The position of the attachment of the lower lateral frenulum varies considerably and may be attached high on the attached gingiva or in the alveolar mucosa of the vestibule. Inspection and palpation of these frenula are best accomplished when the lips and cheeks are retracted (Fig. 7-17). Their position and attachment may be studied on stone models when function impressions are taken. As will be pointed out later, the attachments are of significance in periodontics, orthodontics, and prosthodontics.

The cheek should be reflected and the buccal mucosa inspected for color, texture, and lesions (Fig. 7-18). The cheeks should be retracted sufficiently to give the examiner a clear view of their entire mucosal surface. The examiner should then traverse the buccal mucosa from the vestibular reflection of the mucous membrane to the alveolar processes and posteriorly to the fornix of the vestibule opposite the maxillary tuberosity. The mucous membrane is normally pink in members of the Caucasian race, while in the Negro it is more bluish or bluish gray. This bluish color may have an

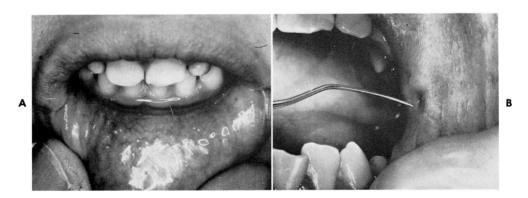

Fig. 7-16. Labial mucosa. **A,** Vestibular glands. **B,** Developmental pit at commissure.

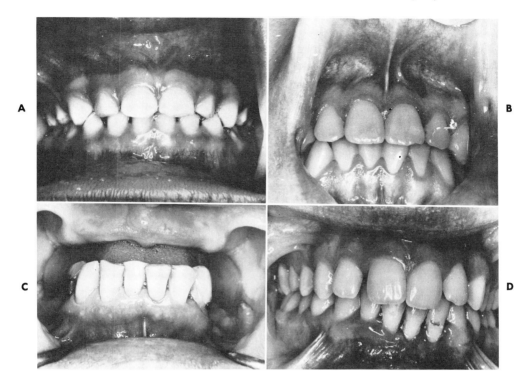

Fig. 7-17. *Frenula.* **A,** In primary dentition. **B,** In young adult. **C,** Maxillary lateral and midline mandibular frenula. **D,** Mandibular lateral frenula.

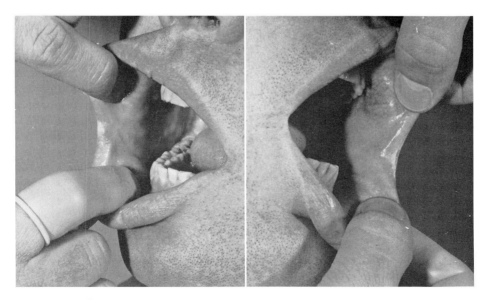

Fig. 7-18. *Buccal mucosa.* Reflection and inspection; note position of examiner's fingers and manipulation of lip for an adequate field of vision.

uneven or patchy distribution. Brown pigmentation may normally be present in buccal mucosa in the Negro.

Quite commonly isolated or confluent ectopic sebaceous glands are present adjacent to the corner of the mouth and extending

to the molar region. In front of the anterior border of the masseter muscle, there may be a rounded eminence containing fat tissue. This is called the buccal fat pad of Bichat. The eminence is variable in size and is seen most prominently in the new-

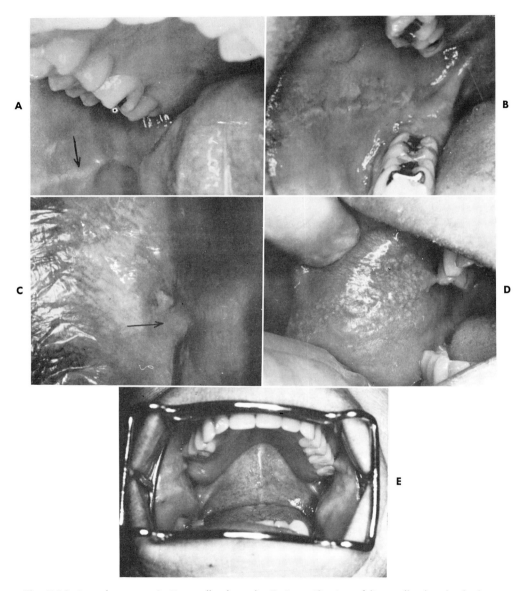

Fig. 7-19. *Buccal mucosa.* **A,** Linea alba buccalis. **B,** Intensification of linea alba by cheek chewing. **C,** Caliculus angularis. **D,** Fordyce spots. **E,** Persistent bilateral buccal fat pads.

born infant. However, pronounced residual eminences of this fat pad may be seen in the adult (Fig. 7-19, *E*).

At the occlusal line in most individuals there is a longitudinal fold of tissue that extends from a point near the angle of the mouth to just anterior to the fold created by the elevation of the pterygomandibular raphe (Fig. 7-19, *A*). This may appear as a thin white line or as a rather thickened elevation. It has been called the linea alba buccalis or torus buccalis. It may be seen infrequently in young children, but it is seen most commonly in adults. It is a thickening of the mucosa resulting from pressure of the cheek into the line of occlusion. It may become accentuated from trauma of biting (Fig. 7-19, *B*). The white color is

caused by surface keratinization. Near the anterior termination of the linea alba buccalis there is often found a projection of the mucosa called the caliculus angularis (Fig. 7-19, *C*). The linea alba buccalis and the caliculus angularis are not important except in the presence of injury and irritation.

The cheek should be examined also by bimanual palpation (Fig. 7-20, *A*). By this method both the underlying structures and the surface of the mucosa can be felt. The examiner should be especially careful in his palpation of the deep structures in the cheek because lesions may be present in this type of loose tissue without showing externally or being noticed by the patient.

Opposite the second maxillary molar is an

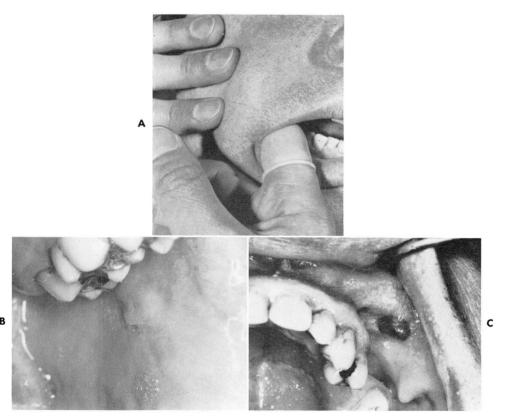

Fig. 7-20. *Buccal mucosa.* **A,** Bimanual palpation of cheek. **B,** Parotid papilla. **C,** Hemangioma anterior to pendulous parotid papilla.

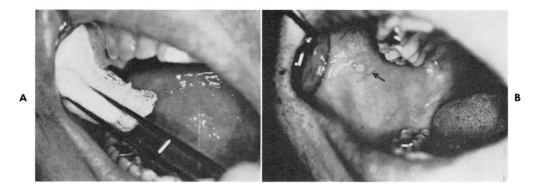

Fig. 7-21. *Inspection of parotid papilla.* **A,** Drying of mucosa to observe flow and character of saliva. **B,** Note drop of saliva at orifice of duct.

eminence of the mucous membrane called the parotid papilla, which marks the opening of Stensen's duct (Fig. 7-20, *B*). The size of the papilla varies considerably and in some instances may extend into the interproximal surfaces of the molar teeth. Many persons (even dental students) seeing this papilla for the first time view it with alarm, believing it to be a tumor of some kind (Fig. 7-20, *C*).

The parotid papilla is soft in consistency on palpation, and if the parotid gland is manipulated, a quantity of serous, somewhat clear fluid may be expressed from the papilla (Fig. 7-21). Careful bimanual palpation may serve to demonstrate the hard firm cordlike Stensen's duct just in front of the anterior border of the masseter muscle (Fig. 7-20, *A*).

The mucous membrane in the fornix of the vestibule is thin, and the many small venules that traverse this tissue are easily seen. It is not unusual for students who see these vessels for the first time to be unnecessarily concerned. The reflection of the cheek tissue onto the alveolar process is characterized by a change in the consistency and attachment of the mucous membrane. The alveolar mucosa covering the alveolar process is attached loosely to the underlying bone. The juncture of the alveolar mucosa and the gingiva is indicated by

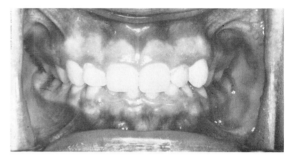

Fig. 7-22. *Buccal mucosa.* Note sharp demarcation of color at junction of alveolar mucosa and gingiva.

a sharp scalloped line that vaguely parallels the free margin of the gingiva. The alveolar mucosa appears dark red in color when compared to the normal pale pink color of the gingiva. The sharpness of the color contrast between the two tissues varies considerably from one individual to another. In general, the more pale the gingival tissues, the greater the contrast in color (Fig. 7-22).

Behind the most distal molars of the upper and lower arches are soft tissue prominences that are called retromolar papillae. In the maxilla these papillae are continuous with the gingiva that covers the termination of the maxillary tuberosity and alveolar tubercle. In the mandible the retromolar papilla is an accentuation of the free gingival margin and is continuous with the retromolar pad. The reflection of the attached gingiva and the cheek mucosa in this region is the site of an aggregation of buccal glands. The prominence caused by the glands gives the tissue a padlike appearance and has been called the retromolar pad, although more commonly the term has been used to designate collectively the prominence caused by both the retromolar papilla and the retromolar pad. The retromolar papillae and the retromolar pads are of significance in periodontal therapy and in the placement and wearing of dentures. Considerable normal variation exists in the form and consistency of the retromolar papilla and the retromolar pad. The form of the retromolar papilla is dependent to a certain extent upon the position and the eruption of the most distal molar teeth and the form of the alveolar process. In older individuals there is a tendency for atrophy of the mucous glands in the retromolar pad so that this prominence becomes more firm than in younger individuals and, as a result, the color appears to be more pale pink or white than previously. With the extraction of the most distal molars there is a new retromolar papilla established behind the remaining molars, but the retromolar pad remains in its original position. With the loss of the most distal molar teeth, movement of the pad under palpation is generally found. This is especially true when the pad is located somewhat to the lingual aspect of the mandible.

Findings in disease. Inspection and palpation of the labial and buccal mucosa, frenula, retromolar papilla, and retromolar pad should be routine procedure in the examination of the mouth. The oral cavity is the special field of the dentist and more often than not patients with disease in a portion of this area will consult their dentist before they consult a physician. Even though the dentist may direct his attention to the diagnosis, prevention, and treatment of diseases of the teeth in an adequate

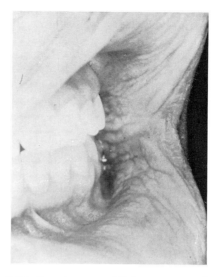

Fig. 7-23. *Buccal mucosa.* Thick, opaque, and somewhat firm folds involving much of buccal and vestibular mucosa throughout mouth. Opacity is not caused by hyperkeratosis but by deposition of amyloid in submucosa.

manner, he has a tendency to view passively other areas of the mouth even when confronted with signs and symptoms of disease. It must be remembered that many diseases show their symptoms in the labial and buccal mucosae (Fig. 7-23). All too often signs of disease, whether related to the teeth or not, are simply overlooked in the routine dental examination. This is unfortunate because most patients and physicians, who generally observe the mouth only when they are looking at the tonsils or the throat, are aware that the dentist is better equipped by training to evaluate abnormalities in any part of the oral cavity.

The *color* of the labial and buccal mucosae may be altered by keratinization, pigmentation, scarring, inflammatory changes, and changes in the amount of reduced hemoglobin and red blood cells and their hemoglobin content. Thus the examiner's attention during an inspection of this tissue may be directed toward any of these factors whenever changes in color are noted. Inasmuch as the labial and buccal mucosae normally are not generally keratinized, localized, or diffused, keratinization may be detected by gray-white or silver-appearing lesions. The most frequent deviation from the normal pink color is related to varying degrees of white associated with lichen planus, focal hyperkeratosis, chronic cheek biting, chemical burns, and leukoplakia. Therefore, when white-appearing lesions with varying degrees of hyperkeratinization are found in these areas, the examiner should be prepared to use his knowledge of the history of the lesion and his findings in the examination as to size, location, distribution, and other characteristics, and relate these findings to a descriptive knowledge of such lesions. Illustrative cases demonstrating the technic of making a differential diagnosis can be found in Chapter 15.

The pallor of anemia and the yellow tint of jaundice may be noted in the labial and buccal mucosae and may be used as positive correlative data. However, it must be remembered that pallor and yellow pigmentation are only symptoms of disease and when present should suggest the need for evaluation and for a search for their cause. When the examiner notes pallor of the mucous membranes, he should search for pallor in other areas and should also rely on other positive correlative findings before making a presumptive diagnosis of anemia. Pallor of the lips and oral mucosa is not sufficient evidence in itself to refer a patient for blood studies, nor is the report of 13.8 mg. percent hemoglobin in the blood sufficient evidence to suggest any type of anemia, let alone start that patient on iron therapy. Thus, pallor of the mucosa, lips, fingernails beds, and conjunctiva is only suggestive of anemia, whereas the additional findings of papillary atrophy of the tongue, exacerbations and remissions of burning and tingling sensations of the tongue, paresthesias of taste, systemic symptoms of dyspnea, palpitation, irritability, abdominal discomfort, dysmenorrhea, and a low-grade fever all strongly suggest the tentative diagnosis of some type of anemia. Even so, the final diagnosis cannot be rendered until the patient has had a complete study of the blood and a complete examination of the body.

Hyperpigmentation of the labial or buccal mucosa should be evaluated for recent onset, distribution, change in intensity, and relationship to pigmentation elsewhere in the mouth and the body. Melanin pigmentation, which may vary in intensity from a light brown to a dark blue-black and be localized to very small islands or be diffuse through large areas, is especially significant when it is of recent onset in normally blond individuals. Increased pigmentation may be exogenous or endogenous in character and systemic or local in origin. Normal physiologic pigmentation increases in intensity with age. In Addison's disease brown to brownish black dots of pigment or a diffuse bluish black pigmentation may occur on

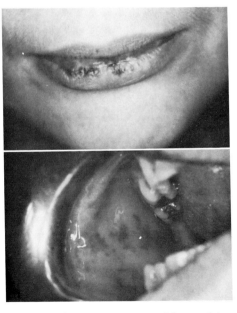

Fig. 7-24. Melanin pigmentation of lips and buccal mucosa in Addison's disease.

the buccal and labial mucosae, palate, lips, gums, or tongue (Fig. 7-24). Heavy metal intoxication may also cause pigmentation in these areas.

It is not unusual for the petechiae of emboli in subacute bacterial endocarditis to be present here as well as on the inferior surfaces of the tongue and in the conjunctiva. The labial and buccal mucosae may also show the petechial hemorrhages and ecchymoses of purpuras and leukemias (Fig. 7-25). It is not uncommon for trauma to produce ulcerations, traumatic fibromas, and mucous retention cysts (Fig. 7-26). A tentative diagnosis of the nature of the lesion may be based upon the clinical history and the appearance and consistency of the lesion. In many instances the history and the clinical examination of the lesion are sufficient to make an adequate diagnosis. However, the final diagnosis of those lesions whose diagnoses are not obvious should be based upon a biopsy. Indications for biopsy are reviewed in Chapter 13. Where a tentative diagnosis of a traumatic ulcer is made in light of the clinical examination and history of the lesion, the examiner should recall the patient 3 or 4 days after the source of the trauma has been removed for a reevaluation of the lesion. This a a mandatory procedure in view of the tendency of many lesions to show later neoplastic change. If the ulcerative lesion fails to heal

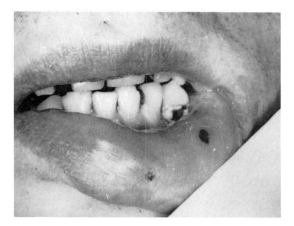

Fig. 7-25. *Vestibular mucosa.* Dark spots in lower vestibular mucosa are petechial hemorrhages caused by idiopathic thrombocytopenic purpura.

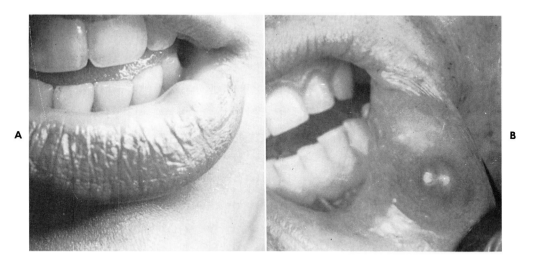

Fig. 7-26. *Labial mucosa.* **A,** Smooth, nodular swellings of vestibular areas may be produced by salivary gland tumors, lipoma, or mucous retention cysts. Palpation and other information determined that this was salivary gland tumor. **B,** Smooth, elevated, translucent, fluctuant swelling in lower vestibular mucosa that arises on erythematous base. Mucoceles of this type frequently are demonstrated in this location.

within a reasonable length of time after the traumatic agent is removed, then the examiner should do a biopsy. Though ulceration of the labial and buccal mucosae may be caused by chronic irritation such as sharp edges of teeth, rough dental fillings, or ill-fitting dentures, traumatic ulcers may also have a superimposed malignancy present.

The orifices of the parotid ducts should be inspected and palpated. Palpation of the parotid papilla and Stensen's duct should be carried out by palpation between the index finger of one hand placed inside of the mouth and the index finger of the other hand, which is placed on the outside of the cheek. Inflammation of the incisive papilla, expression of a purulent type of saliva, and the presence of a hard mass in Stensen's duct suggest the presence of a stone or sialolith in the duct (Fig. 7-27, *A*). Inflammation of a parotid papilla, coupled with a turbid saliva expressed from a duct, and the signs and symptoms of swelling and pain of a parotid region suggest inflammation of a parotid gland. Enlargement of the gland with or without visible signs or symptoms of changes of the saliva or of the parotid papilla, especially in the absence of systemic symptoms, suggests the possibility of a tumor or neoplasm.

Changes in the flow of saliva as evidenced by a dry mouth or excessive salivation should direct the examiner's attention to the cause of the changes. Xerostomia, or dry mouth, may be local or systemic in origin. Sialorrhea, or excessive salivation, may be psychogenic, systemic, or local in origin. Generally an obstruction of only one of the ducts of the parotid glands is not sufficient to cause obvious signs of dry mouth Dry mouth may be related to fear, dehydration, drugs, dentures, and so on. Excessive salivation may be associated with faulty dentures, pain in the mouth, metal intoxications, substances giving an unpleasant taste, and so on. To evaluate the sign of dry mouth, the examiner should determine the duration and degree of incapacitation and review the history, which might reveal the etiologic agent. Ordinarily an excessive flow of saliva is normal for anyone undergoing dental procedures; however, the amount varies from one individual to another. Sialorrhea is of significance to the operator, since it tends to slow down dental procedures since a dry field of working and vision is necessary. Sialorrhea coupled with a metallic taste should be evaluated for the possibility of metal intoxication. Xerostomia and sialorrhea are only symptoms of disease, and they must be evaluated the same as other symptoms of disease. Therefore, the time and mode of onset, character of the dysfunction, presence or absence of contributory signs and symptoms, and the etiology factors producing the symptoms must be determined before an attempt is

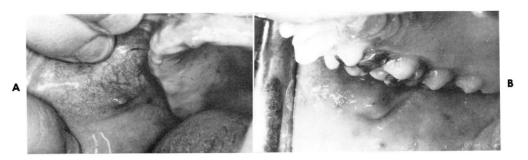

Fig. 7-27. *Parotid papilla.* **A,** Stone in orifice of parotid duct. **B,** Recurrent herpetic ulcers, one involving parotid papilla.

made to make a diagnosis by a comparison with a description of the diseases either known by the examiner or those which may be located in reference material. Thus, the examiner should collect his facts and evaluate his findings and then compare them with a descriptive knowledge of the disease before attempting to make a diagnosis.

Occasionally the persistence of a large buccal fat pad may be of significance to the dentist (Fig. 7-19). Although it cannot be considered as pathologic and is within the range of normal, in many instances its prominence does affect dental procedures. It is of concern to the prosthodontist in the placement and the wearing of dentures, inasmuch as it tends to be chronically irritated by cheek biting. This is especially true in the natural dentition where extractions without replacements have occurred with drifting and extrusion of the remaining teeth. A loss of alignment and an overjet of the maxillary teeth and the presence of sharp edges from abnormal wear or carious lesions, together with a persistent large buccal fat pad, predisposes to chronic irritation of the mucosa overlying the buccal fat pad. Thus the diagnosis of chronic cheek chewing must take into consideration not only the alignment of the teeth, the correct amount of maxillary overjet, and sharp edges of the teeth, but also the prominence of a persistent buccal fat pad.

The position of the attachment of the labial and lateral frenula may be of pathologic significance when the position of the frenula interferes with the normal eruption

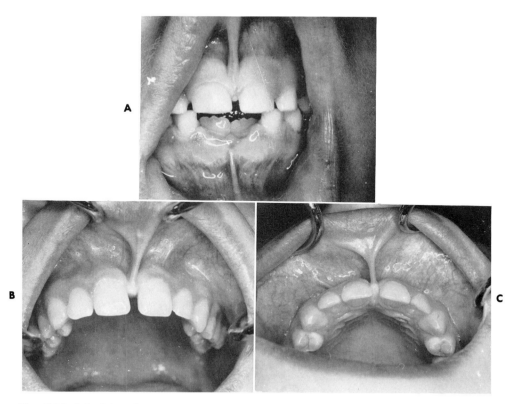

Fig. 7-28. *Labial frenula.* **A,** Persistent labial frenulum in deciduous dentition. **B** and **C,** Persistence of labial frenulum attached to incisive papilla with associated spacing of permanent teeth.

of the teeth or when the relative position of attachment is changed because of periodontal disease. Occasionally a space associated with a persistence of the tectolabial frenulum exists between the maxillary central incisors. In these instances the superior labial frenulum is not reduced to a vestige but remains as a large fibrous band of tissue that may extend even across the free border of the gingiva to the palatine or incisal papilla (Fig. 7-28). This is of significance to the orthodontist when the fibrous band is not eliminated and prevents the closure of the diastema between the central incisors even after the lateral incisors and cuspids have erupted. It is also possible that the abnormally large and attached frenulum does not in itself cause or maintain the diastema between the central incisors but may be secondary to other factors such as congenital absence of lateral incisors and to various types of bone patterns in the midline of the maxilla that are of genetic and familial origin.

An attachment of the inferior labial frenulum above the junction of the alveolar mucosa and the attached gingiva becomes of significance when periodontal disease and recession of the gingiva involves the attachment of the frenulum. When there is a deep labial or interproximal pocket between the two lower central incisors and the attachment of the labial frenulum is in or near the marginal edge of the gingiva, stretching and movement of the lip cause an extension of the margin of the pocket and correct toothbrushing is impossible (Fig. 7-29, A). This arrangement of the margin of the periodontal pocket and the attachment of the labial frenulum makes proper deflection of food impossible and prevents the proper stimulation of the tissues by toothbrushing. This may also occur in the maxillary midline frenulum and in the lateral frenula (Fig. 7-29, B). The presence and location of the lateral frenula are also of significance in the preparation of the mouth for partial and full dentures.

The retromolar papilla of the mandibular arch is of significance to the periodontist, when the most distal molar is only partially erupted and the pericoronal tissues fail to completely obliterate with the formation of a normal retromolar papilla. In other instances, the most distal molar may be fully erupted yet the gingival crevice around the distal aspect of the molar be greater than 2 to 3 mm. in depth because of hyperplastic of the retromolar papilla. Abnormal pericoronal flaps and a hyperplastic retromolar papilla are conducive to pathologic processes (Fig. 7-30). The pericoronal flap is especially prone to the production of a pericoronitis and acute necrotizing inflamma-

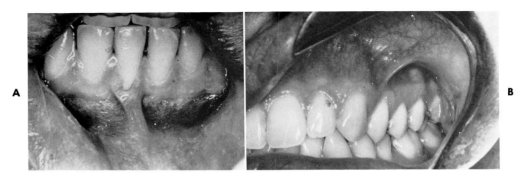

Fig. 7-29. *Frenula.* **A,** Inferior labial frenulum attached to gingival margin of mandibular incisor, producing gingival recession. **B,** Superior buccal frenulum attached to gingival margin of maxillary bicuspid; note associated recession.

tion. The hyperplastic retromolar papilla is conducive to the production of a periodontal pocket on the distal aspect of the most distal molar because the increased depth of the gingival crevice precludes the possibility for adequate cleansing of the area.

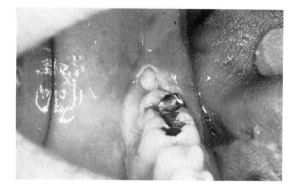

Fig. 7-30. *Mandibular third molar pericoronal flap—operculum.*

Palate

After inspecting and palpating the lips and labial and buccal mucosae, the examiner should examine the hard and soft palates. The numerous membrane of the hard palate is firmly attached to the underlying bone and presents some degree of keratinization; these factors give it a pale pink color often with a bluish gray hue. The peripheral zone of the hard palate is firm but somewhat resilient and connects the tissue of the palate proper to the teeth; this tissue makes up the palatine gingiva and is firmly attached to the underlying bone and teeth. In the midline of the palate there is a narrow whitish streak that is termed the palatine raphe (Fig. 7-31, *A*). It extends from a small projection, the incisive papilla, posteriorly over the entire length of the hard palate. It is often ridge-like in shape in the anterior portion and make take the form of a groove posteriorly. Radiating from the in-

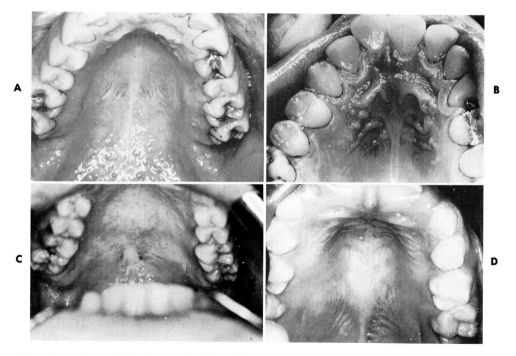

Fig. 7-31. *Palate.* **A,** Palatine raphe. **B,** Palatine rugae. **C,** Foveae palatinae. **D,** Incisive papilla; note foveae palatinae.

cisal papilla and the anterior portions of the palatine raphe are irregular branching ridges termed the "palatine rugae" (Fig. 7-31, *B*). On each side of the raphe, at the junction of the hard and soft palates, fre-

quently a small depression is visible; these are the palatine foveas, into which merge the opening of the excretory ducts of the palatine glands (Fig. 7-31, *C*). In the lateral portions of the tissue between the palatine

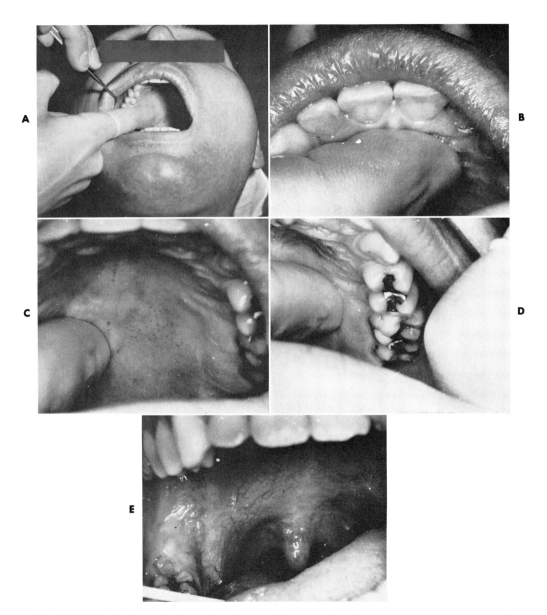

Fig. 7-32. *Examination of palate.* **A,** Palpation of posterior border of hard palate; note position of head and approach to the area to be examined. **B,** Palpation of incisive papilla. **C,** Palpation of palatine suture. **D,** Palpation of lateral palatine space. **E,** Inspection of soft palate.

raphe and the alveolar gingiva are palatal glands, nerves, and blood vessels; these elements are fairly extensive between the periosteum and the submucosa in the molar region but much less extensive anteriorly.

The compressibility of these tissues is of significance in the design of dentures, and their compression when taking an impression is to be avoided; otherwise errors in the impression will result. This is the only area in the hard palate into which a large amount of fluid can be injected without causing tissue damage (Fig. 7-32). Palpation of the tissues in this region shows them to be softer and more resilient than the adjacent alveolar mucosa or the medial portion of the hard palate. A rather thick band of firm tissue, continuous with the maxillary retromolar papilla, may sweep across the alveolar tubercle and give the distal termination of the gingiva a cleft appearance where it meets the hard palate (Fig. 7-33). This cleft is especially prominent where the pterygomandibular raphe fits into the groove when the mouth is opened. On palpation this band of gingiva is firm but somewhat movable. With the extraction of the adjacent molars this tissue may become less pronounced or may increase in size. It is significant in the treatment of periodontal disease and in the placement of partial or full dentures. This hyperplastic tissue prevents adequate treatment of deepened gingival crevices around the maxillary molars by conservative means. Surgical removal of the tissues is usually necessary for proper treatment and removal of periodontal pockets even when shallow. The form of this

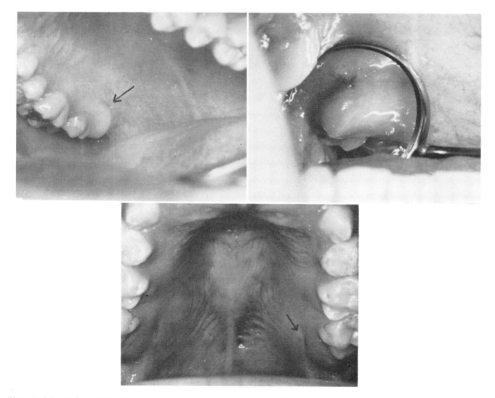

Fig. 7-33. *Palate.* Gingivopalatal groove associated with prominent tuberosity and pterygomandibular raphe.

tissue in relation to the crown of the teeth prevents adequate passage of food over the tissues, and not infrequently the gingival crevice accumulates debris. Occasionally the eminence is primarily dense fibrous tissue. After removal of the teeth the persistence of this band of fibrous tissue may cause complications with the adequate adaptation of dentures. Not infrequently the tissue become flabby and even more hyperplastic than originally; this further complicates the proper seating of the dentures.

The soft palate is covered with a mucous membrane that is thin compared to that of the hard palate; no cornified epithelium is normally present. Numerous mucous glands and blood vessels are present in the soft palate; their structural arrangement gives

the soft palate a darker red color than the hard palate. The boundary between the hard and soft palates may be readily seen by noting the change in position of the soft palate when the patients says "ahhh." This boundary is extremely important in the proper retention of dentures. Bilateral elevation of the soft palate occurs when the patient says "ahhh" or when the palatal reflex is elicited by touching the soft palate and causing the patient to "gag."

The palate should be palpated and inspected for changes in color, density, and texture and for variations in the form that may present problems in denture construction (Fig. 7-34). The junction of the hard and soft palates and the location of the loose mucous membranes should be determined since the design of full dentures and

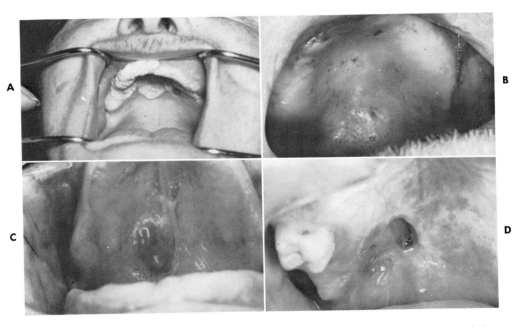

Fig. 7-34. *Examination of palate.* **A,** Plaque of white, verrucal tissue covering large part of denture-bearing area of palate—low-grade squamous cell carcinoma. **B,** Purpura secondary to myelogenous leukemia. **C,** Lobulated, elevated, soft, purplish lesion in posterior hard palate and anterior soft palate having a history of progressive enlargement; lesion is typical of salivary gland tumors that arise from palatal glands. **D,** Perforating lesion of hard palate, which may be produced by gummas, squamous cell carcinoma, or salivary gland tumors. This one is a squamous cell carcinoma.

palatal bars is directly related to so-called denture-bearing areas where there is firm and dense attachment of the mucosa.

Findings in disease. The color of the hard and soft palates may be changed by a localized or diffuse increase in pigmentation, a change in the integrity and the permeability of the blood vessels, a change in the hemoglobin content of the blood or an increase in the amount of reduced hemoglobin present, a change in the character of the epithelium of the mucosa, and changes in the density and attachment of these tissues (Fig. 7-35). The most common change in color is associated with the process of inflammation from traumatic agents. This may be localized or may involve the whole soft and hard palates. Pressure from full dentures or palatal bars may be seen frequently (Fig. 7-35) and may produce color changes from bluish white to brilliant red.

The color of the soft palate may show varying degrees of red resulting from engorgement of the blood vessels that traverse it. This active hyperemia, frequently accompanied by petechiae and ecchymosis (Fig. 2-1, *A*), is seen quite often in association with colds and coughing episodes and allergic manifestations. The soft palate is also a common site for traumatic injuries, herpetic ulcers, and purpuric manifestations, and a large ulcer may be found on it (Fig. 2-12, *D*) in Vincent's angina.

Excessive smoking may produce hyperkeratinization of the palatal mucosa and metaplasia of the ducts of the mucous glands. The palatal appearance is characterized by a diffuse silver-white color from the hyperkeratinization and scattered punctate red areas indicating the orifices of the ducts of the mucous glands. A brown staining of the keratinized surfaces may occur, especially in the area in which a pipestem or a cigar rests. This has been called the smoker's patch. The extensive keratinization of the palate with involvement of the orifices of the mucous glands is called nicotine stomatitis (Fig. 2-8). The areas of hyperkeratinization feel somewhat less resilient and are coarser textured than the surrounding tissues. When there is significant involvement of the orifices of the mucous glands, they may be felt on palpation.

Fairly often the middle portion of the palatine raphe will show a firm bony enlargement. The color of the mucosa on the surface of this enlargement is usually pale pink to white unless inflammation from trauma is present. The size and form of the enlargement may vary from a slight flat elevation of the median portion of the palatine raphe (this is usually considered to be a variation of normal) to a large nodular mass that may reach the proportions of a walnut (Fig. 2-6). On palpation, the mass is hard, firm, bonelike in consistency, and

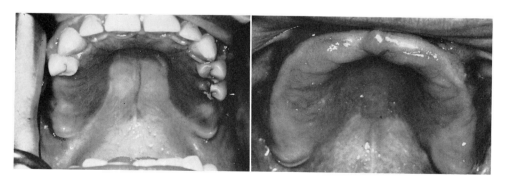

Fig. 7-35. *Palate.* Hyperemia associated with wearing of partial denture and complete denture.

nonmovable. This is a torus palatinus and is of clinical significance because of its relationship to the construction of full dentures and palatal bars on partial dentures and because of its blastomatoid characteristics. It is not a neoplasm and is only of significance to the patient when it interferes with mastication, speaking, and swallowing or when the patient has a cancer phobia. All types of primary and secondary lesions may occur in the palate as elsewhere in the mouth; however, the most frequent type of lesion is ulceration, and it is generally the result of traumatic injury. The most frequently offending etiologic agents appear to be hard toast, chicken bones, and toothbrush bristles. Inflammatory changes of the incisive papilla are fairly frequent and may be associated with any of the traumatic agents previously mentioned. The extensive enlargement of the incisive papilla may result from a cyst (Fig. 7-36). In these cases there is no radiographic evidence of bone involvement. Sometimes malocclusion of the anterior teeth may result in impingement of food and of the mandibular central incisors upon the incisive papilla. Chronic trauma of this nature may give rise to a hyperplastic enlargement of this tissue.

In many instances of partial denture and full denture construction and periodontal disease, the significance of hyperplastic tissue in the anterior palatine region is overlooked. Deep gingival crevices and periodontal pockets are difficult to treat by conservative means because of the tendency of this tissue to persist. The construction of dentures over tissue that is soft and edematous and presents some degree of inflammatory hyperplasia may well lead to additional inflammatory hyperplasia when patients attempt to wear dentures, irrespective of how well the prosthesis may have fit originally. Inspection and palpation of these tissues prior to denture construction will avoid this complication.

Occasionally an ill-fitting denture will produce an inflammatory hyperplasia of the palate that is characterized by localized or diffuse small red nodular elevations of the mucosa. These lesions are within the boundaries or at the periphery of the denture (Fig. 7-37). The elevations may be polypoid or papillomatous in form. This has been termed "palatal papillomatosis" or "polypoid hyperplasia of the palate." Many inflammatory and neoplastic diseases may involve the palate, and it is suggested that the student consult reference works for a comprehensive description of them. The underlying principles governing the approach to the diagnosis of abnormalities of

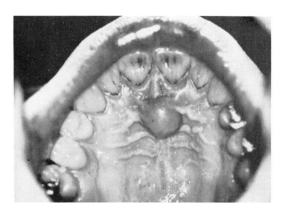

Fig. 7-36. *Cyst of incisive papilla.*

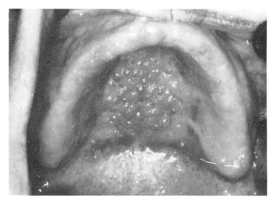

Fig. 7-37. *Palatal papillomatosis* associated with wearing of ill-fitting dentures.

the hard and soft palates are the same as apply elsewhere in the mouth except in instances in which the anatomic and functional relationships present may, in themselves, orient the examiner's attention toward specific items of diagnostic interest. The movement of the soft palate is dependent on the function of the ninth and tenth cranial nerves. In the presence of paralysis, the soft palate will sag on the affected side, and the uvula will be pulled to the unaffected side. It is not uncommon for people with unilateral paralysis of the soft palate to have difficulty in swallowing food, and in some instances water and food may enter the nose upon deglutition. The absence of a palatal reflex is common in hysteria, paralysis of the palate, and in anesthesia resulting from disease of the second division of the fifth cranial nerve. The degree of gagging that accompanies the palatal reflex varies considerably from one individual to another. The palatal reflex is of significance in the construction of full dentures and in many other dental procedures. There are many individuals in whom the palatal reflex is so hypersensitive that the least manipulation of the tissues in the posterior portion of the mouth, especially those adjacent to the soft palate, will produce gagging. In such persons only a few dental procedures can be accomplished without topical anesthetics.

Clefts of the roof of the mouth and the lip may present serious phonetic, esthetic, and functional problems. Although the diagnosis of cleft palate does not present a problem in itself, the evaluation of functional incapacitation and of the structures involved may require an extensive physical and radiographic examination. These procedures are outside the scope of this book. Of significant importance to the general practitioner is the early referral of the patient to the proper specialist for consultation. The treatment of clefts requires the close cooperation of the prosthodontist and the oral surgeon. Of equal importance is the periodic examination and maintenance of the teeth and supporting structures that may be involved in the retention and stabilization of extensive prosthetic appliances

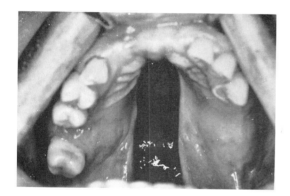

Fig. 7-38. *Cleft palate.* Complete cleft with surgical closure of lip and ridge tissue.

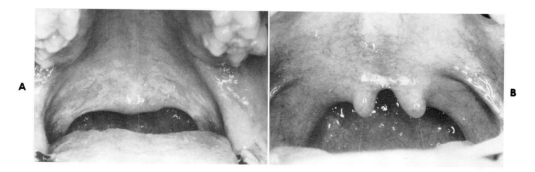

Fig. 7-39. *Soft palate.* **A,** Absence of uvula; after tonsillectomy. **B,** Bifid uvula.

required to cover a cleft. Fig. 7-38 shows an extensive cleft of the soft and hard palates; the maxilla and lip have been surgically closed. A cleft of this magnitude requires all the dental support that can be gained. A loss of teeth in the patient shown would make it very difficult to provide an adequate prosthetic appliance.

The uvula may vary considerably in size from one individual to another. It may be barely present or may extend almost to the tongue. It may be congenitally absent or lost by surgical removal (generally an accident); rarely it may be bifid and represent a mild form of cleft palate (Fig. 7-39).

Oropharynx

The tonsillar area and the oropharynx (Fig. 7-40) usually must be inspected by the use of a tongue depressor. Since there is a tendency for the tongue to retract and obscure the examiner's vision, it is necessary that the depressor be applied properly. Its tip should be placed back of the junction of the horizontal and vertical portions of the tongue; by using this point as a fulcrum to maintain a constant forward and downward pressure, the examiner can hold the tongue out of the line of vision. Unless this technic is followed, gagging will result, and the oropharynx will be obscured.

Tonsils may vary greatly in size; in children they tend to be large and to project toward the midline of the tonsillar fossa. If they have not been removed, they tend to atrophy during the latter part of the third and fourth decades so that in older age the lymphoid tissue may have regressed to such a degree as to appear as if a tonsillectomy had been done. In the plane with the soft palate and on the posterior wall of the pharynx is a ridge of tissue called Passavant's bar. This functional landmark is of significance in the closing off of the nasal cavity during deglutition. In the presence of a cleft palate, the location of this ridge is of significance to the prosthodontist in the construction of obturator bulbs.

The size and form of the oral cavity and the oropharynx may vary considerably and are often related to the character of the facies. A broad-faced child usually has a broad and rather large oropharynx, whereas the narrow-faced child has a narrow and small oropharynx. Anatomic varia-

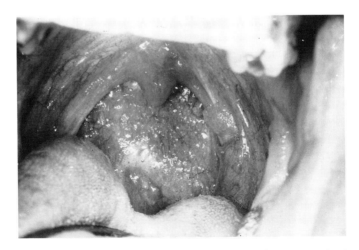

Fig. 7-40. *Inspection of soft palate and posterior pharyngeal wall.* Note lymphoid tissue on posterior pharyngeal wall and paralysis of left side of soft palate.

tions of the form and size are great. Though the normal appearance of the pharynx is hard to define, in general it is moist and bright pink, and a few dilated veins and nodular prominences are present. The true size and form of the normal oropharynx is difficult to establish because of the variation in the quantity of the lymphoid tissue that surrounds the pharynx in the area designated as Waldeyer's ring. In general there is a physiologic enlargement in childhood and a diminution in adults. Normal age changes are not well known, and a clinical standard for normal lymphoid tissue is difficult to establish. The tonsils in healthy children may enlarge considerably in the absence of disease, presumably in response to unknown demands.

Findings in disease. It has been said that enlarged pharyngeal and palatine tonsils cause mouth breathing by blocking the nasal pharynx and that this may give rise to an acquired swallowing reflex, causing an undesirable thrusting of the tongue. It must be remembered that mouth breathing is related not only to obstruction of the pharyngeal air passages by hypertrophied pharyngeal lymphoid tissue, but also to para-

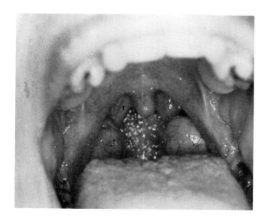

Fig. 7-41. *Fauces.* Tonsils appearing as two oval structures on lateral aspect of fauces showing intense lymphoid hyperplasia. In children this enlargement is caused by repetitious and persistent upper respiratory infections.

nasal sinus infection, engorged turbinates, and septal deviations. It is obvious that nasal obstruction, resulting in difficult nasal breathing, may induce habitual mouth breathing, which continually dries out the gingival tissues and contributes to gingival disease. It has been suggested also that chronic mouth breathing interferes with normal development of the dental arches and face in susceptible individuals because of the influence of malfunctioning muscles. Further, it has been suggested that inflamed and enlarged tonsils produce an involuntary and reflex muscle action of the tongue and adjacent muscles, whereby the mandible and tongue are moved forward (tongue thrusting) to increase the space around the inflamed tonsil and give relief from pressure upon it. Thus chronic tongue thrusting, resulting either from enlarged tonsils or reflex muscle action, can produce malocclusion of the teeth in susceptible individuals.

Since the palatine tonsils are those most easily observed by the dentist, gross enlargement is usually used as a criterion for the diagnosis of encroachment upon the oropharyngeal space (Fig. 7-41). However, the diagnosis of inflamed and infected tonsils should not be made on the basis of enlargement alone. The chief characteristics of a chronically infected tonsil are persistent redness of the tonsil and adjacent mucosa with repeated attacks of tonsillitis and the presence of lymphadenopathy of lymph nodes draining the tonsils. The diagnosis of infected or inflamed tonsils and a rationale for the removal of tonsils and adenoid tissue when related to the prevention or treatment of malocclusion require considerable rapport and understanding between the dentist and the physician. The referral of a patient to a physician for evaluation and treatment of mouth breathing or tonsil abnormality should not be predicated with a diagnosis of the abnormality; rather, the referral should be based on the dental examiner's findings and its significance to the patient's oral health.

Floor of the mouth

The structures that occupy the floor of the mouth include the sublingual glands and ducts, the superior part of the submaxillary glands and ducts, the lingual nerves and branches, and various lymph nodes along the inferior border of the mandible. The sublingual sulcus is traversed in the midline by the lingual frenulum, which attaches to the inferior surface of the tongue and reaches forward to the mandibular alveolar process. Close to the lingual frenulum and on each side of it lies a small round nodule called the sublingual caruncle. This papilla contains the openings of the submaxillary gland duct and often those of the sublingual gland duct. Sublingual folds containing the sublingual glands extend posteriorly and laterally in the floor of the mouth from the vicinity of the sublingual caruncle to the molar region (Fig. 7-42). The ridges

over the sublingual glands contain the openings of the minor sublingual ducts.

Examination of the floor of the mouth can be best accomplished by inspection and palpation. The former is carried out by having the patient elevate his tongue while the examiner retracts the tissues away from the mandible with a mouth mirror (Fig. 7-43). The examination should start with inspection of the color of the tissues and observation of the position of the structures in the floor of the mouth during functional movements of the tongue. Any inflammatory changes about the caruncle or enlargements of the sublingual ridges should be noted. The position of the attachment of the lingual frenulum on the mandibular alveolar process, best observed when the patient places the tip of his tongue on the palate or the lingual aspects of the maxillary incisors and pushes against them, should

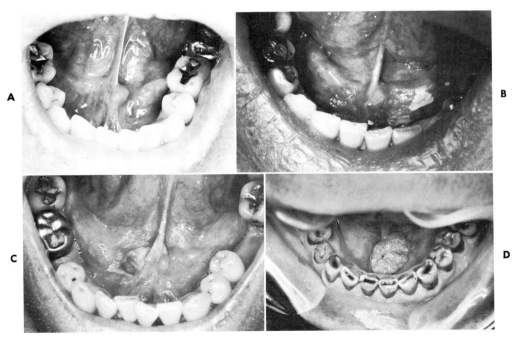

Fig. 7-42. *Floor of mouth.* **A,** Normal floor of mouth, lingual caruncles. **B,** Focal hyperkeratosis and early carcinoma. **C,** Ulcerated carcinoma in area of hyperkeratosis. **D,** Exophytic carcinoma arising from area of lingual frenum.

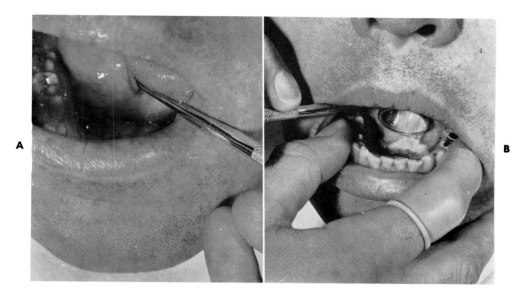

Fig. 7-43. *Inspection of floor of mouth.* **A,** Retraction of tongue. **B,** Reflection of light into floor of mouth.

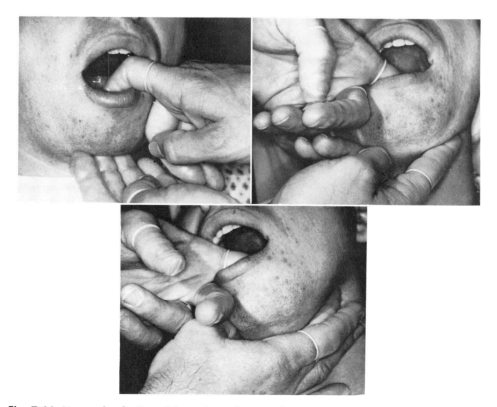

Fig. 7-44. *Bimanual palpation of floor of mouth.* Note altered head position to facilitate examination of each area.

also be noted, especially if partial dentures or full dentures are contemplated. This same maneuver allows the examiner to determine the relationship of the floor of the mouth to the alveolar ridge and to note any encroachment of the tissues of the floor of the mouth into edentulous spaces.

Palpation of the floor of the mouth is best done bimanually. The examiner should face the patient, who should be in an upright position with his head and jaw turned slightly downward in order to get maximum relaxation of the muscles of the floor of the mouth. When possible the examiner should use the first finger of his left hand for intraoral palpation of the left side and the first fingers of his right hand for the right side. The structures should be palpated against the examiner's other fingers, which are placed extraorally and, where necessary, against the mandible (Fig. 7-44). The lingual aspects of the mandible can be best palpated when the floor of the mouth is being examined. For the examination to be successful, it is necessary that the patient remain relaxed.

Palpation of the floor of the mouth should begin in the midline and traverse the soft tissues posteriorly as far as the examiner can go without causing undue discomfort to the patient. At the same time he should palpate the lingual surface of the mandible for the presence of exostoses, areas of tenderness, and loss of firmness. In a normal mouth he should be able to feel the soft nodular tissue of the sublingual glands and the submaxillary duct. He should also be able to feel the firm mass of the muscles in the floor of the mouth and occasionally the mental spine. The contents of the sublingual fossa and the submaxillary fossa should be palpated (Fig. 7-45). The examiner can usually follow the external oblique line of the mandible from the area of the bicuspid teeth to the ascending ramus. The bony prominence on the lingual aspect of the mandible made by the bone over the apices of the molar teeth, as well as the mylohyoid muscle attachment, should be palpated. In this area just posterior to the last mandibular molar, the lingual nerve can occasionally be palpated just beneath the mucosa as it enters the floor of the mouth in the posterior lingual region.

Findings in disease. Changes in the color of the floor of the mouth are unusual,

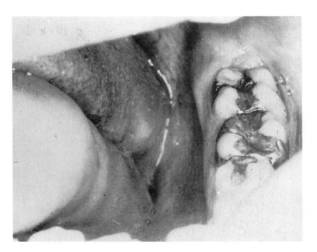

Fig. 7-45. *Bimanual palpation* of contents of sublingual and submaxillary fossae. Note retraction of tongue from the mandible to gain access to the fossae.

but they may be present in association with inflammatory changes, hyperkeratotic changes, and retention cysts. Sometimes ulcerations will occur as a result of trauma or in association with primary or secondary herpes. A swelling in the floor of the mouth should be palpated to determine its consistency and its extent. Soft fluctuant masses are probably cystic in nature, and hard boardlike manifestations may be associated with cellulitis of the sublingual space; hard, firmly attached enlargement associated with the sublingual glands may be inflammatory or neoplastic in origin. Neoplastic change may involve the mucosal surface or the glandular structures. Occlusal radiographs are sometimes helpful in determining the presence or absence of stones in Wharton's duct. One must remember, however, that stones are not always associated with the formation of cysts in the floor of the mouth (Fig. 7-46). Enlargements of the floor of the mouth associated with cystic lesions may often be associated with periods of remission, related to an increased flow of saliva, which generally occurs at mealtime. Cellulitis of the floor of the mouth is usually associated with pulp disease.

Lesions of the floor of the mouth that present enlargement, induration, and infiltration but do not involve the mucosa are difficult to evaluate without an adequate history and biopsy. In general, cystic lesions of the floor of the mouth present sufficient evidence in the history and in the examination to strongly suggest their char-

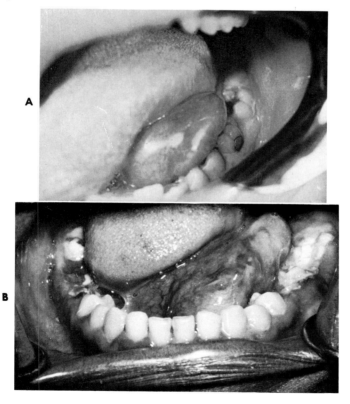

Fig. 7-46. *Ranula.* **A,** Note enlargement of floor of mouth and displacement of tongue. **B,** Dermoid cyst and adjacent hyperkeratosis of gingiva.

acter. However, it is not infrequent that neoplastic diseases of the floor of the mouth, especially those involving the salivary glands, show the signs and symptoms of a cystic structure as well as those of a neoplasm. Therefore, it is necessary to palpate completely the floor of the mouth for the presence of disease in the glandular structures as well as the ducts. In the presence of neoplastic disease, the examiner should be able to feel the loss of the normal contour of the gland, its hard, firm, nodular consistency, and its attachment to surrounding structures if invasion has occurred. If the examiner has had sufficient experience in palpation of a normal gland, he should have no difficulty in determining whether the consistency, form, character, and function are abnormal. In those cases where sufficient inflammation has produced fibrosis, scarring, and an obliteration of many of the glandular elements, the changes presented may be sufficiently confusing to require a biopsy for an adequate evaluation. Any hyperkeratotic lesion, persistent ulcerative lesion, or enlargement of the floor of the mouth should be biopsied. Recent induration and swelling of the floor of the mouth associated with the signs of inflammation, especially pain and tenderness, should direct the examiner's attention to a history of pulp disease and the possibility of an alveolar abscess draining into the sublingual space.

Tongue

In the past, many indications of health and disease have been attributed to the tongue. However, it cannot be said that all were based on sound principles. This structure was considered especially sensitive to gastrointestinal disturbances, but, since the development of the fluoroscope, electrocardiography, and other forms of diagnostic aids, the use of the tongue as an indicator of general systemic health has been largely dropped. Thus, because of the lack of scientific evidence, the idea that a coated tongue represents constipation and other gastrointestinal disturbances should be considered misleading and of no significance. A certain degree of coating is normal; the amount may vary from day to day and from morning to afternoon in the same individual. Probably of more significance is the absence of any coating. However, even this finding is a rather nonspecific manifestation.

Clinical examination of the tongue should include visual inspection of as much of the surface as is possible to see. The tongue should be observed in its normal position in the mouth and in an extended position. To ensure as much inspection of the surface as possible, the tip should be grasped in a piece of gauze between the examiner's index finger and thumb and gently pulled forward so that the lateral surface, base, and dorsal surface can be inspected (Fig. 7-47). The anatomic landmarks to be considered are the papillae (filiform, fungiform, circumvallate, and foliate), the foramen cecum, the lingual tonsil or tissue, the lingual veins, and the anterior lingual glands and ducts (Fig. 7-48).

The largest of the papillae are the circumvallate. They number from six to sixteen and are situated almost parallel to and in front of the terminal sulcus, forming a V or Y. Their size and number vary considerably from one individual to another and may cause the student some apprehension when he sees them for the first time. The foramen cecum is usually a small depression at the junction of the terminal sulcus; it is located just behind the circumvallate papillae at the apex of the V formed by these papillae.

The lingual tonsils are accumulations of lymphoid tissue on the root of the tongue. They may extend as far back as the epiglottis and laterally through the palatine tonsil. Lymphoid tissue is seen commonly on the posterolateral borders of the tongue associated with the foliate papillae (Fig. 7-48). Patients may complain of soreness of these areas. Generally the soreness is on

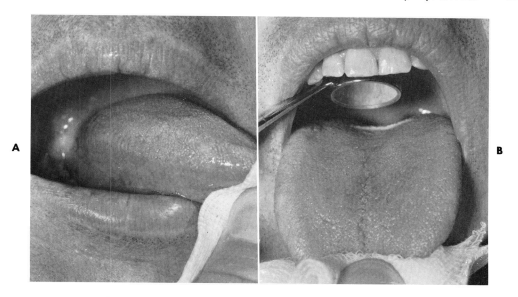

Fig. 7-47. *Inspection of tongue.* **A,** Lateral border. **B,** Dorsum.

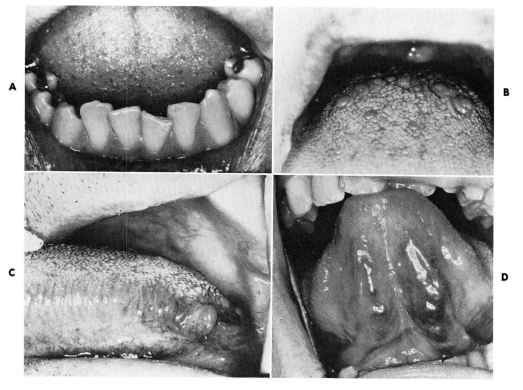

Fig. 7-48. *Tongue.* **A,** Fungiform papillae. **B,** Circumvallate papillae. **C,** Foliate papillae. **D,** Varicosity of sublingual vein.

one side, and the patient attributes it to rubbing the tongue against sharp tooth surfaces. Though sharp teeth may aggravate this tissue, inflammatory lymphoid hyperplasia is the main factor. Because the soreness may last from several days to a week, many patients become concerned with the possibility of cancer. Most are unaware of the existence of lymphoid tissue in this area and do not associate the soreness with a cold or sore throat that they may have at the time or have had in the immediate past.

The anterior lingual gland (gland of Blandin and Nuhn) lies close to the inferior surface and the tip of the tongue. Its ducts, of which there are from five to seven, open on small protuberances of the mucous membrane under the tongue on the plica fimbriata. The glands occasionally give rise to mucoceles. On the inferior surface of the tongue in the median plane and extending from the inferior surface of the tongue to the gums or the alveolar ridge, there is a fold of tissue called the lingual frenulum.

An abnormally broad lingual frenulum may result in tongue-tie (ankyloglossia).

Generally in the median plane of the tongue, there can be seen on the dorsal surface a shallow groove called the median lingual sulcus. Occasionally the tongue is furrowed on its dorsal surface. The furrow may vary in extent from an exaggeration of the median lingual sulcus to a network of irregular grooves. A furrowed tongue is generally of no clinical significance. It is considered to be of developmental origin, but the grooves appear to be more pronounced with advancing age. Infrequently, deep grooves may accumulate food debris and produce unpleasant odors and inflammation (Fig. 7-49, *A*).

Two other rather common variations of the tongue that may be seen are phlebectasia linguae and median rhomboid glossitis. The former is merely a dilatation of the lingual veins seen on the inferior surface of the tongue. Some forms of these blood vessel varices may be seen in the

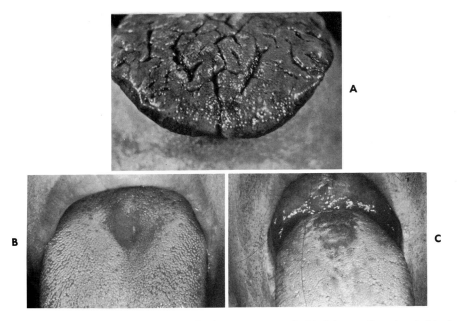

Fig. 7-49. *Tongue.* **A,** Furrowed tongue with glossitis migrans. **B,** Nodular median rhomboid glossitis. **C,** Flat median rhomboid glossitis.

skin and mucous membranes as a hereditary hemorrhagic telangiectasia; lingual varicosities may be related to this defect provided that there are other areas of involvement. However, in general, lingual varicosities are quite common in older individuals, are of local origin, and are of no particular significance. Median rhomboid glossitis is a term used to describe a minor developmental disturbance of the tongue located just anterior to the foramen cecum in the middle third of the dorsal third of the tongue (Fig. 7-49, *B* and *C*). It has a rhomboidal and red appearance and is often mammillated on its surface. It differs from the surrounding surface of the tongue in color and in surface appearance. The appearance is related to the absence of papillae. This disturbance is of no clinical significance, is not an inflammatory lesion as the term implies, is seen infrequently, and is considered within the range of normal. It may be mistaken for carcinoma; however, carcinoma is rare in this location.

The tongue should be palpated as well as visually inspected. Since most of it is muscle, it should have the resilient characteristics of muscle tissue and, depending upon the thickness at the particular area of palpation, should have a uniform consistency. The position of the tongue in its normal position in the mouth is of special clinical significance to the orthodontist and the prosthodontist. At rest, the tip of the tongue and its lateral borders approximate the edges of the teeth. Though indentations of the teeth may be seen on the tongue, this does not necessarily mean undue pressure nor is it characteristic of any particular disease. However, when the tongue appears to more than fill the area allotted it and extends over the surfaces of the teeth, it should be evaluated for macroglossia or displacement by such factors as enlarged tonsillar tissues. An extremely large tongue or one that is habitually placed forward of its normal position to compensate for an air passage that has been encroached upon

by enlarged tonsils may cause generalized diastemas of the anterior teeth or undue labially directed force on them.

The tongue should be examined during its action to determine whether there are asymmetrical functions; it should also be studied during swallowing to determine whether abnormal swallowing habits are present. The normal position of the tongue and its functional movements are important for the stability of both partial and full dentures. The size, shape, and control of the tongue is especially important to the stability of lower dentures. When much of the posterior alveolar ridge has been lost, there is a tendency for the tongue and the sublingual fold, which runs from the lingual frenulum to the glossopalatinus arc, to overflow onto the remaining alveolar ridge. This tissue may prevent the taking of an adequate impression unless it is recognized and the impression tray altered to block it out.

The normal position of the tongue is such that it lies lax in the floor of the mouth. The apex lies slightly below the incisal edges of the mandibular incisors, and the dorsal surface is visible above the teeth in all parts of the mouth. Some tongues appear to assume a low level and some a high level. The edges in the low-level position tend to rest on the posterior mandibular teeth, whereas in the high-level position they rest on the maxillary teeth. A retraction of the apex of the tongue downward and backward or upward, and a depression of the tongue into the floor of the mouth, represents an unfavorable position during function and is undesirable for denture stability (Wright and others). Many tongues assume upward retracted positions in response to encroachment upon the normal tongue space.

Findings in disease. The clinical examination of the tongue should include inspection and palpation for size, function, and lesions. Disturbances may be congenital, traumatic (Fig. 7-50), infectious, meta-

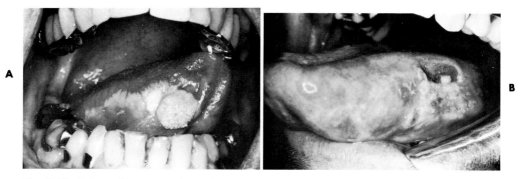

Fig. 7-50. A, Hyperkeratosis and exophytic nodular squamous cell carcinoma. **B,** Mottled atrophic mucosa with area of ulceration that is carcinomatous. Changes are secondary to irradiation.

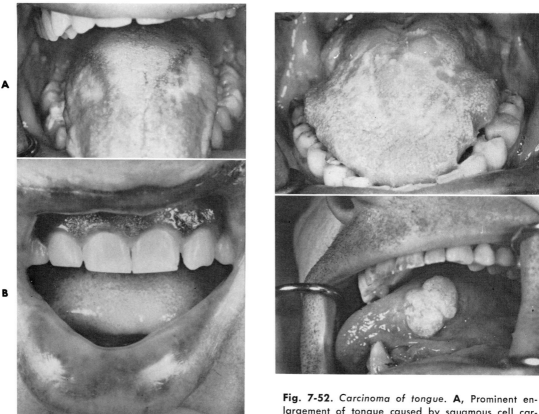

Fig. 7-51. *Pigmentation.* **A,** Intense addisonian pigmentation of tongue; note that pigment shows symmetrical bilateral distribution. **B,** Pigmentation of lip associated with Addison's disease. (Courtesy Dr. S. Fajans.)

Fig. 7-52. *Carcinoma of tongue.* **A,** Prominent enlargement of tongue caused by squamous cell carcinoma developing in a syphilitic glossitis. Secondary infection is superimposed with development of abscesses; note lateral indentations on tip and left border of tongue. **B,** Exophytic, lobulated, sessile, white lesion attached to lateral border and extending onto inferior surface. Appearance of lesion plus induration indicates a squamous cell carcinoma.

bolic, hormonal (Fig. 7-51), allergic, hematologic, neuromuscular, and neoplastic (Fig. 7-52) in origin. Of these, trauma is the one most common cause of lesions. It must be remembered that to effectively diagnose any lesion of the tongue, a history must be taken first in a systematic way so as to uncover all existing symptoms of the disease. This history cannot be limited merely to a review of the tongue itself; it must be an entire systems review since the presenting lesions may be oral manifestations of a systemic disease. A thorough history of the tongue should be taken, and those salient features of the history that might orient the direction of the examination should be kept in mind during the examination procedure.

The examiner who is aware of the normal size, texture, and resiliency of the tongue and has a knowledge of the normal anatomy of the tongue and its variations should be able to detect any disturbances of this organ. It must be remembered that the tongue goes through an intricate developmental period, and occasionally growth disturbances will be found. The history and duration of the disturbance and the absence of traumatic agents will serve to orient the examiner toward a developmental disturbance. The most common are bifid tongue, tonguetie, furrowed tongue (Fig. 7-49, *A*), median rhomboid glossitis (Fig. 7-49, *B*), thyroglossal duct cysts, and macroglossia. Macroglossia, in the absence of systemic disease such as cretinism and infantile myxedema, may be considered to be developmental in origin if there is no change in the resiliency and texture of the tongue. Macroglossia associated with neoplastic, inflammatory, or retrogressive changes will usually show changes in resiliency, texture, function, and sensation.

Changes involving the surface of the tongue and papillae but not involving deep-seated lesions or induration should alert the examiner's attention to drug reactions, vitamin-deficiency manifestations, anemias, dermatologic diseases, or geographic tongue. Chronic infective granulomas, traumatic lesions, and neoplasms usually produce pronounced changes in the consistency, function, and sensations of the tongue. Rarely are the manifestations of dermatologic disease confined to the tongue, and the examiner can usually orient his diagnostic thinking in the direction of a dermatologic disease when he finds lesions present in the mouth and also on the skin. This does not mean that lesions of the mouth and skin have to be related; however, the relationship should be evaluated. Traumatic lesions are usually painful on palpation, and a positive history of trauma can be obtained. Lesions associated with infective granulomas are usually deep seated, change the consistency of the tongue, give rise to functional problems, and are likely to be of long duration. Primary lesions of the chronic infective granulomas such as syphilis are of short duration and produce little change in sensation of the tongue unless the lesions is in an advanced stage and the patient has a history of contact with syphilis (Fig. 7-52, *A*).

Of special significance to the dentist are the mucous patches of secondary syphilis. These may occur on the tongue as well as other areas of the mucous membranes. The patch may arise as a macule, papule, or vesicle that frequently may ulcerate to form a lesion not unlike a canker sore except for the absence of an erythematous halo and pain. Most often it appears as a grayish white, slightly elevated lesion comparable to the papule of the skin (Fig. 7-53). The membranelike surface can be removed easily. The mucous patch is highly infective.

To make a diagnosis of any lesion of the tongue, one needs to have an adequate history, the results of the clinical examination showing the character and extent of the lesion, and a descriptive knowledge of the disease that may be producing the lesions. In general, it is possible to classify the par-

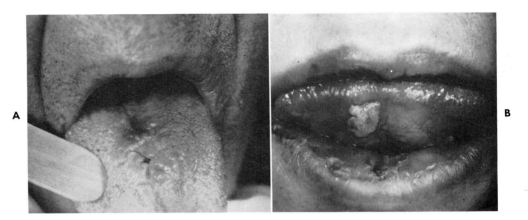

Fig. 7-53. *Tongue.* **A,** Tuberculous ulcer. **B,** Mucous patch of syphilis.

ticular zone of pathology to which the examiner must orient his thinking simply by determining the general characteristics of the lesions that are present.

Developmental disturbances are fairly characteristic because of their location (such as the lines of fusion), failure of embryonic structures to obliterate, and uncomplicated anomalies of size. Traumatic lesions tend to be recognized because of a positive history of trauma. However, chronic traumatic ulcers can be a diagnostic problem because of their tendency to resemble carcinoma, and biopsy may be necessary. Dermatologic lesions generally have skin manifestations, and the diagnosis usually can be made on the basis of skin involvement. Single lesions are usually of traumatic or local neoplastic origin, whereas multiple lesions are more likely to be manifestations of systemic disease, dermatoses, or allergic disorders. Changes in the resiliency, density, function, and sensation of the tongue should suggest to the examiner the possibility of chronic infective granulomas and neoplasms. The history and system review are significant prerequisites for making a diagnosis of this type of lesion. When there is no positive history of trauma or disease to account for a lesion, a neoplasm of the tongue should be suspected,

especially if the lesion is deep seated and of long duration and there is a positive history of progressive growth.

Superficial lesions of the tongue that are either localized or diffuse in nature, accompanied by changes in the papillae and changes in the size and consistency of the tongue as a result of edema, suggest the possibility of anemias, vitamin deficiencies, and drug reactions. A review of the history or inquiry into the patient's use of drugs may serve to orient the diagnosis of the lesions. Sensitivity reactions can arise from antibiotic therapy. The manifestations of drug sensitivity can arise from ingestion of the drug or contact with the drug. Drug reactions, vitamin deficiency, and anemias all produce some degree of change in the tongue sensations.

Sensitivity changes of the tongue may vary from a mild burning sensation to deep pain. The pain may be localized, diffuse, deep seated, or superficial. A burning sensation is the most commonly encountered pain of the tongue. This generally involves the lateral borders and the tip; however, it may be general in coverage or even vague in localization. Inability to localize pain is common when neurosis is a factor. The examiner must be careful not to classify readily those patients with obscure

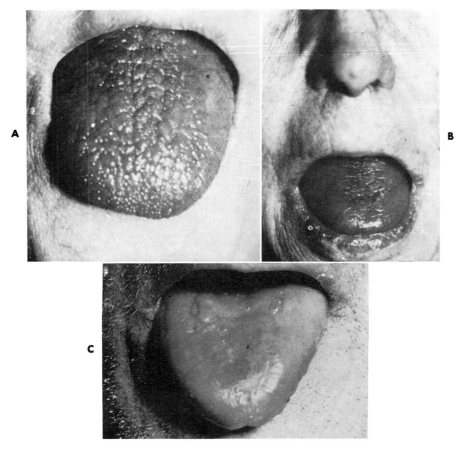

Fig. 7-54. *Tongue.* **A,** Pellagra. **B,** Cheilitis and glossitis of vitamin B deficiency. **C,** Pernicious anemia.

tongue pain as psychoneurotic individuals. The most common cause of pain of the tongue is traumatic injury such as biting. Traumatic injuries are easily determined because of their history. Burning tongue may be associated with dentures, anemias, or menopause, and the burning is generally intensified by irritation. Occasionally occlusal disharmony will result in a burning sensation and hyperesthesia of the tongue. The mechanism for this is unknown, but this relationship should be investigated. An occlusal adjustment will relieve many of these patients, especially when the pain also involves the face and ear region.

In macrocytic anemia the tongue may be painful and red. The whole tongue, or just the lateral borders, may be affected. The papillae are atrophic or absent, with the result that the tongue has a bald, glassy, slick, or glazed appearance (Fig. 7-54). These changes may also reflect some form of anemia that is a secondary expression of some other state, such as sprue, Plummer-Vinson syndrome, pregnancy, and vitamin B deficiency. It should be pointed out that the tongue manifestations seen in some of the diseases just mentioned are not particularly characteristic; the diagnosis of anemia certainly cannot be made on the

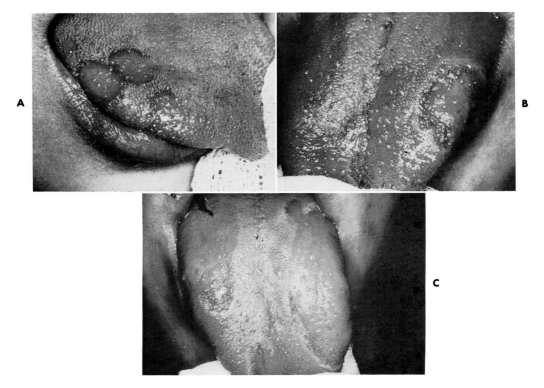

Fig. 7-55. *Geographic tongue.* Same tongue at 1-week intervals showing so-called migration of lesion.

basis of tongue changes alone. Such changes should alert the examiner to the possibility of the presence of concomitant systemic disease and the need for additional positive correlative data. The same reasoning applies to the so-called magenta-colored tongue of riboflavin deficiency and the red, beefy, painful, swollen tongue of pellagra (Fig. 7-54).

The two most common ulcerative lesions of the tongue are traumatic ulcers from biting and the shallow, painful lesions associated with primary and secondary herpetic stomatitis (canker sores). There is generally no difficulty in making a differential diagnosis of these lesions. The history of onset, the character of the lesion, and the multiplicity of the herpetic lesions tend to make their recognition relatively easy.

Another fairly common disturbance of

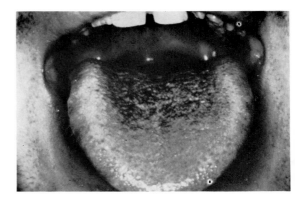

Fig. 7-56. *Black hairy tongue.*

the tongue is the so-called geographic tongue. It is also commonly called glossitis migrans and wandering rash of the tongue. It is a chronic and transient more or less circinate mucosal atrophy or desquamation of the superficial epithelium of the tongue. The lesions are red in those areas in which atrophy of the papillae has occurred and white in those areas in which hyperplasia of the filiform papillae has occurred prior to their atrophy and loss. In general, the degree of redness depends on the relative color of normal areas and the degree of desquamation. In many instances no white elliptic borders will be present. Occasionally the areas will appear as small areas of red depapillated islands, especially if the tongue is heavily coated or the filiform papillae are hyperplastic (Fig. 7-55). The character and location of these lesions change from day to day. The cause is unkown. They are of no significance except to apprehensive persons.

An overgrowth of the filiform papillae in the presence of pigment-producing mold or fungus gives the appearance of a hairy tongue. This condition is usually caused by the use of hydrogen peroxide, sodium perborate or, in some instances, antibiotics. A positive history of prolonged use of these drugs in the presence of an overgrowth of the filiform papillae suggests a diagnosis of black hairy tongue (Fig. 7-56).

REFERENCES

Atterbury, R. A., and Vazirani, S. J.: Examination procedure for oral cancer, J. Oral Surg. **26**:80-86, 1968.

Bowen, C. M., and Engleman, M. A.: Oral cancer detection and prevention, J.A.D.A. **74**:971, 1967.

Beam, W. B.: The changing incidence of certain vascular lesions of the skin with ageing. In Ciba Foundation Colloquia on Ageing. Boston, 1955, Little, Brown & Co., Vol. 1, pp. 80-87.

Dempster, W. T.: Selected dissections of the facial regions for advanced dental students, Ann Arbor, Mich., 1956, The Overbeck Co.

Pullon, P. A., and Miller, A. S.: Survey of tissue diagnostic services in U. S. dental schools, J.A.D.A. **83**:1097, 1971.

8

Examination of the periodontium

The examination of the periodontium includes a visual evaluation of the gingiva, probing of the gingival sulcus for pathologic deepening associated with periodontal disease, and a review of full-mouth radiographs and posterior bite-wing radiographs for loss of continuity of the lamina dura and height of the alveolar crest bone. The use of a periodontal chart is a valuable and informative record of the level of the free gingival margin, depth of periodontal pockets, and level of the bone around the teeth. Tooth mobility, malposition of teeth, and loss of teeth may also be incorporated in the findings on the periodontal chart. Some charts are used to record dental caries, a plaque and calculus index, and the status of the periodontium as well.

Gingiva

The gingival tissues should be examined for color, form, density, level of attachment, and depth of crevice. The examination should be systematic and should start with the gingiva in the third molar region and extend around the buccolabial and lingual surfaces of the arches to the opposite side. It should consider both the attached and free gingivae. An appreciation for normal gingivae at different ages is necessary (Figs. 8-1 to 8-3).

The normal and healthy attached and free gingivae are uniformly coral pink in color throughout the mouth. The color of the gingiva is dependent upon the vascularity of the mucosa, the hemoglobin content of the blood, the amount of reduced hemo-

globin in the blood, the density and attachment of the connective tissue, the width of the epithelium, the degree of keratinization and pigmentation of the epithelium, and the presence or absence of inflammation. The shade and intensity of the normal color varies from one individual to another. The gingiva in the primary dentition period is usually uniformly pale pink throughout the mouth but tends to show more the vascular pattern of the subpapillary venous plexus. This is probably true because of the absence of keratinization and chronic inflammation.

Physiologic pigmentation, either diffuse or localized in character, may alter the shade and uniformity of the color of both the primary and adult dentitions (Fig. 2-1). Localized pigmentation may cause a variation from light brown to dark blue. Diffuse or generalized pigmentation modifies the shade of the gingiva in direct proportion to the color of the skin. In general, the gingiva of the primary and mixed dentition periods will show less diffuse or generalized pigmentation than does the adult dentition. This follows the normal physiologic development of pigmentation with age. The gingiva is usually a pale coral pink in the primary dentition but may show areas of whiteness (blanching) and redness (erythema) associated with eruption of teeth during the mixed dentition period. Though one of the signs of a healthy gingiva is a coral pink color, this color may be present even though there is a hyperplastic alteration of the form of the gingiva associated with inflammation deep in the gin-

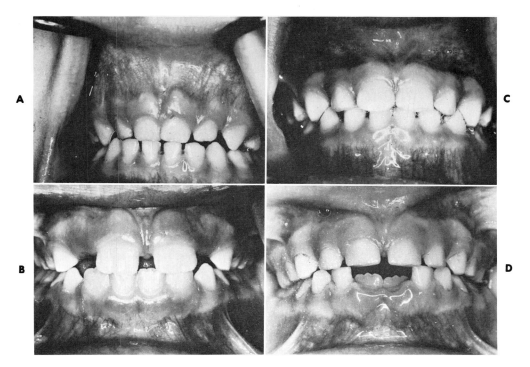

Fig. 8-1. *Normal gingiva.* **A** and **B,** Note form of gingiva and uniform shade in primary dentition. **C** and **D,** Changes in form and uniform shade in mixed dentition.

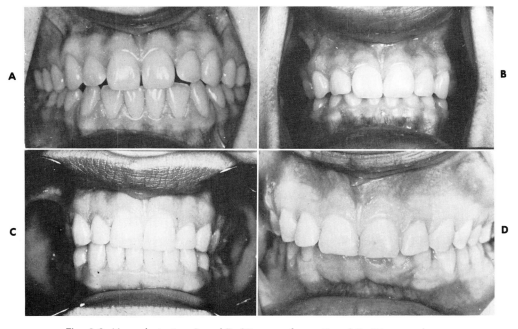

Fig. 8-2. *Normal gingiva.* **A** and **B,** 20 years of age. **C** and **D,** 35 years of age.

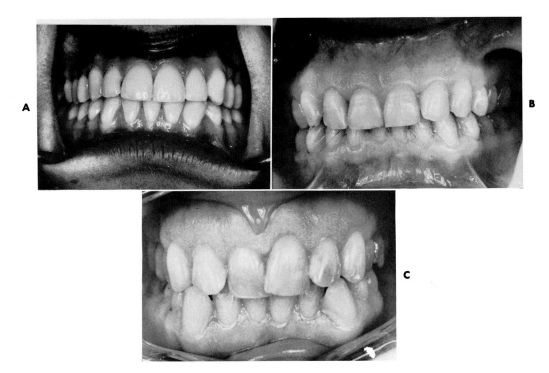

Fig. 8-3. *Normal gingiva.* **A** and **B**, 45 years of age. **C**, 55 years of age; note uniform shade, stippling, and adaptation of gingiva to the teeth.

gival crevice. It is also pale pink with gingival fibromatosis. In general, however, the pale pink color that turns to white on pressure (blanching) denotes a healthy gingiva.

The form or contour of the interdental papillae, free gingival margin, and the attached gingivae is related to the morphology of the crown of the tooth, the spacing of the teeth, the contour of the roots of the teeth, and the presence or absence of disease. In a normal healthy mouth the gingiva fills the interproximal spaces and ends in a knifelike edge and is closely adapted to the surfaces of the teeth. The form of the interproximal space is especially significant to the form of the interdental papilla. Where the width of the crown of the tooth at the cervical area is not much less than that at the contact area, the height of the interproximal papilla will be shorter than

in those instances where the width at the cervical portion of the crown is considerably less than that of the width at the contact area. It is to be expected that attrition of the contact areas, physiologic atrophy of the gingiva, and passive eruption will give rise to variations in the form of the gingiva. The contact areas between adjacent teeth are subject to wear, and the consequent loss of the tooth structure brings about a movement of the teeth in a mesial direction (mesial drift) that compensates for the decrease in mesiodistal width of the teeth. Thus, the space below the contact area (interproximal space) varies with the type of tooth, the position of the tooth, and the position of the adjacent tooth. The form of the gingival tissue that fills this space is thus related to these factors and to the presence or absence of disease. Where diastemas are present, the interdental papilla will follow

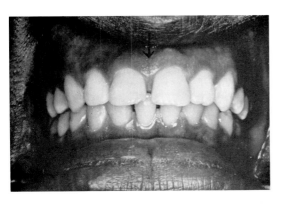

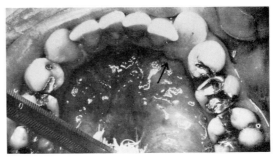

Fig. 8-5. *Retrocuspid papilla.*

Fig. 8-4. *Gingival contour associated with diastema and spacing of the lower incisors.*

the contour of the alveolar ridge (Fig. 8-4). Where the diastema is large or where there is absence of teeth, there will be little suggestion of a papillary contour in the usual sense; however, a modified type of papilla may be found on the mesial or distal proximal aspect of the teeth. This can be readily observed on the distal aspect of the mandibular bicuspids and mesial aspect of the mandibular molars where intervening teeth have been lost. Though this condition cannot be considered as normal, it can be considered as healthy when the relative contour of the gingiva is favorably related to the contour of the crowns of the teeth. In these instances the gingiva should be closely adapted to the surface of the tooth and end in a knifelike edge.

The surface of the attached gingiva, including the interdental papilla, is generally stippled, whereas that of the free gingival margin and the borders of the interdental papilla is smooth. The texture of the surface can be more readily appreciated when the gingiva is dry. There is considerable variation in the degree of stippling even in the absence of disease. The surface may vary from a light stippling to that not unlike velvet and somewhat analogous to that of the surface of an orange. Stippling and keratinization of the gingiva are generally considered to be a protective adaptation to function. They are not well developed in the primary or mixed dentition but become more prominent in the young adult and progressively more apparent in the older adult. In older persons there appears to be decrease in gingival keratinization with advancing age associated with atrophy of the oral epithelium and concomitantly a decrease of gingival stippling. This is difficult to evaluate because of the difficulty of separating those changes caused by aging from those caused by disease of the periodontium that is almost universal in patients of the older age group. A small papule is often present on the lingual aspect of the gingiva adjacent to the mandibular cuspid. It is called the retrocuspid papilla and is of no pathologic significance (Fig. 8-5).

The density or consistency of the gingiva depends upon its location, its attachment, and the presence or absence of disease. Normally it is firm and resilient and tightly bound down to the alveolar process and teeth except at the free gingival margin and the borders of the interdental papilla. On palpation of the attached gingiva, the examiner should be able to feel primarily the contour of the underlying bone and only slight movement or resiliency of the interposed attached gingiva. Palpation of the free margin should yield slightly more to pressure and should give a sense of slight movement. Surface palpation and light rubbing will reveal the degree of stippling and to some extent the degree of keratinization.

Palpation of the attached and free gingivae will be found especially helpful in relating their contour to the underlying bone and tooth structure. Thus, palpation of the gingiva and the underlying bone and tooth structure will serve to determine the true size and form of the gingiva and will relate the form to bony prominences.

The depth of the gingival crevice or sulcus in the adult is considered to be normal if it does not exceed 1.5 to 2 mm. The position of the gingival margin on the crown of the tooth varies with the age of the individual and with the degree of eruption of the tooth. The depth of the crevice may vary considerably during the active eruption of the teeth. This may be readily appreciated by probing it in the mixed dentition. Quite often the crevice of the erupting permanent maxillary incisors will be very deep, especially where the free gingival margin is located high on the enamel. This usually represents a transitory stage, and with the completion of the eruption of these teeth and the completion of the growth of the alveolar bone the depth of the gingival crevice reaches normal limits.

In the normal adult mouth the level of the epithelial attachment should be on the enamel or at the cementoenamel junction. In the presence of simultaneous atrophy of the alveolar crest and marginal gingiva, without an increase in the depth of the crevice, migration of the attachment apical to the cementoenamel junction is considered to be physiologic. However, this recession of the gingiva probably does not occur in the mouth that has been free of disease. The position of the epithelial attachment in the young adult is usually on the cervical one-third of the teeth. Since the establishment of occlusion cannot be considered to be final at this time, changes in the position of the gingival margin and epithelial attachment are to be expected. Within certain limits the compensatory eruption of the teeth for wear or physiologic attrition will, to a certain extent, determine the later position of the gingival margin and the epithelial attachment.

Inasmuch as the form of the gingiva is intimately related to the form of the teeth, this relationship is best served for the protection and stimulation of gingiva and supporting structures when the epithelial attachment is at or above the cementoenamel junction. Any recession below this level must be considered as abnormal. It is possible, however, for the gingiva to be healthy even though it is attached below the cementoenamel junction. This is frequently seen in elderly individuals, but the problem of maintaining the health of the gingival tissues and of the exposed cementum is exceedingly more difficult than when the gingival tissue and attachment are in their normal positions. The main difficulty arises because of the loss of the normal and physiologic relationship between the gingivae and the contours of the teeth. When the teeth and gingiva are in the normal position, the convexity of the labial, lingual, and buccal surfaces of the teeth prevents food from being forced into the cervice and at the same time allows the food to pass over the gingiva and provides stimulation and massage of the tissues. The following is a list of clinical signs of normal gingiva.

1. Color—uniform pale pink except for physiologic pigmentation when present
2. Form—should fill the interproximal space and end in a knifelike edge closely adapted to the surfaces of the teeth
3. Density—interdental papillae and free and attached gingivae should be firm and dense in all areas
4. Crevice—should not exceed 2 mm. in adults
5. Attachment—the epithelial attachment should be on the enamel or at the cementoenamel junction in children and adults; may be on the cementum in elderly individuals; however, it

should not be more than 1 mm. below the cementoenamel junction

The difference between normal and healthy gingiva is important for the recognition of normal tissue in contrast to that which is abnormal in form and attachment but healthy. This distinction becomes important in the recognition of the effects of past disease and in evaluating the success of periodontal therapy. The color and density of healthy gingiva are the same as for normal gingiva; however, the form and level of the epithelial attachment are not the same. The depth of the gingival crevice is the same for both normal and healthy gingivae. Gingivectomy, necrotizing gingivitis, periodontitis, gingivitis, and gingival recession may permanently alter the form of the gingiva; therefore, the gingiva is no longer normal. However, if the gingival tissue is free of inflammatory and other abnormal changes of color, form, and density, and the gingival crevice does not exceed 2 mm., the gingiva may be considered to be healthy although not normal. The following list gives the clinical criteria for healthy tissue.

1. Uniform pale pink color except where physiologic pigmentation exists
2. Contour and relationship of the gingivae to the teeth functional
3. Tissues firm and dense
4. Depth of the gingival crevice should be less than 2 mm.
5. Level of the epithelial attachment irrelevant

Findings in disease. Changes in the color of the gingiva may result from any alteration of those factors that are responsible for its normal pink color. Changes may be related to the mucosa of the rest of the mouth or may be localized to particular areas of the gingiva. Thus the alteration of color may involve simply the free gingival margin of one or more teeth or involve all the attached gingiva and extend itno the alveolar mucosa. The examiner should determine the areas that show the alteration of the color and make a record of these findings.

The significance of the change in color from the normal is important not only for a diagnosis of disease in these tissues, but also for an evaluation of periodontal therapy. The changes may be transitory or of long duration. When observing an abnormal color, one must remember that the color that is seen at that particular time may not be the same as that which existed at a prior time. Where a color other than pale coral pink exists throughout all of the gingivae, the examiner should relate this apparent change to the rest of the oral mucosa and the skin since an alteration of the color may be associated with a more generalized dis-

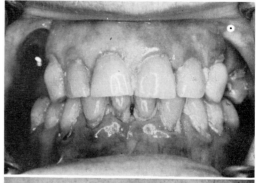

A

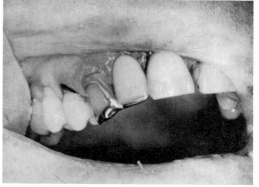

B

Fig. 8-6. *Gingival pallor associated with severe anemia.* **A,** Note absence of the change in color (shade) that exists normally at the junction of the alveolar and gingival mucosa. **B,** Hemorrhage about central incisor and bicuspid secondary to leukemia.

ease (Fig. 8-6). For example, a paleness of the gingiva, buccal mucosa, palate, lips, conjunctiva, and fingernail beds may be related to an anemia; a generalized redness of the gingiva, buccal mucosa, palate, and tongue may be related to a sensitivity manifestation or, when this redness also includes the face, hands, and neck, may indicate the presence of such a condition as polycythemia; a melanosis of the gingiva, buccal mucosa, and palate may indicate Addison's disease; or a bluish cast to the gingiva, buccal mucosa, palate, tongue, hands, and face may indicate the presence of a central or peripheral cyanosis. Therefore, the examiner in his inspection of the gingiva for changes in color must consider the possibility of changes also existing elsewhere.

The most frequent change in the color is associated with chronic inflammation. The alteration of the normal color as the result of inflammation is related to the chronicity of the injurious agent and to the response of the tissues to this irritation. Inflammation is a physiologic response of the tissues to injury and is accompanied by changes in the vascular bed, maturation of the epithelium, pigmentation of the gingiva, and alteration of the activity of the connective tissue of the submucosa. Changes in the vascular bed that alter the color of the gingiva are capillary dilatation, and active hyperemia, increased capillary permeability with exudation, hemorrhage per diapedesis, passive congestion with a reduction in the rate of capillary flow, and a reduction in lymph flow. Active hyperemia with capillary dilatation and engorgement of the vessels, especially associated with acute inflammation, gives rise to a bright red erythematous discoloration. Where the capillary bed is obvious and where the epithelium is thin, as in the alveolar mucosa, buccal mucosa soft palate, and pharyngeal wall, the examiner may see evidence of a relative increase in the number of capillaries; this effect is from a complete

utilization of the capillary reserve. The engorgement of an increased number of capillaries tends to give the tissues an erythematous discoloration with a netlike appearance. This is seldom seen in the gingiva proper because of the masking of the changes by hyperplastic epithelium and the depth of the subpapillary venous plexus. However, it may be readily observed where the epithelium is atrophic, ulcerated, and thin and where the inflammatory reaction extends to the alveolar mucosa.

Although an initial bright red erythematous discoloration usually signifies active hyperemia and acute inflammation, such a discoloration may also be present in chronic inflammation where the epithelium is thin and atrophic and the underlying capillaries are near the surface (Fig. 8-7). In general, however, in the presence of chronic inflammation and where the surface epithelium is intact, an excessive amount of reduced hemoglobin in the vessels will give the tissues a bluish red discoloration. Increased permeability of the vessels in inflammation results in an edema, with the result that fluid in the tissues tends to mask the discoloration present. The loss of red blood cells from the capillaries either by diapedesis or rhexis into the connective tissue results in a breakdown of the hemoglobin into hemosiderin and other pigments. Where

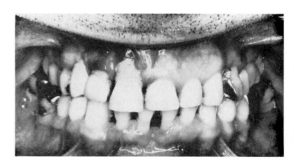

Fig. 8-7. *Localized intense redness (indicated by dark shade) around the maxillary central and lateral incisors. This is a response to the materia alba present.*

history of gingivectomy, and for those local factors that may produce recession of the gingiva. Necrotizing gingivitis (Vincent's infection) and chronic periodontitis are the primary causes for the loss of interdental papillae. Traumatic occlusion, improper toothbrushing, and orthodontic movement of the teeth may produce gingival recession. It must be remembered that the alignment and form of the teeth and the form of the alveolar arches may in themselves predispose to gingival recession (Fig. 8-11).

A systematic appraisal of the form of the gingiva is necessary for the formulation of a diagnosis since the descriptive knowledge of specific diseases of the periodontium is based upon alteration of the color, attachment, density, and form of this tissue. A generalized bluish cyanotic discoloration, together with a generalized soft and spongy enlargement of the tissues, should direct the examiner's attention toward those factors that produce local or generalized gingival hyperplasia. These factors may be local, dysfunctional, or systemic in origin. Simple hyperplasia is generally related to local irritants such as calculus, soft debris, poorly adapted margins of restorations, and mouth breathing. The enlargement may be associated with a modification of the normal inflammatory response of the tissues to irritants because of hormonal imbalance in puberty and pregnancy, and with the use of therapeutic agents such as diphenylhydantoin (Dilantin Sodium).

Clinical manifestations of changes in the consistency of the gingiva can be best evaluated by digital palpation. The examiner should differentiate changes of the gingiva itself from those arising from changes in its surface texture and underlying bone. The changes in consistency are usually related to the alteration in form. Palpation with slight pressure may be utilized to discover

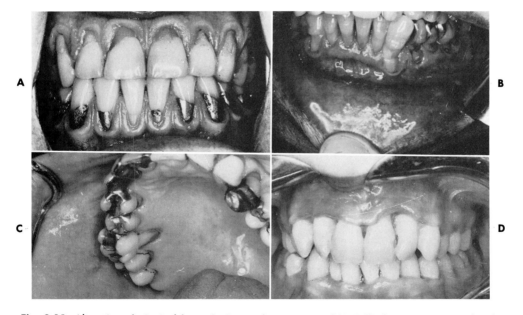

Fig. 8-11. *Alteration of gingival form.* **A,** Gingival recession and McCall's festoons associated with traumatic occlusion. **B,** Gingival recession resulting from improper toothbrushing. **C,** Gingival recession associated with orthodontic movement. **D,** Change in gingival contour produced by recurrent Vincent's infection.

edema, pitting, fluctuance, induration, and friability of the tissues.

Soft spongy gingival tissues that pit on slight pressure may be associated with an accumulation of intercellular fluid in the mucosa and submucosa. Localized edema of the gingival tissues may be found as a result of an obstruction of the venous or lymphatic return either by tumors or inflammation; it also may be mechanical or allergic in origin. By far the most common cause of edema is that associated with chronic inflammation. This local type is produced by those factors that favor filtration, such as increased capillary permeability and obstruction of the venous return. Exaggerated sponginess and pitting edema are seen frequently in certain types of leukemia. Neoplastic disease, such as carcinoma, may result in tissues that are extremely soft and friable. Fluctuance may be associated with intercellular and intracellular edema of the mucous membranes of the gingiva and may also be found with periodontal abscesses. When palpation reveals fluctuance, the examiner must be sure to rule out crepitus and changes in the underlying bony structure. Fluctuance involving the surface of the gingiva may be associated with bullae and vesicles whose margins are well defined. Fluctuance associated with periodontal abscesses is of a somewhat different character than that associated with vesicles or bullae because of the nature of the fluid present. Vesicles and bullae have a rather thin covering and tend to rupture easily. Tenderness is a prominent feature of periodontal abscess and a thick serosanguineous purulent material may be expressed provided there is a drainage site.

Palpation of an enlarged gingiva characterized by a firm, hard, and leathery consistency should suggest fibrosis associated with chronic inflammation, gingival fibromatosis, or neoplasia. Firm, smooth, nodular circumscribed lesions of the gingiva may be related to bony protuberances or exostoses (Fig. 8-12). Localized enlargements

may be reactive (inflammatory) or neoplastic in origin. The final diagnosis of this type of lesion is best made by a gingival biopsy. Occasionally a small, firm, movable, discrete yellowish white lesion may be found on the attached gingiva, especially in the area of the mucobuccal fold in the posterior part of the mouth. Such lesions are generally confluent ectopic sebaceous glands and their true identity may be established by a gingival biopsy if necessary.

Changes in the texture of the surface of the gingiva is a common finding in gingival disease. The loss of the normal stippled surface results in a smooth glossy surface. A

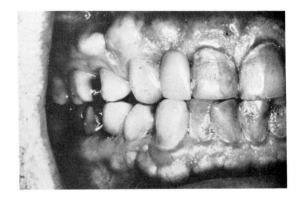

Fig. 8-12. *Alteration in gingival contour. Exostoses.*

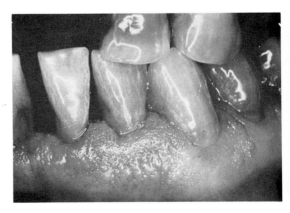

Fig. 8-13. *Gingival texture. Persistent stippling in the presence of periodontal disease.*

smooth surface may be presented when there is atrophy of the gingival epithelium, desquamation of the superficial layers of the epithelium, and stretching of the epithelium from underlying edema or scar tissue. Although stippling is utilized as one of the criteria for a healthy gingiva, it may be present in chronic periodontal disease. It is related to superficial tissues and not necessarily to deeper portions of the periodontium. Thus, with gingival massage, it may exist in the presence of deep intrabony periodontal pockets (Fig. 8-13).

The surface texture of the gingiva associated with hyperkeratosis may vary from a slightly rough or pebbly texture to an elevated circumscribed verrucous nodular leathery texture. A verrucous texture is generally related to the degree of hyperkeratosis. Friability, ulceration, and induration are important features of hyperkeratosis to be evaluated by inspection and palpation. The differential diagnosis of hyperkeratotic lesions includes leukoplakia, focal hyperkeratosis, and lichen planus. Although all of these lesions appear clinically as white, lichen planus does not present the rough nodular surface texture that leukoplakia and focal hyperkeratosis do. It is possible, however, that these lesions may present a diagnostic clinical problem in their early stages because of the slight degree of hyperkeratinization. In these instances a history and clinical examination may not be sufficient to arrive at a diagnosis, and a biopsy is indicated. Focal hyperkeratosis, beginning leukoplakia, erosive lichen planus, and desquamative gingivitis frequently present diagnostic problems even to clinicians who are well versed in examination procedures and oral diagnosis. However, such problems may be minimized by proper attention to the history and by understanding the characteristics of these lesions and the principles and indications for biopsy. Thus, focal areas of hyperkeratosis associated wth chronic trauma alone may suggest to the examiner the tentative diagnosis. How-

ever, in view of the tendency for leukoplakia and focal hyperkeratosis to break down into malignancies, a clinical diagnosis without microscopic examination is of doubtful value, especially in older individuals.

The clinical evaluation and diagnosis of lichen planus of the gingiva depends to a large extent upon the configuration of this lesion and the texture of its surface (Fig. 2-7, *A*). The surface of lichen planus is usually only slightly rough and hyperkeratotic. Its borders may be well defined by inspection because of its white color, but it may be difficult to palpate because of the absence of a well-defined elevation and lack of roughness of the surface. When present, linear striations, nodule points, and involvement of other areas such as the tongue, buccal mucosa, and flexor surfaces of the extremities aid in making the clinical diagnosis of lichen planus. The history is of considerable significance here since lichen planus may be somewhat transitory in nature; the history of onset is usually vague and not usually related to traumatic agents.

The location of the epithelial attachment and the depth of the gingival crevice should be determined in all areas of the mouth since alteration of the normal level of attachment and depth of gingival crevice is a positive sign of gingivitis and periodontitis. An increase in the depth of the crevice and associated apical migration of the epithelial attachment and resorption of alveolar bone are signs of a periodontal pocket, An increase in depth may be related to gingival hyperplasia. In this instance the level of attachment is on the enamel or at the cementoenamel junction, and there is no loss of bone.

Any increase in depth over 2 mm. must be considered as a sign of disease. Usually other signs of disease such as altered color, form, and density will also be present. In some instances a significant increase in depth will be present without apparent signs of inflammation; however, the deeper portions of the crevice will be involved. Thus the active inflammatory reaction of the surface tissues may subside, leaving these tissues to appear clinically as relatively healthy. However, the inflammatory process deep in the crevice still has active chronic inflammation present. This may be easily overlooked if inspection and palpation of all the gingival crevices are not carried out routinely by probing.

When the epithelial attachment is located on the cementum, disease is then present or has been present. This means that the presence of the epithelial attachment on the cementum is a positive sign of present or past disease. In either case it is an abnormal position. If the disease has been arrested and the color, form, and density reflect good function, the gingiva is healthy even though it cannot be considered normal.

Excessive mobility of the teeth may be caused by loss of bone support, root resorption, or traumatic occlusion. In chronic destructive periodontal disease the loss of bone may allow the teeth to become so mobile that movements of 1 to 2 mm. or more are possible. In other instances the same quantitative loss will show no increase in the mobility of the teeth. Resorption of the roots of teeth from orthodontic movement, occlusal trauma, or unknown cause may increase the mobility of the teeth so involved. Here again the teeth may show no excessive mobility. Teeth in traumatic occlusion may show extreme mobility without an increase in the width of the periodontal membrane space.

Increased mobility of the teeth is an important sign of periodontal disease, and the examination should include palpation of all the teeth for evidence of this condition. The prognosis of treatment and treatment planning may depend to a large degree on the amount of mobility present, the cause of the mobility, and the possibility of its limitation.

One of the most significant findings in peroidontitis is the presence of periodontal pockets involving bifurcation and trifurcation areas. Such areas cannot be kept free of irritants in most instances and are prone to the formation of periodontal abscesses. Actual pocket formation into these areas generally spells a poor prognosis for the teeth so involved. Treatment is difficult, if not impossible, because of the anatomic form of the areas. The presence of periodontal pockets involving bifurcation and trifurcation areas cannot be determined adequately without the use of a periodontal probe. Radiographic evidence is not conclusive—only suggestive. In many instances involvement may be present without radiographic evidence of their presence. The radiographic signs of periodontal disease will be found in Chapter 12.

It is important not only to recognize that disease exists, but also to determine the cause of the disease. By far the most important causes of periodontal disease are local factors. These consist of local irritants such as bacterial plaques, soft debris, calculus, overhanging margins on restorations, food impaction, and carious lesions. Dysfunctional factors such as unilateral mastication, lack of stimulation of the tissues, malposed teeth, mouth breathing, traumatic occlusion, and lack of function are also important in the etiology of periodontal disease. Systemic disease such as diabetes mellitus may affect the resistance of the individual to local irritants; it does not in itself produce periodontal disease. The response of the tissues may be modified or adversely affected by pregnancy, puberty, and leukemia. Thus periodontal disease is largely inflammatory in nature and the result of local injury. The following outline of periodontal disease may serve to summarize the clinical findings in the examination of the periodontium.

CLASSIFICATION OF PERIODONTAL DISEASE

1. **Simple gingivitis**

    This is an acute or chronic inflammation caused by poor oral hygiene or local irritations. Alteration of color, form, and density of the tissues is related to response of the tissue to injury. Some degree of gingival enlargement is present but is not extensive. The changes may involve only a few areas of the free gingival margins (Fig. 8-14).

2. **Infective gingivitis**
   A. **Vincent's infection (necrotizing ulcerative, ulceromembranous)**
   The color, form, density and attachment of the gingivae may be significantly altered. Alteration is characterized by necrosis of the gingival margins and interdental papillae, which leaves punched-out craterlike depressions. The surfaces of the lesions are covered with a gray or grayish-yellow pseudomembrane that is easily removed, leaving a bleeding ulcerated surface. The margins of the lesions present a pronounced erythematous appearance. The lesions may involve only a few areas on all the teeth. Symptoms include pain of varying degrees, sialorrhea, wedging sensation of the teeth, and foul breath. Local lymphadenopathy is likely to be present. Fever, malaise, an-

orexia, and other systemic manifestations may be present (Figs. 2-12, 8-9 and 8-15).
   B. **Herpetic gingivostomatitis**
   This is an acute process caused by the initial invasion of any or all of the oral mucosa by the herpes simplex virus. Early features include regional lymphadenopathy, fever, malaise, and "sore throat." The latter is generally dysphagia rather than typical sore throat. There are generalized gingival hyperemia, tenderness, and usually vesicles. The lesions generally follow the initial systemic phase; they arise as vesicles that soon rupture to form shallow ulcers with an erythematous halo. Lesions may involve only the gingiva but generally involve all of the oral mucosa. The disease is self-limiting, lasting from about a week to 10 days (Figs. 8-16 and 2-13, *C*).

3. **Hyperplastic gingivitis**
   A. **Simple hyperplastic gingivitis**
   This is a simple enlargement of the gingival tissues, especially the free gingival margin and the interdental papillae, resulting from chronic irritation. Alteration of color, form,

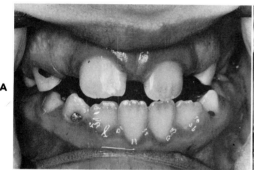
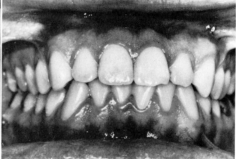

Fig. 8-14. *Gingival disease.* **A,** Eruption gingivitis. **B,** Simple marginal gingivitis.

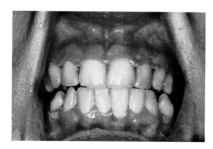

Fig. 8-15. *Gingival disease.* Acute necrotizing ulcerative gingivitis (NUG, acute Vincent's infection).

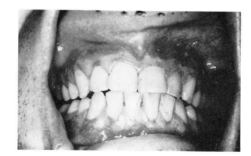

Fig. 8-16. *Gingival disease.* Acute herpetic gingivostomatitis; note lesions on free gingival margins of all maxillary incisors.

and density is related to the inflammatory response of the gingiva. The proliferative response of the tissues is more pronounced than in simple gingivitis. Thus, altered form is a constant and characteristic finding. The chronicity of the irritant is also an important factor. The tissue is soft and spongy. The color is bluish-red (Fig. 8-17).

B. **Hereditary gingival fibromatosis**

This is a progressive proliferative process in which the normal contour and form of the gingiva are altered. The tissue is generally pale pink, firm, and very dense. The enlargement may be so pronounced as to completely cover the teeth. Local irritation may be superimposed. The tissues tend to return progressively after surgical removal even in the absence of local irritation (Fig. 8-18).

C. **Gingivitis modified by systemic factors**

(1) **Dilantin hyperplasia**

This is a progressive proliferation of the gingiva associated with Dilantin therapy. Clinical signs and symptoms are the same as those of simple hyperplastic gingivitis. To make the diagnosis of Dilantin gingivitis, it is necessary to know the patient is taking Dilantin Sodium. Local irritants cause the inflammatory response; Dilantin only exaggerates this response, with resultant gingival enlargement (Fig. 8-19).

(2) **Pubertal gingivitis**

This is gingival enlargement that is thought to be associated with hormonal imbalance at the time of puberty. The color, form, and density changes are the same as in simple hyperplastic gingivitis. The color is intense, and the gingiva tends to bleed readily. This is a nonspecific inflammatory hyperplasia. Local irritation is the cause of the inflammatory response; the hormonal imbalance appears only to modify the response (Fig. 8-20).

(3) **Pregnancy gingivitis**

This is gingival enlargement showing all the signs and symptoms of simple hyperplastic gingivitis plus a greater tendency to bleed. It is a nonspecific inflammatory response of the tissues to local irritants; the response is modified by hormonal imbalance that occurs during pregnancy. Unless the physical state of pregnancy exists, the diagnosis relative to the signs and symptoms present would be simple hyperplastic gingivitis (Fig. 8-21).

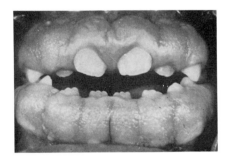

Fig. 8-18. *Gingival disease.* Hereditary gingival fibromatosis.

A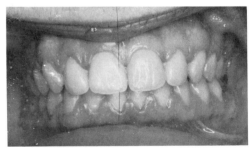

B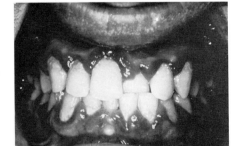

Fig. 8-17. *Gingival disease.* **A,** Simple hyperplastic gingivitis; mild. **B,** Severe.

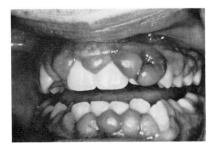

Fig. 8-19. *Gingival disease.* Pronounced Dilantin hyperplasia.

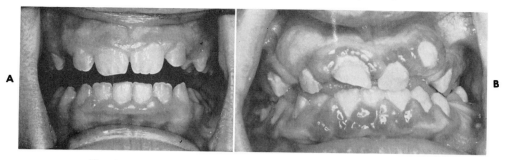

Fig. 8-20. *Gingival disease.* Pubertal gingivitis. **A,** Mild. **B,** Severe.

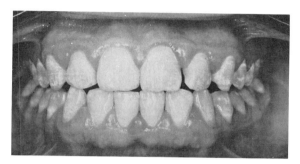

Fig. 8-21. *Gingival disease.* Pregnancy gingivitis.

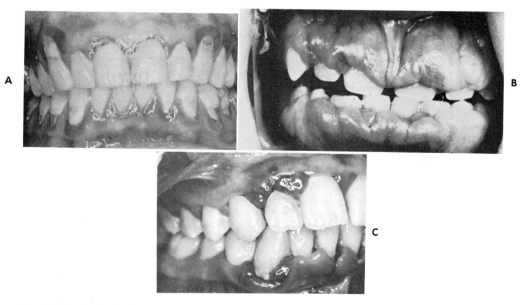

Fig. 8-22. *Gingival disease.* **A,** Leukemic gingivitis (granulocytic). **B,** Leukemic gingivitis (monocytic). **C,** Gingivitis caused by cyclic neuropenia.

(4) **Leukemic gingivitis**

This type of gingivitis is characterized frequently by pronounced gingival enlargement. The enlargement is primarily caused by the infiltration of the gingival tissues by neoplastic blood cells, which produces a peculiar thickening of the gingival margins, which have a tendency to stand away from the teeth. The color may be bluish-red to pink. The tissues are generally soft and spongy. Spontaneous and persistent hemorrhage occurs frequently. The gingival enlargement in some forms of the disease may cover the surface of the teeth. Regional lymphadenopathy may be present. A complete history and examination are necessities. Areas of ulceration suggestive of Vincent's infection may be present (Fig. 8-22).

4. **Hormonal gingivitis**

A. **Chronic desquamative gingivitis**

This is a type of gingivitis associated with altered premenopausal hormonal stimulation. It is occasionally seen in males. Desquamation of the epithelium is the most constant feature; this may be limited or diffuse throughout the gingiva. The color of the gingiva varies from one location to an-

other from grayish blue to brilliant red. The overall appearance of the gingiva may show a patch of speckled discoloration. In same forms the entire gingiva may be erythematous. The density of the gingiva is soft, and digital palpation may be attended by peeling of the epithelium. Stippling is absent, and the gingiva is not tightly bound down to the underlying tissues. Some degree of hyperplasia is present, and the surface of the epithelium is easily stripped or peeled off in severely affected areas. Pain is a common symptom and varies in intensity according to the severity of the process (Fig. 8-23).

B. **Chronic atrophic senile gingivitis**

This type of gingivitis is related to postmenopausal hormonal stimulation. It is also occasionally seen in males. The gingival tissues are thin and atrophic and are easily traumatized. Thus many of the changes seen are secondary to the lack of protective adaptation of the gingiva to trauma. Not infrequently even well-fitting dentures cannot be tolerated. Clinically the cheek mucosa may have a milky appearance and irregular grayish white areas that can be mistaken for leukoplakia. In general, the tissues are pale and grayish white. In some

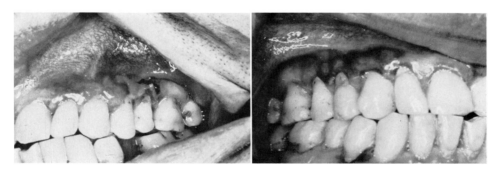

Fig. 8-23. *Gingival disease.* Chronic desquamative gingivitis.

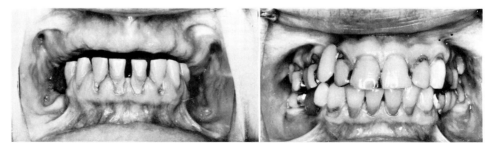

Fig. 8-24. *Gingival disease.* Chronic atrophic gingivitis.

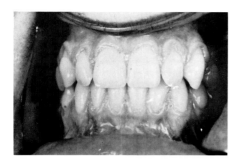

Fig. 8-25. *Gingival disease.* Atrophic gingivitis resulting from trauma.

areas a mild degree of hyperkeratinization may be present (Fig. 8-24).

C. **Atrophic gingivitis**

This refers to gingival recession excessive for age. The gingiva is usually free of inflammation unless the exposed cementum is hypersensitive and for this reason is not kept clean. The soft tissue recedes at an equal rate with the loss of alveolar bone. Atrophy may be caused by poor toothbrushing habits, hyperfunction, bruxism, or hypofunction. Generalized recession in young individuals may be related at times to large teeth and an inadequate bony support (Fig. 8-25).

5. **Periodontitis**

This is an inflammatory disease, usually the sequela or untreated gingivitis, characterized by

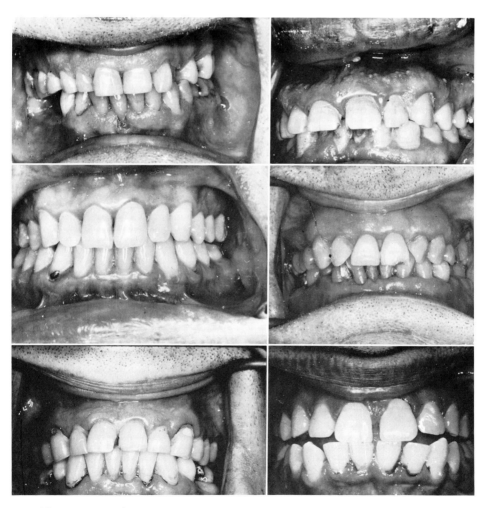

Fig. 8-26. *Periodontitis.* Gingival appearance with periodontitis of varying severity.

an extension of the inflammatory process into the deeper structures of the periodontium. The color, form, and density are all expressions of chronic inflammation. Periodontal pockets are present, and the teeth may or may not show hypermobility. Clinically the gingiva is red or bluish red and soft and spongy, and the margins are thick and rolled. The interdental papillae are soft and spongy and may overfill the interproximal spaces. There is generally supragingival and subgingival calculus present throughout the mouth (Fig. 8-26).

The clinical evaluation of color, form, density, and attachment is an important step in the formulation of a diagnosis, and careful collection of the facts will serve to orient the examiner to the proper field of reference. It is impossible for the student or general practitioner to know all the ramifications of periodontal disease or to have the descriptive knowledge necessary to make a diagnosis of obscure or differential diagnostic problems. He must remember, however, that his reference to the literature must be based upon his orientation to the correct field and his ability to relate his findings to those descriptions in the reference material that are couched in terms of abnormalities of color, form, density, epithelial attachment, and depth of the gingival crevice.

Examination procedure. The examination of the gingiva should begin with a systematic inspection from the junction of the alveolar mucosa to the free gingival margin. Any alteration of the normal color should be recorded. The location, extent, and coloration should be given in detail. An attempt should be made to determine the cause of the alteration, for example, pigmentation, cyanosis, or desquamation. All information should become a part of the patient's permanent record, since it is valuable in making the ultimate diagnosis and in determining the progress of therapy. The inspection should also include observation of the signs of altered form. The form may be altered by disease or past therapy. Gingival enlargement may be diffuse or localized; the areas involved should be recorded.

For example, the gingival form may be described thus: "The free gingival margins of the maxillary central incisors are blunt, rolled, and enlarged; the interdental papillae of this area are swollen and overfill the interproximal spaces; the gingiva is enlarged sufficiently to cover half of the labial surface of these teeth."

The teeth should be examined for the presence of soft debris, plaques, stains, and calculus. The type, location, and amount should be noted and recorded. This should be done prior to the examination of the teeth for dental caries since it is necessary to clean the teeth thoroughly before effective evaluation of the presence of carious lesions can be accomplished. Discoloration of the teeth from exogenous causes can be evaluated best before the teeth have been cleaned, whereas discoloration associated with endogenous causes can be best appreciated after the cleaning.

Many colored substances that are introduced into the mouth or substances that are broken down in the mouth may stain the teeth or produce soft plaques upon them (Fig. 8-27). Such extrinsic stains may be green, yellow, orange, brown, or black. The origin of many of these colors is not well understood, but they probably arise from sulfides formed in oral putrefaction or from pigment-producing bacteria. A green stain frequently appears on the necks of children's teeth, especially on the maxillary incisors. This appears to be associated with the remains of Nasmyth's membrane but may also be associated with penetration of the surface of the enamel beneath the membrane. A thin line of black pigment, "mesenteric line," may occur about the necks of the teeth of individuals, usually females, who often exhibit very good oral hygiene. It is most often seen on the lingual aspects of the maxillary teeth in the form of a fine black line following the gingival margin (Fig. 8-27, *C* and *D*). It can be removed but tends to recur in a few days despite adequate home care. The etiology of this stain is not known. It appears to be of no pathologic significance and cannot be used as an indication of the patient's oral hygiene. Orange to orange-red stains may be seen either as thin lines or diffuse plaques around the necks of the teeth, and their etiology has been attributed to the action of chromogenic bacteria. These stains are of no pathologic significance, but they do give some indication of the oral hygiene of the patient. Tobacco stains may either be deposited upon the surfaces of the teeth or penetrate into the substance of the enamel and dentin. This type of staining is dependent primarily upon the presence of mucinous plaques on the teeth. It is not neces-

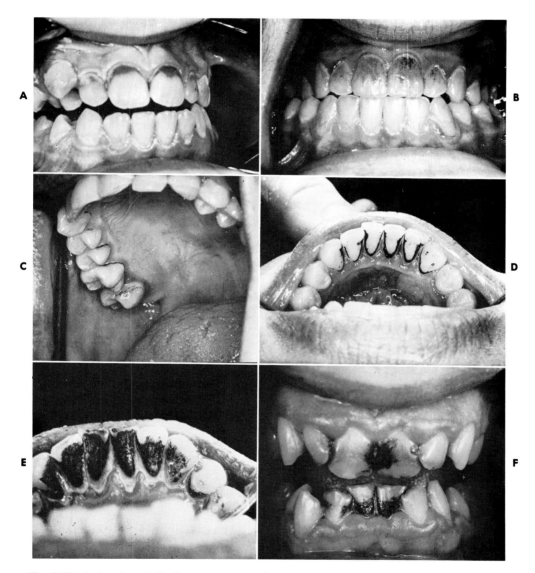

Fig. 8-27. *Stains.* **A** and **B**, Green stain. **C** and **D**, "Metabolic" black stain. **E** and **F**, Tobacco stains.

sarily dependent upon the amount of tobacco used. Persons who chew tobacco or smoke cigars appear to be more prone to have penetration of tobacco juices into the pits and fissures of the teeth. The amount of staining that occurs is directly proportional to the presence of lamellae, cracks, and poorly calcified areas.

Palpation of the gingiva (Fig. 8-28) should be systematically carried out to determine the resiliency, texture, and status of the underlying tissues. Areas of tenderness, friable tissues, loss of normal texture, exuded pus, and soft spongy tissue should be noted.

Charting. The level of the attachment

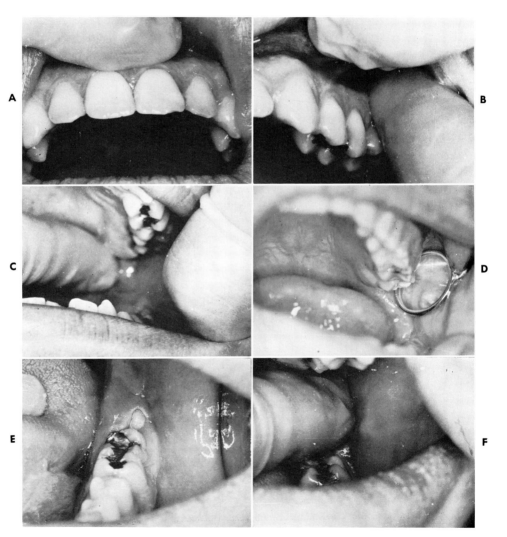

Fig. 8-28. *Examination of gingiva.* **A,** Palpation of free and attached gingiva over eminences produced by roots of central incisors. **B,** Palpation of gingiva over the roots of molar teeth. **C,** Palpation of gingiva over tuberosity. **D,** Inspection of the alveolar and gingival mucosa of the tuberosity. **E,** Inspection of retromolar papilla, pads, and flaps. **F,** Palpation of retromolar area.

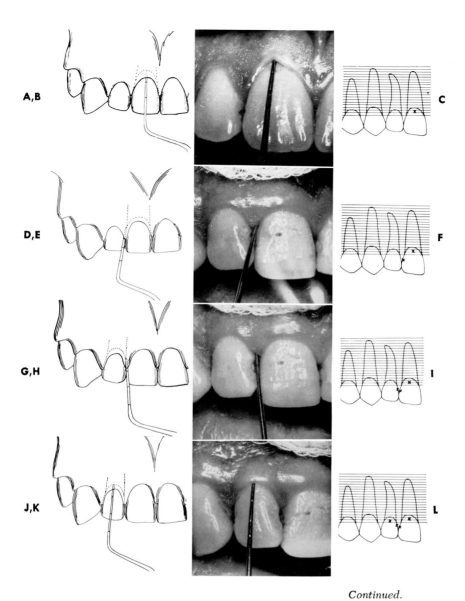

Continued.

Fig. 8-29. *Charting.* **A** to **R**, Location of free gingival margin in relation to the cementoenamel junction and recording it on the chart. The drawings to the left are schematic representations of measuring the free gingival margin in relation to the cementoenamel junction. The pictures in the center show the measurement clinically. The schematic drawings to the right show the measurement recorded on the chart. **S** and **T** show completion of the free gingival margin on chart. **W** to **Z**, After the free gingival margin has been determined in relation to the cementoenamel junction and recorded on the chart, the location and depth of gingival sulci over 3 mm. are recorded. The drawings to the left are schematic representations of the probe in periodontal pockets. The pictures in the center indicate the position of the probe clinically. The schematic drawings on the right show the depth of the pocket on the chart as measured from the free gingival margin. The depth of the periodontal pocket is measured from the free gingival margin to the base of the pocket. This measurement is indicated by a vertical line placed on the involved side of the tooth drawn apically from the free gingival margin to the measured depth of the pocket. **ZZ,** Completed chart showing free gingival margin and location and depth of periodontal pockets; chart indicates pockets on distal surface of incisor and mesial surface of the cuspid.

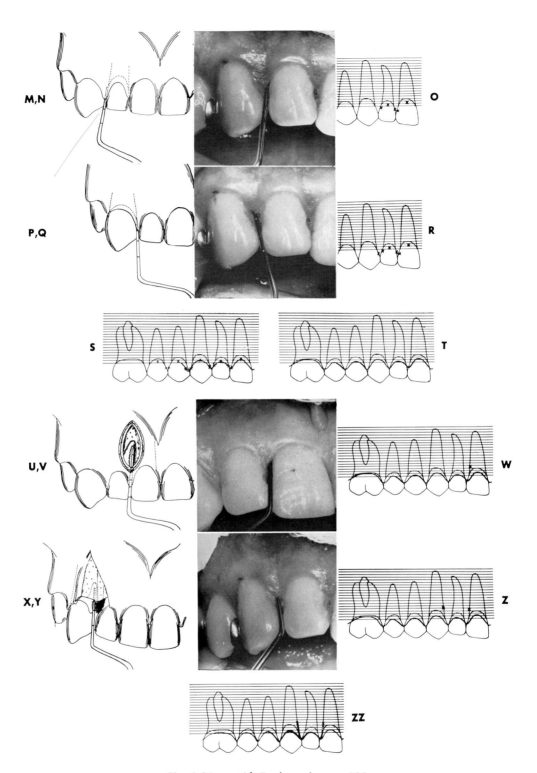

Fig. 8-29, cont'd. For legend see p. 185.

and the position of the free gingival margin should be measured relative to the cementoenamel junction and a record made of these measurements. The initial measurements are made by ascertaining the cementoenamel junction and measuring the height of the gingival margin from this position (Fig. 8-29). This procedure is followed throughout the mouth, and these measurements should be made at four points: the mesial and distal aspects of the buccal or labial surfaces and the mesial and distal aspects of the lingual surfaces of each tooth. The free gingival margin is then drawn on a dental chart that has been ruled with 1 mm. gradations. When this has been accomplished, the examiner then should probe the depth of all the gingival crevices to determine where the crevices exceed the normal limits of 2 to 3 mm. in depth. This will serve to determine the position of the epithelial attachment relative to the cementoenamel junction. The actual measurement is made from the free gingival margin to the base of the crevice or periodontal pocket. This measurement of the depth of periodontal pockets is recorded on the chart as demonstrated in Fig. 8-29.

Although certain clinically evident changes in the color, form, and density of the gingiva and radiographic evidence of bone resorption may suggest the presence of periodontal pockets, the only reliable method for detecting their presence and extent is to probe the gingival crevices with a suitable periodontal instrument. The most suitable for measuring the depth of periodontal pockets is a very thin calibrated probe. It should be straight, resilient, and marked at 3, 6, and 8 mm. (Fig. 8-30). From a practical standpoint, probes that are marked for every millimeter are somewhat confusing. The probe must be carefully inserted to gain the deepest penetration possible without penetrating the gingival tissue or epithelial attachment. The examiner must know the anatomy of the root surfaces of the teeth well and must be able to detect alterations in the surfaces of the roots so that the probing can be accurately accomplished. Calculus, enamel pearls, variations in the cementoenamel junction, and interradicular areas require special attention.

Full delineation of periodontal pockets may at times be difficult because of malpositioned teeth, overhanging restorations, carious lesions, tortuous pockets, tender gingiva, hypersensitive cementum, and gingival bleeding. Because of the convexity of the anatomic crown, the examiner should attempt to measure the depth of the pockets always at the same angle and as nearly parallel to the long axis of the tooth as possible (Fig. 8-31). Pockets involving interradicular areas are at times difficult to measure because of the relationship between the roots and crowns of the teeth. The measurement of the depth of pockets involving bifurcation and trifurcation areas is not so important as establishing that the involvement of these areas does exist. Probing for bifurcation areas of the mandibular molars does not present too much difficulty, especially when a "cowhorn" explorer is used Although this explorer cannot be used to measure the depth of periodontal pockets, it is of considerable aid in determining the extent of bifurcation involvement (Fig. 8-32). The area in which it is most difficult to ascertain the extent of periodontal pock-

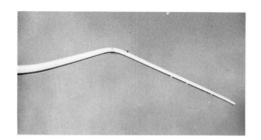

Fig. 8-30. *Gingival probing.* Gingival probe with 3, 6, and 8 mm. markings.

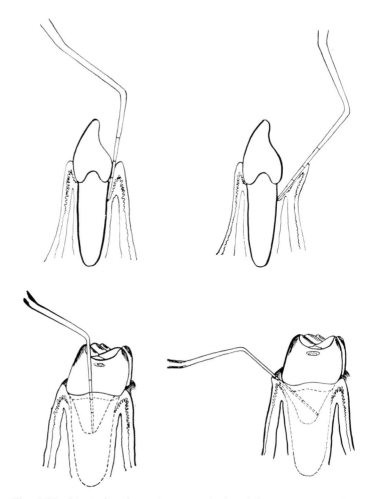

Fig. 8-31. *Gingival probing.* Correct method on left; incorrect on right.

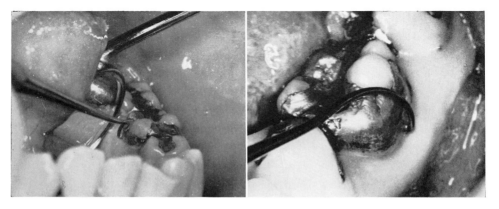

Fig. 8-32. *Clinical probing.* Examination of bifurcation area with "cowhorn" explorer.

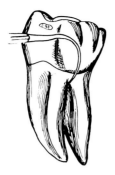 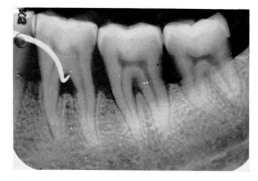

Fig. 8-32, cont'd. For legend see opposite page.

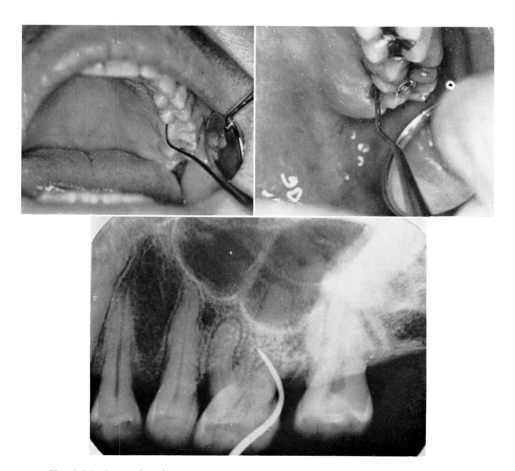

Fig. 8-33. *Gingival probing.* Examination of trifurcation area with periodontal probe.

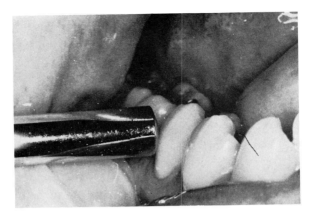

Fig. 8-34. *Detection of mobility.* Note placement of finger on lingual aspects of tooth to detect displacement caused by handle of explorer.

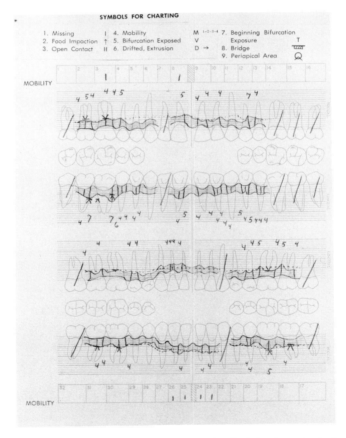

Fig. 8-35. Periodontal charting. Most coronal line is the level of the free gingival margin relative to the cementoenamel junction. Shaded area is crevice area. Solid lines running from free gingival margin to base of crevice are periodontal pocket measurements. Dotted line is estimation of bone level taken from radiographs (Fig. 8-36).

ets in the trifurcation area of the maxillary molars. Because of the anatomic arrangement of the roots, the convexity of the distal aspect of the crowns, and the angle at which the probe must be inserted, the probing of intrabony pockets involving the trifurcation area on the distal aspect of maxillary molars may be quite difficult (Fig. 8-33). Radiographs are especially helpful for determining the anatomic features of the interradicular area and help the examiner to probe these areas more effectively. It is important to record the depth of the periodontal pockets in these areas; however, it is more important to know whether actual involvement of the interradicular area has occurred. The examiner must fully delineate the extent and depth of the periodontal pockets and determine how much alveolar process has been lost on the mesial and distal aspects of the teeth and on the lingual, buccal, or labial aspects.

Periodontal pockets involving long fused roots of molars are usually of less significance than those involving teeth with divergent roots. Thus it is very important that the examiner not only attempt to measure carefully the extent and depth of periodontal pockets, but also to relate the morphology of the pocket to the length and form of the roots. Information relative to the morphology of the root will not only aid in more efficient probing of the periodontal pockets, but will also be useful in determining the prognosis and treatment of the teeth involved.

The mobility of all the teeth should be tested and the degree of mobility indicated in terms of a numerical reference (Fig. 8-34). The use of 1, 2, 3, and 4 will facilitate recording the degree of mobility; 1 may be used to indicate minimal lateral movement and 4 to indicate extensive lateral and intrusive movement of the teeth. Excessive mobility of the teeth may not be

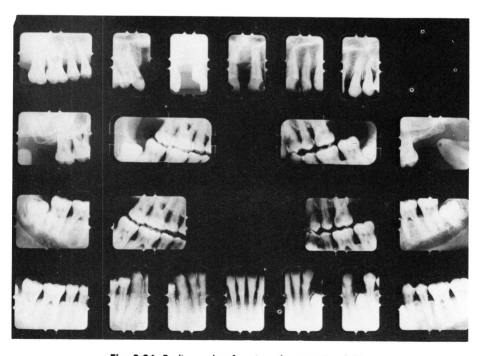

Fig. 8-36. Radiographs of patient shown in Fig. 8-35.

associated with periodontal pockets, and conversely periodontal pockets involving trifurcation and bifurcation areas will not necessarily cause increased mobility. Although bifurcation and trifurcation exposure and excessive mobility of the teeth are common clinical features of periodontal disease that are used in making a diagnosis, their significance to the prognosis and treatment planning varies considerably with individual cases. This is discussed in further detail in Chapter 15. Inasmuch as the treatment of periodontal disease is based upon the history and findings of the clinical examination, it is necessary that the examination of the periodontal structures be as complete as possible.

A clinical chart for recording periodontal as well as other dental findings is shown in Fig. 8-35. The charting shown represents most of the periodontal facts that might be recorded in a given case. The ruled lines are representative of 1 mm. The symbols that may be used on the chart are not necessarily exhaustive; however, the ones given are those that are used most often.

The chart represents a complete record of the location of gingival margins, epithelial attachment, and the location of periodontal pockets. Radiographs for the same patient as charted in Fig. 8-35 are shown in Fig. 8-36.

REFERENCES

Ash, M. M.: Physiology of the mouth. In Bunting, R. W. (editor): Oral hygiene, Philadelphia, 1957, Lea & Febiger.

Björn, H., Halling, A., and Thyberg, H.: Radiographic assessment of marginal bone loss, Odontol. Revy **20**:165, 1969.

Dummett, C. O., and Barens, G.: Pigmentation of oral tissues, J. Periodont. **38**:369, 1967.

Kerr, D. A., and Ash, M. M.: Oral pathology, Philadelphia, 1971, Lea & Febiger, pp. 209-244.

Ramfjord, S. P., Kerr, D. A., and Ash, M. M. (editors): World workshop on periodontics—1966, Ann Arbor, Mich., 1966, The University of Michigan Press.

Schroeder, H. E., and Listgarten, M. A.: Fine structure of the developing epithelial attachment of human teeth, Basel, 1971, S. Karger, pp. 100-116.

Theilade, J.: An evaluation of the reliability of radiographs in the measurement of bone loss in periodontal disease, J. Periodont. **31**:143, 1960.

Wentz, F. M., Maier, A. W., and Orban, B. J.: Age changes and sex differences in the clinically "normal" gingiva, J. Periodont. **23**:13, 1952.

9

Examination of the teeth

The examination of the teeth should be preceded by a careful prophylaxis so that calculus, stains, and soft debris will not interfere with exploration and inspection. For this reason stains, oral hygiene, and the location and character of calculus should be considered during the examination of the gingivae.

The examination should be systematic and always begin and end in a definite locality. Methods of examination include inspection with the naked eye using a mouth mirror, exploration with suitable sharp explorers, and percussion with the end of the handle of the mouth mirror or single-ended explorer. Radiographic examination and vitality testing should also be considered part of a thorough examination.

The examiner should remove any debris and dry the teeth before attempting to examine them for carious lesions. The use of a saliva ejector will facilitate the examination procedure. The patient should be instructed to rinse the mouth thoroughly before the examination is begun. A mouthwash of water containing a few drops of 28 percent ammonia may be provided to aid in removing thick mucous saliva from the mouth.

The following should be considered in the examination of the teeth: color and stains; size, form, structure, and number; erosion, abrasion, and fractures; vitality; functional contours; carious lesions; contact relationship.

Color and stains. The color of the teeth may show considerable normal variation; the primary teeth are generally bluish white, whereas the permanent teeth are generally more opaque and show variations of gray and yellow hues as the individual becomes older. The inherent color is determined by the translucency and thickness of the enamel and by the thickness and color of the underlying dentin. Alteration may be physiologic or pathologic and intrinsic or extrinsic in origin. As the individual grows older the enamel becomes worn and thinner, and unless it is lost entirely and wear of the dentin takes place, the dentin becomes thicker because of the deposition of secondary dentin. Because of the thinness of the enamel and the thickness of the dentin, the teeth of older persons are generally more yellowish or grayish-yellow in color than those of younger persons.

Discoloration may result from developmental disturbances whereby the normal pattern of enamel prisms and dental tubules are disturbed. Examples of this type may be seen in amelogenesis imperfecta, dentinogenesis imperfecta, brown hereditary teeth, and dental fluorosis or mottling.

Discoloration can also result from intrinsic pigments formed at the time of the development of the teeth or after the teeth have fully formed (Fig. 9-1). Pigments arising from hemolysis of blood cells or associated with jaundice may discolor the teeth. Discoloration associated with blood-borne endogenous pigments usually disappears with the termination of the disease process. The color of the teeth in these conditions may be considerably green, yellow-brown, or orange-yellow in appearance. With the death of the pulp, degeneration

193

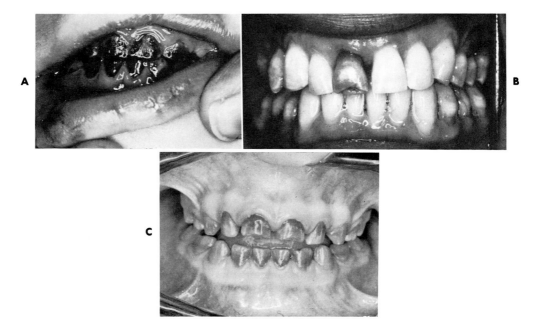

Fig. 9-1. *Teeth—altered color.* **A,** Discoloration associated with porphyrinuria. **B,** Devital tooth. **C,** Pigmented teeth that vary in both degree and distribution of pigment. The pigmentation is complete in the anterior teeth but involves only the cervical areas of the molars. The color in the anterior teeth is purplish brown; in the posterior teeth it is canary yellow. This is the type of pigmentation produced by tetracycline.

and decomposition products from the iron and proteins in the pulp tissue may diffuse into dentin, and the teeth will be stained gray, yellow-brown, or black. A dark gray color may indicate devitalization; however, this finding should be supplemented with vitality tests before the final diagnosis is made (Fig. 9-1, *B*). Internal resorption of the dentin may produce a pink or black discoloration of the teeth. These teeth give a positive response to vitality tests.

Discolorations may arise from the introduction of medicaments into the root canals and pulp chambers during endodontic therapy. Staining may also occur from permeation of medicaments into the dental tubules when sterilizing a cavity preparation. Metallic staining may arise from the ingestion or inhalation of metals or their salts. This occurs most often from the use of drugs but may be an occupational haz-

ard. In most instances these metals or their salts are deposited in plaques or films upon the teeth; however, they may penetrate the enamel and dentin. This is especially true of teeth that are porous and have extensive cracks and lamellae. A history of the patient's occupation is extremely important in making a differential diagnosis of stains of the teeth. The use of tobacco is the most frequent cause of staining. This is especially true when abrasion has exposed dentin and the patient chews tobacco. In general, cleaning will only remove the external tobacco stains, and tobacco stains of dentin, fissures, pits, and lamellae will be difficult, if not impossible, to remove.

From the foregoing description of exogenous and endogenous stains it is apparent that the diagnosis is dependent upon an adequate history and a descriptive knowledge of a few characteristic stains. The

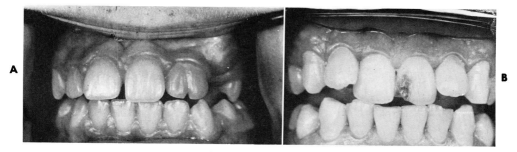

Fig. 9-2. *Teeth-altered form.* **A,** Fusion, **B,** Hypoplasia of central incisor (Turner's tooth).

diagnosis of most of the stains is dependent upon a history of the conditions that may be responsible for the staining such as occupation (for example, an industrial worker may be inhaling copper, brass, or bronze particles), developmental disturbances associated with defects in the dentin and enamel, serious diseases such as hepatitis or erythroblastosis fetalis, restorative or endodontic procedures, use of drugs containing iron, mercury, or other staining elements, use of colored dentifrices, use of tobacco, and a history of pulp disease. The rather characteristic location and color of green stain, black linear stain, and red-orange stains associated with chromogenic bacteria make their diagnosis more dependent upon a descriptive knowledge than upon the history. However, the history is of value in the sense of negative correlation.

Size, form, structure, and number. The examiner should pay particular attention to the size, form, structure, and number of teeth, since developmental disturbances are frequently manifested by an alteration of these factors. This is especially true of the developing dentition because the size of the teeth play an important role in occlusion. The size of the crowns, the length and configuration of the roots, and the space presented by absence of teeth are all important to restorative procedures. Edentulous area should be evaluated for the presence of impacted or unerupted teeth.

Anomalies of size include macrodontia and microdontia. Anomalies of number include supernumerary teeth and complete or partial anodontia. Developmental disturbances of form include geminated teeth, fused teeth, concrescence, enamel pearls, dens in dente, Turner's teeth, odontomas, Hutchinson's teeth, mulberry molars, accessory cusps and roots, and hypoplastic defects (Fig. 9-2). Hereditary alteration of form includes hypoplasias, dentinogenesis imperfecta, dentin dysplasia, and amelogenesis imperfecta. Both hereditary and developmental defects show an alteration of structure. Extrinsic or environmental alterations that are responsible for variation in form after the teeth have fully formed may be manifest as erosion, abrasion, caries, or excessive attrition.

Enamel dysplasia refers to hypoplasia and hypomaturation of the enamel. Enamel hypoplasia is a defect that occurs as a result of any disturbance in the formation of the enamel matrix. Enamel hypocalcification occurs as a result of any disturbance that interferes with normal deposition of calcium, whereas hypomaturation occurs from incomplete crystallization of the enamel. These types of enamel dysplasia can result from local, systemic, or hereditary disease.

Local factors that can produce defects in the teeth include periapical inflammation, trauma, and surgical procedures. Periapical inflammation of a deciduous tooth may pro-

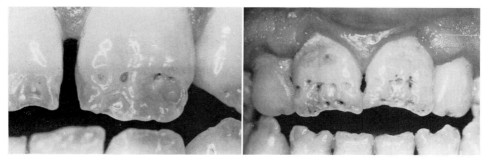

Fig. 9-3. *Teeth—altered form.* Hypoplasia; note rhythmic character of defects.

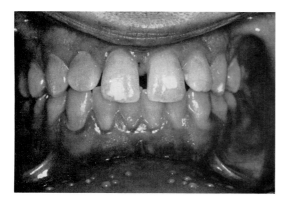

Fig. 9-4. *Teeth—altered color and texture.* Opaque spots caused by hypomaturation of enamel.

duce hypoplasia and hypomaturation of a succedaneous tooth if the inflammatory process occurs at the time of amelogenesis and maturation. Nutritional deficiencies, endocrine disturbances, and other systemic diseases have been suggested as etiologic agents in hypoplastic defects of the enamel. Enamel hypomaturation can be produced by ingestion of an excess of fluorine. Various hereditary defects of the enamel are seen, such as amelogenesis imperfecta, hereditary brown teeth, and other hypoplasias of the enamel. Some hereditary enamel defects appear quite similar to those of local or unknown origin.

Enamel hypoplasia may appear as a localized alteration of one or several teeth or involve all the teeth. It may consist of the absence of enamel and dentin or of only the enamel. Its clinical appearance will depend upon the stage of amelogenesis at which the disturbance occurred and the external or environmental factors that have altered the enamel. Frequently enamel hypoplasia of the central incisors will show rather well-defined horizontal lines of pits and grooves (Fig. 9-3). The levels at which the defects occur represent an expression of the rhythmic or intermittent character of the interference in the development of the tooth structure. A comparison of levels of hypoplasia from one area of the mouth to another serves to point out the chronologic period or stage of development that various teeth were in during the period of disturbance. Though the time period for the defect may be established, it is only rarely that a history of systemic disease will correspond to this time period. A recent study by Witkop indicates that many forms of enamel defects loosely classified as amelogenesis imperfecta may be distinct clinical and genetic entities. Thus a history of similar hypoplastic and hypomaturation defects of the enamel and dentin in other members of the patient's family should be determined.

Single or multiple chalky-white opaque spots may be present on the teeth. These spots are most obvious on the central incisors (Fig. 9-4). With eruption of teeth and recession of the gingiva, they may ap-

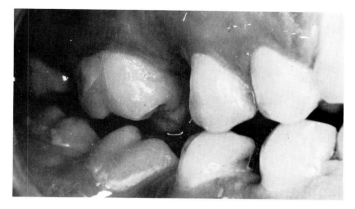

Fig. 9-5. Teeth—altered texture and color. Cervical decalcification.

pear to the patient to be of recent origin; however, the defect actually occurs during the formation of the enamel. Clinically the enamel in an opaque spot may be soft and can be penetrated by an explorer if the surface is worn away; however, if the overlying enamel has remained intact, the surface will be granular but hard, and the explorer will not penetrate into the opaque spot. Not infrequently removal of the surface for restoration purposes reveals for the first time that the underlying enamel is softer than normal. Opaque spots may also be caused by faulty matrix apposition, which changes the index of refraction.

The greatest difficulty in arriving at a diagnosis of opacity of the enamel appears to be centered around the difference between hypocalcified and decalcified enamel. Clinically both appear white and opaque in character. No difficulty arises if the surface of the opaque spot is glazed and smooth since the defect of decalcification results in a granular, rough, and soft surface that can be penetrated with a sharp explorer. However, if both surfaces have a similar texture, some difficulty may arise. The white opaque areas of decalcification associated with the early phases of dental decay are usually found beneath soft masses of materia alba along the cervical one-third of the crowns of teeth adjacent to the free

gingival margin and in areas that are not self-cleansing (Fig. 9-5). Opaque spots caused by hypomaturation, hypoplasia, or altered pigmentation may be found anywhere on the teeth, including self-cleansing areas.

Endemic dental fluorosis (mottled enamel) is an acquired form of enamel hypoplasia resulting from the consumption of water containing an excess of fluorine. Mottled enamel may be mild or severe in character. Unless the concentration of fluorine is high, enamel apposition will proceed normally. The clinical manifestation will consist of cloudy opaque areas or of yellow or brown areas if extrinsic material has pigmented the areas (Fig. 9-6). Since mottled enamel is only one of the signs by hypomaturation, the unequivocal diagnosis of mottled enamel cannot be made without a positive history of excessive fluoride ingestion.

The differential diagnosis of Hutchinson's teeth, mulberry molars, and hypoplastic defects may be the most difficult. The difficulty involved in making a diagnosis of Hutchinson's incisors and mulberry molars can usually be attributed to an inadequate understanding of the morphologic and histologic characteristics of these manifestations of congenital syphilis. The most common error regarding Hutchinson's incisors occurs when the examiner attributes the notching of the incisor teeth to an under-development of the central developmental lobe rather than to the loss of tooth struc-ture from trauma. It must be remembered that the characteristic shape of a Hutchin-son's incisor results from the underdevel-opment of the central developmental lobe

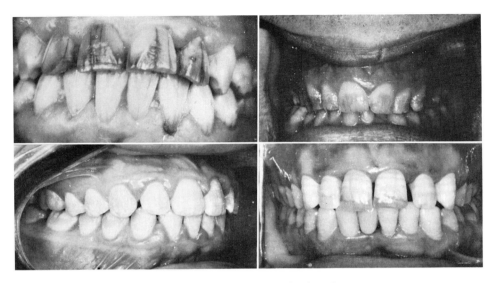

Fig. 9-6. *Teeth—altered texture and color. Fluorosis.*

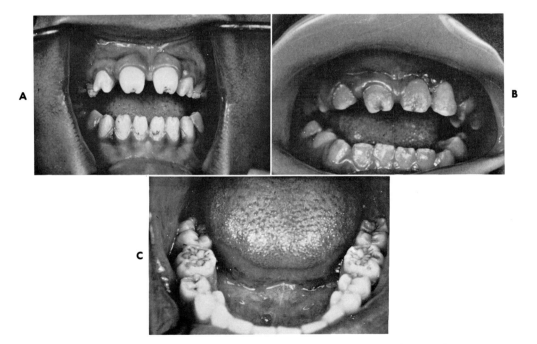

Fig. 9-7. *Teeth—altered form.* **A** *and* **B,** *Hutchinson's incisors.* **C,** *Mulberry molars.*

with a collapse of the lateral developmental lobes. This causes the incisal edge to be narrower than the cervical portion of the tooth, thus giving it a characteristic screwdriver shape (Fig. 9-7, *A* and *B*). Therefore, the examiner should not consider notching of the incisal edge of the incisors as evidence of the absence of the middle developmental lobe unless the width of the incisal edge is less than that of the cervical portion of the tooth.

Mulberry molars are also suggestive of congenital syphilis (Fig. 9-7, *C*). They are characterized by normal buccal and lingual surfaces but have occlusal surfaces analogous to a mulberry. A variation of this type of molar has pinched-in buccal and lingual surfaces and is called a bud molar. Localized defects of the occlusal surface of the molar teeth have at times been incorrectly diagnosed as mulberry molars. These dental stigmas do not occur in all cases of congenital syphilis, and the final diagnosis of congenital syphilis cannot be made purely on the basis of hypoplastic defects that are suggestive of Hutchinson's incisors and mulberry molars. In a few instances, Hutchinson's triad of notched incisors, deafness, and interstitial keratitis may be present.

Another form of enamel dysplasia is amelogenesis imperfecta. This designation has been loosely applied to many disturbances of the enamel involving hypoplasia, dysplasia, hypocalcification, hypomaturation, altered pigmentation, and defects involving hereditary or genetic linkages. Most of these defects are generalized throughout the teeth; however, they also may be localized. The involvement in amelogenesis imperfecta may vary from a complete lack of enamel to an immature enamel matrix. The enamel, where present, is soft, poorly calcified, and easily abraded (Fig. 9-8). A form of amelogenesis imperfecta in which the enamel is apparently normal in thick-

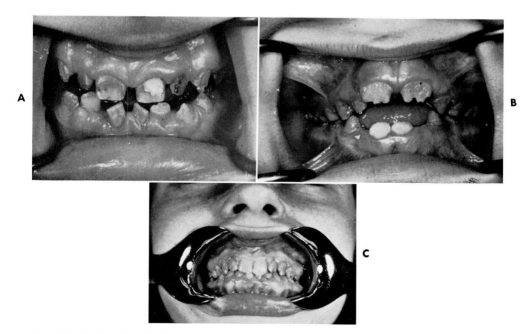

Fig. 9-8. *Teeth—altered color, form, and texture.* **A** and **B**, Amelogenesis imperfecta; note small area of enamel remaining on left maxillary central incisor in **A** and complete absence of enamel of maxillary incisors in **B**. **C**, Hereditary brown hypoplasia.

ness and surface consistency is hereditary brown teeth (Fig. 9-8, *C*). The enamel is not as hard as normal and tends to chip on the incisal and occlusal surfaces. Extension of the brown color throughout the enamel and involvement of all the teeth are rather characteristic. The absence of enamel, poorly formed enamel, hyperpigmented enamel, and a hereditary background of amelogenesis imperfecta are the points to be remembered in a differential diagnosis.

Defects of the dentin that are distinct genetic and clinical entities include dentinogenesis imperfecta and dentin dysplasia. Dentinogenesis imperfecta is characterized by opalescence, abnormal coloration, absence of pulp canals, poorly calcified dentin, and constricted roots (Fig. 9-9, *A*

to *C*). The enamel tends to chip away from the dentin and leaves a surface that is easily abraded. The clinical and radiographic findings are typical with little alteration in the usual pattern. Once this defect is seen, usually no diagnostic problems occur.

Dentin dysplasia is clinically manifested by wandering and malposed teeth. Radiographically the teeth affected show absence of pulp canals, decreased density of dentin, and short narrow roots. Radiolucent apical areas are also frequently present (Fig. 9-9, *D*). Chevronlike areas may appear radiographically in the remaining portion of the pulp chamber.

It is important to determine the number of teeth that are present because of the

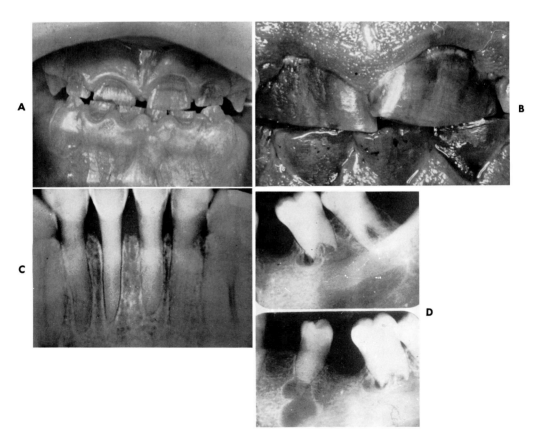

Fig. 9-9. *Teeth—altered color and form.* **A to C,** Dentinogenesis imperfecta. **D,** Dentin dysplasia.

significance of supernumerary teeth and the congenital absence of teeth in diagnosis and treatment planning. The clinical absence of teeth should always be verified by radiographic examination.

The maxillary lateral incisors and the mandibular second bicuspids are congenitally absent more often than any teeth except the third molars. The congenital absence of teeth is usually bilateral. Congenital absence is an important consideration in orthodontic treatment and space management. Anodontia may be associated with other ectodermal defects such as anhidrosis, asteatosis, hypotrichosis, and defects of the salivary glands. One such defect is anhidrotic ectodermal dysplasia (Fig. 9-10, *A* and *B*). Partial anodontia is seen frequently in this ectodermal defect.

Supernumerary teeth refer to an increase in the normal number of teeth present in the dentition (Fig. 9-10, *C*). The presence of extra teeth, whether normal or abnormal in form, is an important factor in disturbances of occlusion. Supernumerary teeth may interfere with normal eruption of the teeth, may erupt outside the normal line of the dental arch, and may occasionally give rise to dentigerous cysts.

Numerous unerupted supernumerary teeth can be seen radiographically in persons with cleidocranial dysostosis, although clinically such patients may not show obvious signs of unerupted teeth. Since this disease is often associated with a failure of permanent dentition to erupt, the kind and number of teeth present may suggest to the examiner simple delayed eruption or partial anodontia. However, radiographs will show the presence of supernumerary teeth. In addition to the dental defect, defective ossification of the clavicles and bones of the skull can be noted. It is not uncommon for these persons to completely lack clavicles.

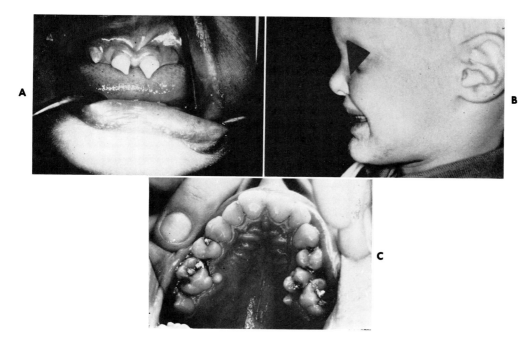

Fig. 9-10. *Teeth—altered number.* **A,** Anhidrotic ectodermal dysplasia; note congenitally missing teeth, abnormal form of those present. **B,** Note absence of eyebrows and coarse hair. **C,** Supernumerary teeth.

Erosion, abrasion, and fractures. The examiner should note the presence of defects caused by abrasion and erosion and, if possible, the etiologic agent should be determined. Erosion results from a chemical process, and the defects are usually limited to the labial and buccal surfaces of the teeth. These defects vary in shape from saucerlike depressions to deep wedgelike grooves. The base presents a hard, polished surface. The lesions are seen most often on the labiocervical portions of the maxillary incisors (Fig. 9-11). They differ from those caused by decalcification in that their base is hard, smooth, and polished and their cause cannot be determined.

Abrasion may occur anywhere on the enamel surfaces or the cervical area of the root and is related to mechanical wearing of the tooth structure by physical agents such as toothbrushes, abrasive powders, hairpins, nails, clay pipestems, glass, tooth-

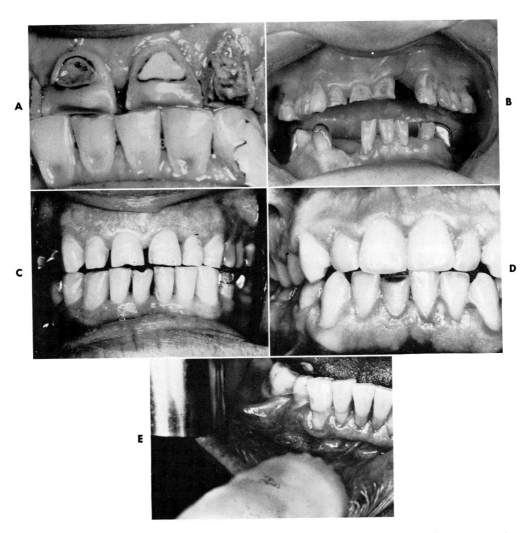

Fig. 9-11. *Teeth—altered form.* **A,** Idiopathic erosin. **B,** Lemon juice erosion. **C,** Abrasion caused by thread biting. **D,** Abrasion caused by biting pipestem. **E,** Toothbrush abrasion.

picks, dental tape, sand, thread, and so on (Fig. 9-11). Abrasion may affect any hard dental structures, whereas erosion is generally limited to the enamel surface. Abrasion of the cementum and dentin in the cervical area is frequently encountered in the presence of gingival recession. The location and character of the lesions produced by abrasion are related to the type of mechanical agent that produces the defect. Exposure of the cementoenamel junction and the cementum by recession of the gingiva may give rise to softening and brown discoloration of the cementum or exposed dentin. The softening is associated with decalcification or maceration of the cementum or dentin by the fluids of the mouth. Changes in color are associated with exogenous pigments. Exposure of the cementum and dentin of the cervical area by erosion frequently leads to cervical decay and hypersensitive cervical areas.

Fractures of teeth may involve both the crowns and roots (Fig. 9-12). Although coronal fractures are obvious, root fractures require radiographic evaluation. Radiographic examination should be a part of any examination involving traumatic fractures of the teeth. Two factors must be determined in the evaluation of a fractured tooth: whether the fracture directly in-

volves the pulp and whether the pulp has been secondarily involved by injury at the apex. Unfortunately many fractures occur in young individuals when the pulp spaces are large. One must remember, however, that the spaces are generally more open than in an adult, and the pulp is more vulnerable to injury. Many times it is possible to observe that the pulp is involved in a fracture; at other times direct involvement may be difficult, if not impossible, to detect. The presence of hemorrhage is good evidence of direct involvement. The final diagnosis of pulpitis may not be realized in some instances until the pulpal tissues have fully reacted to the injury. One can say that trauma will always produce pulp disease; either directly or indirectly; however, the response of the pulp may vary considerably. In general, the pulps of young teeth respond more favorably than do those of older teeth. Pulp testing immediately after a fracture has occurred would appear to serve no useful purpose since the full extent of pulpal damage will not have had time to manifest itself. Immediately after fracture, most teeth are hypersensitive to electric stimulation.

Vitality. All questionable teeth should be examined for vitality. The state of the pulp may be questioned because of the history given by the patient, radiographic signs of disease, discoloration of the teeth, hypersensitivity of the teeth, and the presence of referred pain. Routine testing of all the teeth should be a part of a thorough and complete examination. This is of particular value when the operator is able to compare several evaluations in a program of periodic examinations. Present methods of pulp testing do not allow any great degree of correlation between the diseased state of the pulp and the clinical evidence of pulp disease. However, when the operator understands the principles of pulp testing and uses standardized methods, a certain amount of useful correlative data may be found. Details of pulp testing by thermal

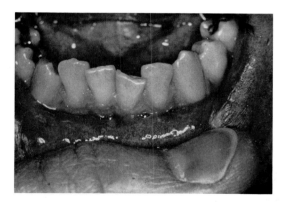

Fig. 9-12. *Teeth—altered form.* Fracture; no change in color of tooth.

and electric means can be found in Chapter 13.

Functional contours. The labial, lingual, and buccal curvatures at the cervical and are related to the protection of the periodontal tissues. When the teeth are in normal position and carious lesions have been properly restored, the convexity of the labial, lingual, and buccal surfaces prevents food from being forced into the gingival crevice and at the same time allows the food to pass over the gingiva to provide stimulation and massage of the gingival tissues. If these curvatures are too convex or too flat or are improperly placed in the dental restoration, normal cleansing action may be lost or food may be forced into the gingival crevices. The examiner should give careful attention to these factors since the health of the supporting structures is directly related to the form and function of the teeth. The apparent absence of disease

of the supporting structures does not necessarily indicate that poor form of the contact areas, marginal ridges, and deflection curves will not ultimately produce injury to the tissues.

Carious lesions. A periodic examination of the teeth is indicated for all individuals regardless of their age. The interval of time between examinations depends upon many factors such as rate of development of caries, lactobacillus count, sugar intake, age, and susceptibility to decay. New carious lesions may develop within 6 months or take as long as 1 or 2 years. Extension of the lesion may be rapid in some individuals, whereas in others it may be exceedingly slow. Rampant decay is seen most frequently in children and in older adults (Fig. 9-13). It is obvious that the periodic examination of individuals with a high caries rate should be more often than those with a low caries rate. This does not im-

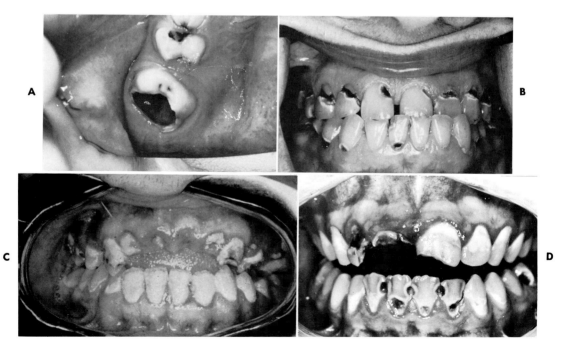

Fig. 9-13. *Teeth—caries.* **A,** Caries of primary teeth. **B,** Rampant caries. **C,** Extensive caries in hemophiliac. **D,** Postirradiation caries.

ply that the rate will be constant; it may increase. It may also be reduced by natural or acquired preventive measures. The evaluation of carious activity can be accomplished by caries activity tests (Chapter 13). In many individuals certain areas of the mouth appear to be more susceptible to decay than others. This may be caused by unknown factors or by acquired factors such as exposure of the cementum, improper extension of restorations for prevention of decay, or malposed teeth. This does not imply that these affect the basic mechanism of dental decay; it does suggest that faulty developmental grooves, overhanging margins, and rough cementum are much more prone to the deposition and maintenance of bacterial plaques than areas that are naturally more self-cleansing or can be reached by home-care methods. All the factors are important in the initiation of dental caries, especially if the sugar intake and lactobacillus count is high. Periodic examinations of the teeth should be based on the need of each individual. All individuals should be examined at least once a year or more often not only for carious lesions, but also for all the other abnormalities that may occur in the oral cavity and contiguous structures.

Carious lesions develop frequently in the pits, fissures, and developmental grooves of the occlusal surfaces of the teeth and in the non–self-cleansing areas such as the interproximal surfaces at or near the contact areas. Areas less commonly affected initially are the buccal, labial, and lingual surfaces, which are generally considered to be self-cleansing areas. Not infrequently, carious lesions may extend to these areas or be initiated in buccal developmental grooves and in the labiocervical and buccocervical surfaces adjacent to the gingival margins. Occasionally carious lesions may initiate in the lingual cervical surfaces of the molar teeth.

Special attention should be given not only to susceptible regions of dental decay, but also to all the tooth surfaces. Those areas that are considered to be non–self-cleansing and the margins of proximal restorations are difficult to assess without the aid of radiographs. The examiner should carry out his clinical examination and utilize dental radiographs. The radiographs are of special value in locating recurrent decay, occlusal caries, and proximal carious lesions. It must be emphasized that clinical examination of the teeth with a mouth mirror and explorer only or by radiographs alone is never sufficiently accurate.

The examination should be done by combining clinical exploration and radiographs. The use of posterior bite-wing films alone cannot be considered to be more effective than exploration, nor can exploration alone be considered more effective than the use of posterior bite-wings since both methods of examination have inherent weaknesses that the examiner must take into consideration. It is not a question of which method of examination is better or which one may be omitted but a matter of using both to their fullest extent for the most effective demonstration of carious lesions. The diagnosis of recurrent proximal caries by radiograph may be difficult in the presence of restorations that hide carious lesions because of the angulation of the central ray at the time the radiographs are taken or because of the location of the caries within the boundaries of the margins of the restoration. Although the posterior bite-wing tends to eliminate much of this error, inaccuracies in positioning of the central ray are frequent. Obviously recurrent caries lying on the buccal or lingual aspect of the restoration may be completely obliterated by the shadow cast by the restoration. There can be no question that combined radiographic and visual inspection and exploration for occlusal decay are superior to the use of radiographic methods of examination alone.

The accuracy of both the clinical and radiographic examinations is limited to some extent by the form and position of the teeth. Those teeth that present large convex approximating surfaces are easier to examine clinically and radiographically than those that present flat approximating surfaces. Broad contact areas in the mandibular bicuspid and maxillary molar regions are especially troublesome at times in the radiographic examination because it is difficult to take radiographs with the central ray exactly parallel to the proximal surfaces of these teeth so that no superimpositioning of the proximal surfaces occurs. The clinical examination may also be complicated because of the difficulty in gaining access to these contact areas with an explorer. The clinical examination may be more effective in these instances especially where separation of the teeth will allow entrance of an explorer tine into the area in question. Thus, the detection of early carious lesions of the contact areas may present difficulties even when both clinical and radiographic examination methods are used.

Even though a radiographic examination tends to be more effective in detecting initial carious lesions of the proximal contact areas, clinical exploration and separation of the teeth may be necessary to remove any question of doubt regarding the presence of recurrent lesions.

An incipient lesion first appears clinically as an opaque white spot that presents a rough surface to the explorer; it may not be sufficiently advanced to cause the exploring tine to catch or hang. When the convexity of the contact area is great and the central x-ray is parallel to its surface, an initial lesion of the proximal surface may appear radiographically to be slightly roughened or etched. With further advance of the lesion, perforation of the enamel can be seen radiographically; clinically the enamel shows discoloration, and upon pressure the exploring tine hangs in the opening of the lesion. Careful consideration of the interproximal surfaces of the teeth should include not only the contact

areas, but also the cervical areas above and below the gingival margin. Not infrequently the initial lesion is on the labiocervical or buccocervical surfaces of the teeth and is manifested as a chalky white area of decalcification that spreads from this area to the proximal and subgingival surfaces of the teeth. Careful attention should be given to this type of carious lesion, especially around the distal, buccal, and proximal surfaces of the teeth.

All restorations should be carefully inspected for secondary or recurrent carious lesions by clinical and radiographic examination. Open margins, overhanging margins, and broken restorations that are found on clinical examination should alert the examiner to the presence of caries, which may not be found on clinical examination alone. The radiographs should be studied in detail, and when necessary new radiographs using a different angulation should be taken. The principles of radiographic interpretation of dental caries is given in Chapter 12.

The examination for carious lesions may require the use of different explorers to adequately examine all the surfaces of a tooth. Those shown in Fig. 9-14 may be used; however, other types may be more desir-

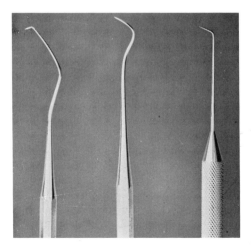

Fig. 9-14. *Explorers for examination of teeth.*

able for some examiners. The main requirements are that the explorer be sharp and be suited to the area to be examined.

The examination should be systematic and include both clinical and radiographic methods. It should begin at a specific location and proceed systematically tooth by tooth throughout the whole mouth and should be made with the aid of a mouth mirror and a fine sharp explorer (Fig. 9-15). The field of observation should be dry and well illuminated. Special attention should be given to variations in shade or color of the enamel and changes in its

texture and hardness; these are significantly changed in the presence of dental decay. The initial lesion of dental decay is generally seen as an opaque or white spot. This area may later become pigmented or stained.

Unless the explorer is fine and sharp, many areas of occlusal decay may be overlooked. Use of posterior bite-wing radiographs will enhance the yield of carious lesions. Manipulation of the explorer and sufficient pressure to push the exploring tine into soft decayed tooth structure will result in a "hang" or "catch" (Fig. 9-16).

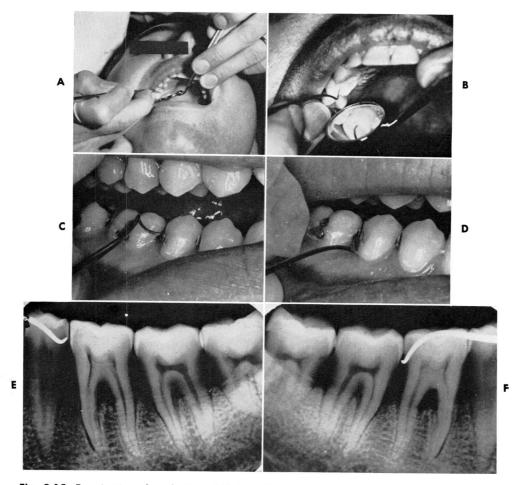

Fig. 9-15. *Examination of teeth.* **A** and **B,** Use of mirror and explorer. **C** to **F,** Exploration for interproximal caries.

The examination should begin with a specific tooth and proceed systematically throughout the arches. All surfaces of a tooth should be examined completely before proceeding to the next tooth. The examination may begin at the occlusal surfaces, proceed to the proximal surfaces, and then proceed to the labial and lingual surfaces.

No examination of the teeth can be considered to be thorough without a complete examination of all the pits, grooves, and fissures that are vulnerable to decay. This is especially true in children, since a significant percentage of the first permanent molars are lost 6 months after eruption and an even greater percentage may be lost before the age of 12 years. Even in the adult a large percentage is lost before the age of 25 years. In effect, the chance of decay occurring in pits, grooves, and fissures is significantly probable. It must be remembered that teeth in fluoride areas will show a significant number of defects in the occlusal developmental grooves. These should not be mistaken for carious

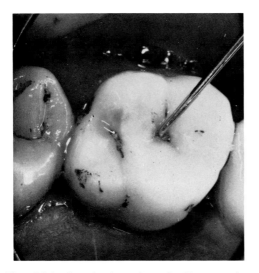

Fig. 9-16. *Examination of teeth.* Mirror and explorer; pit and fissure caries; explorer caught in the carious lesion.

lesions. Special attention should be given to mesial and distal occlusal pits and grooves and to the lingual groove of the maxillary permanent molars; their depth, overhanging edges, and inaccessibility to toothbrushing make them ideal places for the initiation of decay. Similar defects may be present in the occlusal buccal grooves of the mandibular permanent molars as well as in the bicuspids. Careful consideration should also be given the lingual pits in the cingulum area of the maxillary central and lateral incisors. Frequently very deep pits occur on the lateral incisors in this area and can be fully evaluated only with radiographs. The frequency of occurrence of deep pits on the maxillary lateral incisors and cuspids and their relationship to dens in dente are well known.

Gross occlusal decay may be present without obvious clinical signs; therefore, the use of radiographs is necessary for an evaluation of the extent of decay.

The proximal surfaces should be examined next. Since initial decay here may be difficult to detect with only an explorer, radiographs should also be used. The determination of recurrent decay around the margins of restorations requires the use of both explorer and radiographs. The margins of restorations should be explored with a No. 3 or No. 17 explorer to determine the presence of open margins, soft tooth structure, and overhanging margins. The extent of the carious lesion can most generally be determined from the radiographs. In many instances, however, exploration is the only method possible. The removal of calculus and debris is essential before an adequate diagnosis can be made. In some instances gingival packs may be necessary before the evaluation can be made successfully. In rare instances a separation may be required to adequately probe the gingival margins of a restoration. This is true when access is limited and the radiographs do not give conclusive evidence of an open margin. Hypersensitive cervical areas are not in themselves evidence of dental decay. Resorption of the tooth rarely occurs externally or in conjunction with internal resorption. These areas appear to be dental decay radiographically; however, exploration will reveal their true nature. These areas are filled with soft tissue, and the margins are generally firm and hard. This is in contradistinction to carious lesions whose margins and centers are soft.

Examination of the labial, buccal, and linguocervical surfaces is best accomplished wth a No. 3 explorer. It is imperative that the examiner be able to determine the location of the cementoenamel junction. Changes in the texture and hardness of the cementum as compared to the enamel are sometimes confusing to the dental student. This is especially true where recession of the free gingival margin has exposed the cementum to fluids and stains. Cementum so exposed tends to become macerated, soft, and darkly stained. It is not infrequent that this condition is mistaken for dental caries. When decay involves both the cementum and the enamel and the cementum is soft from exposure to the fluids of the oral cavity, the extent of the decay may be difficult to determine without careful attention to the difference between texture and softness of decay and cementum. Smoothing of the surface with periodontal

files may serve to facilitate delineation of the lesion. Opaque and white areas of decalcification on the cervical areas of the molar teeth are frequently mistaken for calculus by dental students. These areas generally follow the line of the free gingival margin and may extend around to distal and mesial surfaces of the teeth involved. The ability to penetrate this area with an explorer generally serves to differentiate decalcification from calculus. In addition, repeated scaling has little effect on removing it, and the curvature of the tooth indicates that the opaque area is a part of the tooth structure.

Contact relationship. Dental floss should be used to determine the tightness of contact areas throughout the mouth. It should be unwaxed and fine enough to pass between the proximal contact without undue pressure (Fig. 9-17). Thick, flat, and waxed dental tape, which is suitable for interproximal cleaning, is not suitable for this test since it does not slide easily and its thickness does not permit an adequate evaluation of the proper contact relationship. Thin round unwaxed nylon has the optimum characteristics for delicate manipulation of the floss between the contact areas. Dental floss should pass through the contact area without being torn or shredded. Tearing or shredding of the tape or obstruction of its

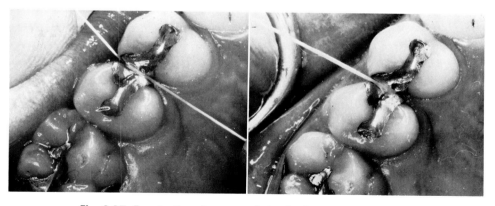

Fig. 9-17. *Examination of contact relationship* **by use of dental floss.**

passage is usually indicative of dental caries or overhanging dental restorations. With radiographs as a guide, overhanging cervical margins of dental restorations should be examined with the tine of a sharp explorer. Careful examination of this area will aid in determining whether these margins can be recontoured or whether the whole restoration must be replaced. Both clinical examination and radiographic examination of the cervical areas of restorations may be necessary for complete evaluation of overhanging margins of restorations.

An improper contact relation is indicated when the floss can be pulled easily through the contact areas. Also, the gingival tissues will show evidence of food impaction—detachment, enlargement, and alteration of normal color. They will also show evidence of disease if contact areas are incorrectly placed, if marginal ridges are faulty, and if a restoration encroaches upon the interproximal spaces. Normally, the form and position of the mesial and distal marginal ridges and the interproximal contact areas of the teeth prevent food from being driven between the teeth. When the marginal

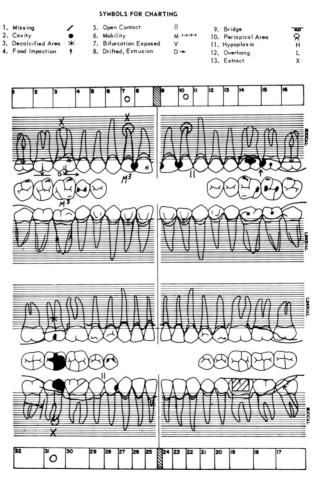

SYMBOLS FOR CHARTING

1. Missing	╱	5. Open Contact	‖	9. Bridge		
2. Cavity	●	6. Mobility	M 1-2-3-4	10. Periapical Area	Q	
3. Decalcified Area	✳	7. Bifurcation Exposed	V	11. Hypoplasia	H	
4. Food Impaction	✝	8. Drifted, Extrusion	D→	12. Overhang	L	
				13. Extract	X	

Fig. 9-18. *Examination of teeth.* Typical chart showing periodontal disease and dental caries. (See also Fig. 9-20 for work sheet.)

ridges and the contact areas are lost from decay or are improperly placed in restoration, food impactions usually occur. Unfavorable alterations of the interproximal space by dental restoration, abnormal tooth positions, and disease are common causes of gingival disturbances.

The examiner should inspect the contact area from the occlusal and incisal surfaces of the teeth and at the same time observe the gingival tissue. Observation of the interdental papillae from the occlusal and incisal views will aid considerably in assessing the health of these tissues in relation to

the contact area, marginal ridges, and lingual, labial, and buccal curvatures of the teeth.

Charting. Charting of teeth may be accomplished by the use of a printed form (Fig. 9-18). This form has been prepared to be used for both periodontal and dental findings. Charting is a useful procedure, since any part of the derived data can be readily seen in relation to the whole picture. The form presented here is only one of the many that might be used. However, most other charting forms do not include provisions for both periodontal and dental

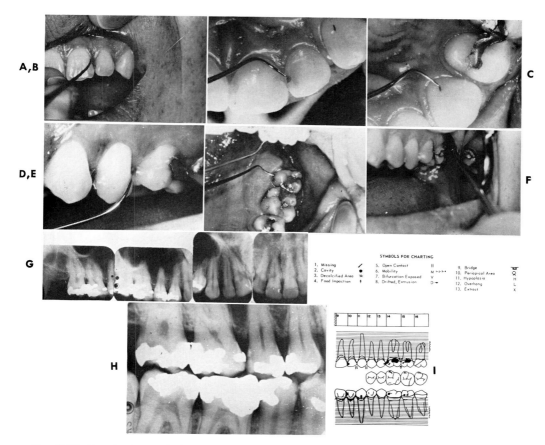

Fig. 9-19. *Examination and charting of teeth.* **A** to **F,** Clinical examination of the teeth in one quadrant of the mouth. **G** and **H,** Corresponding radiographic examination of the same quadrant. **I,** Completed dental chart of the corresponding quadrant showing clinical and radiographic findings.

findings. Combining the results of the examination into a single form greatly enhances the correlation between the teeth and the supporting structures.

The charting of carious lesions, decalcification, and recurrent decay may be accomplished first by clinical examination, with the aid of a mouth mirror and explorer. An example of the examination and charting procedure is given in Fig. 9-19. The results of the clinical examination may be indicated on the chart first. The radiographs should also be examined and the charting completed. The periodontal examination in the example has already been completed. For clarity, carious lesions, decalcified areas, and areas of recurrent decay are first outlined only; those findings derived from the radiographic examination are indicated by blocked-out areas. In the completed chart all initial recurrent carious lesions are indicated by blocked-out areas.

In addition to the chart, a work sheet may be utilized for the listing of carious lesions and the preparation of a tentative treatment plan (Fig. 9-20). One system of indicating a particular tooth is to number the permanent teeth from 1 to 32. Starting with the maxillary right third molar as 1, one numbers the teeth consecutively around the arch to the maxillary left third molar, which is numbered 16. Then dropping down to the mandibular left third molar, which is numbered 17, one gives the teeth consecutive numbers to the mandibular right third molar, which is numbered 32. The primary teeth are lettered in the same sequence using A through T. Another system for symbolic designation of teeth is recommended by the Committee on Nomenclature of the American Dental Association. This plan divides the arches into four quadrants. Each arch is divided into halves by a median plane, and each arch

WORK SHEET

	RADIOGRAPHIC FINDINGS		ORAL FINDINGS	SUMMATION	TREATMENT PLAN
	PBW	FM			
1.					PERIODONTICS
2.					
3.					OPERATIVE
4.			5	4^5	10 E (ENDO.)
5.					15^{1-5} A
6.					15^3 A
7.		1	1-4	7^1 7^4	15^4 A
8.		2	2	8^2	15^6 A
9.		1-2	1-2	9^1 9^2	14^{2-6} A
10.		1	1-4	10^1 10^4	14^3 A
11.					14^4 A
12.					9^1 S
13.					9^2 S
14.	2		3-4-6	14^{2-6} 14^3 14^4	10^{1-4} G (D)
15.	1		3-4-5-6	15^{1-5} 15^3 15^4 15^6	28^{1-5} G (D)
16.					28^6 F
17.					SPLINT
18.					29
19.					
20.					SURGERY
21.					EXTRACT
22.					3,7,31,32
23.					
24.					
25.					PROSTHETICS
26.					BRIDGE
27.					2-4, 6-8
28.	1		5-6	28^{1-5} 28^6	PART. DENT.
29.					CLASS II
30.					
31.	1		5-4	31^{1-5-4}	
32.					

Fig. 9-20. *Examination of teeth.* Treatment plan work sheet. *PBW,* Posterior bite-wings; *FM,* full mouth radiographs. (See also Fig. 9-18 for charting.)

is separated from the other by a horizontal plane. In the permanent dentition, numbering starts with the central incisor on each side of the midline and proceeds with the sequence of 1 through 8. The teeth of the primary dentition are designated by the letters A through E. Thus the symbol $\overline{|6}$ would indicate the mandibular left sixth-year molar and $6|$ would indicate the maxillary right sixth-year molar. The symbol $\overline{|C}$ would indicate the primary mandibular left cuspid and $C|$ the primary maxillary right cuspid. Both this plan and the preceding plan for the symbolic designation of teeth have advantages and disadvantages.

Numbering the teeth from 1 through 32 eliminates the necessity of using brackets and can be used to indicate various surfaces of the teeth involved in dental decay. The surfaces are numbered from 1 through 6; these numbers are added as superscripts to the number of the tooth; for example, carious lesions involving all the surfaces of the maxillary right third molar would be indicated by the symbol $32^{1\text{-}2\text{-}3\text{-}4\text{-}5\text{-}6}$. The surfaces are numbered as follows: 1, mesial; 2, distal; 3, labial or buccal; 4, lingual; 5, occlusal; and 6, distal fossae and pits of the mandibular first bicuspids and the maxillary molars. Thus a carious lesion of the mesial surfaces of the maxillary right central incisor would be indicated by 8^1. Lesions present on the mesial, distal, and occlusal surfaces of the mandibular right second permanent molar would be indicated by $31^{1\text{-}2\text{-}5}$. A lesion involving only the buccal surface of the mandibular left cuspid would be indicated by 22^3.

A temporary work sheet may be used to facilitate the clinical examination and charting procedure. It should not take the place of charting but should be used for summation and treatment planning while the patient is present. It can then be utilized for a more elaborate write-up and treatment plan when the patient is not present. The work sheet shown in Fig. 9-20 is arranged in five columns. The number of the tooth is given at the extreme left. Under radiographic findings and oral findings, only the surfaces involved by carious lesions are listed. In the summation column the number of the tooth is repeated and the surfaces involved are given. The treatment plan column is merely an outline of the treatment to be rendered and the type of restorative material to be used. Letter abbreviations to indicate the restorative material are used as follows: S, silicate; A, amalgam; G, gold; G (D), gold direct; G (I), gold, indirect; F, gold foil; E, emergency treatment.

REFERENCES

American Dental Association: Committee on Dental Education and Hospitals. Tooth numbering and radiograph mounting, Amer. Dent. Ass. Trans. **109**:247, 1968.

Black, A. D.: G. V. Black's work on operative dentistry with which his special dental pathology is combined. Vol. 1. The pathology of the hard tissues of the teeth; oral diagnosis, ed. 7, Chicago, 1936. Medico-Dental Publishing Co.

Committee on Nomenclature: Committee adopts official method for the symbolic designation of teeth, J.A.D.A. **34**:647. 1947.

Hals, E., and Olow, M.: Turner teeth, Odont. Tidskr. **66**:199-212, 1958.

Hazen, S. P., Chilton, N. W., and Mumma, R. D., Jr.: The problem of root caries. 1. Literature review and clinical description, J.A.D.A. **86**:137, 1973.

Jackson, D.: The clinical diagnosis of dental caries, Brit. Dent. J. **88**:207, 1950.

Mitchell, D. F., Standish, S. M., and East, T. B.: Oral diagnosis/oral medicine, Philadelphia, 1969, Lea & Febiger.

Pindborg, J. J.: Pathology of the dental hard tissues, Philadelphia, 1970, W. B. Saunders Co.

Robinson, H. B. G.: Abrasion, attrition, and erosion of teeth, Health Center J., Ohio State Univ. **3**:21, 1949.

Witkop, C. J.: Hereditary defects in enamel and dentin, Acta Genet. (Basel) **7**:236-239, 1957.

10

Examination of the occlusion

One of the most difficult aspects of the oral examination is the evaluation of the occlusion. An occlusal analysis must take into account changes in the occlusion related to growth and development as well as those changes related to extrinsic factors such as extractions, carious lesions, restorations, periodontal disease, and functional disturbances of the masticatory system. Functional disturbances are caused by disharmony between function and structure and include acute and chronic traumatic temporomandibular joint arthritis, altered mandibular mobility, joint sounds, discomfort, pain, muscle dysfunction, bruxism and excessive tooth wear, occlusal instability, and trauma from occlusion to the supporting structures. These disturbances are related to occlusal discrepancies, muscular dysfunction, and environmental or emotional stress.

Functional disturbances reflect a failure of the components of the masticatory system to adapt to structural and functional demands, either demands that are excessive for a normal system or those that become excessive because of the effects of accumulative disturbances, both functional and structural.

In the younger patient the diagnosis and interception or treatment of malocclusion may be of primary importance, whereas in the young adult and older patients the diagnosis and treatment of functional disturbances become the more likely problem to be dealt with in the practice of dentistry. Although occlusal problems are not dependent necessarily on age, the examination of occlusion procedures presented here are divided into the examination of the developing occlusion and the adult occlusion.

Developing occlusion

With the growth of dental specialties, such as pedodontics, orthodontics, and periodontics, the general practitioner has come to regard the recognition of malocclusion and periodontal disease as being in the private domain of these specialties. However, for a general practitioner to fulfill his responsibility in the field of preventive dentistry, he needs to recognize those changes that may be predisposing factors in dis-

eases of the mouth of the adult; he must also be able to recognize the initiation of disease in the child or adolescent so that effective preventive measures may be applied. This is not only true in operative dentistry and periodontics, but also in the field of orthodontics. Preventive dentistry as it relates to malocclusion is based upon the recognition and diagnosis of deviations from the normal pattern of growth and the recognition of factors that may predispose to malocclusion at a later time.

The examination suggested here is of a screening nature and should not be construed as a complete orthodontic examination, since this field of endeavor is outside the objective of this text. The development of occlusion is presented to provide the student and the general practitioner with certain basic landmarks and examination procedures for the early detection of occlusal disturbances. The orthodontic literature is replete with the basic principles of examination for the interception of malocclusion and for efficient and rational referral to an orthodontist. Although this type of examination is primarily screening in nature and is not intended to be a complete coverage of all the diagnostic procedures necessary for complete evaluation, it is hoped that it will alert the general practitioner and student to their responsibilities in the field of preventive dentistry, for example, the prevention and interception of disturbances of the developing occlusion.

The principles for the recognition of incipient malocclusion are based on a knowledge of the normal growth and development of the teeth, jaws, and face and of those etiologic factors that may produce malocclusion. The factors that influence the development of occlusion are genetic or environmental in nature. The latter may be local or systemic in origin. Inasmuch as the development of occlusion is based on genetic, dental, and muscle factors, it may be related to abnormalities in any or all of these. Thus, malocclusion may be skeletal, dental, or functional in origin, and the examination of the young patient should consist of an evaluation of these factors. The examination should begin with a complete history and an evaluation of the patient's past and present health. It has been well established that constitutional factors and systemic disease have an important effect upon general health and upon those tissues that are responsible for the development

and establishment of occlusion. It goes without saying that the general health of the patient must be appraised before an examination can be considered complete.

In addition to the information considered in Chapter 6 on the skull and facies, the examiner must also consider the form of the face as it relates to the occlusion. There is a close relationship between the development of occlusion and the develoment of the face. This is well known to the orthodontist, but the general practitioner has at times failed to fully appreciate this fact. This situation is not without foundation; the pattern of facial growth is complex and the determination of facial disharmony is not generally considered in the usual examination procedures used by the general practitioner.

The development of occlusion does not originate solely from processes in the mouth; it is also derived from the skeletal parts responsible for the development of the face. When a facial disharmony is present, it does not necessarily follow that there will be a disturbance in the development of the occlusion. However, there are certain alterations in the proportions of the face that are considered to be outside the range of normal; these alterations are quite likely to be associated with a disturbance in the development of the occlusion. Thus, when evaluating the occlusion, it is necessary to consider the facial form as well as the alveolar processes and the jaws.

Facial form analysis. An analysis of facial form will serve to appraise the harmony of growth and development of the facial skeleton as it relates to the support of the dentition. The examination should show the presence or absence of abnormal anteroposterior relationships and asymmetries of the dentofacial parts. It should also indicate to the examiner the possibility of a difference in the absolute size of the parts of the dentofacial complex and point out the variations in dental and occlusal relationships that have resulted from the combination of parts of abnormal size and form. It must be pointed out again that the facial form is not entirely dependent upon the facial skeleton; it is also dependent upon the teeth.

One of the difficulties that the general practitioner must face in his examination of a growing child is the fact that the facial form is an ever-changing pattern and that no clearly defined or static standard of dentofacial relationship exists. Thus, the concept of normality or the range of normal is difficult to visualize and even more difficult for the general practitioner to measure without the equipment and training necessary to utilize comprehensive gnathometric and cephalometric indexes of so-called normal relationships between the occlusion, face, and skull. However, it is possible for him to evaluate gross skeletal variations by direct observation of the facial form. He can learn much about the position of the teeth by observing the facial profile and the facial musculature. Though this type of examination fails to give the exact and precise results of a complete facial form analysis, it does keep the examiner from having to evaluate an occlusion on a purely intraoral basis without due regard for other dependent relationships.

The examiner should not base his entire evaluation of malocclusion on the relationship of the first permanent molars or the relationship of opposing arches, since the remainder of the face and muscles are often intimiately related to malocclusion. From a practical standpoint, the occlusion and dentofacial structures should be related to established planes of the face and skull; this relationship then can be used to grossly evaluate obvious variations from the normal. The planes that are used relate to the facial profile and to a division of the face into two equal parts. Abnormalities of the profile are related to the profile plane; abnormalities of asymmetry are related to the midsagittal plane.

An appraisal of the profile may be made by use of the Frankfort horizontal (eye-ear) plane and a plane perpendicular to the Frankfort plane that passes through the nasion, called the anterior facial plane (Fig. 10-1, *A*). An appraisal of facial symmetry may be made by using the midsagittal plane; this plane is perpendicular to a plane through the orbitale and vertically divides the face and head into two equal parts (Fig. 10-1, *B*).

By using these reference planes the examiner can determine the anteroposterior relationships between the dentofacial parts and also the presence of asymmetries of the dentofacial parts. This procedure serves to estimate the difference in size of one facial part as compared with another, to indicate angle variations between the maxillary occlusal and Frankfort planes, and to provide a plane of reference for the evaluation of inclinations of the anterior maxillary and mandibular teeth. Thus, the information may reveal whether the abnormality is symmetrical or asymmetrical, bilateral or unilateral, anterior or posterior; whether the conditions extends beyond the boundaries of the maxilla and mandible or both; or whether a deviation in the anteroposterior relationship involves the upper or lower teeth or both groups of teeth or other parts of the dentofacial structure.

Four points of reference may be used to evaluate changes in the anteroposterior relationship of the parts making up the facial profile. These can only be approximated in the living; however, their determination serves a useful purpose. The points of reference are skeletal areas whose placement provides the basis for the facial profile, and they must be visualized on soft tissues. They are the subspinale for the midfacial region—where the ala of the nose meets the cheek, the prostheon for the maxillary alveolar region, the infradentale for the mandibular alveolar region—deepest point of the mentolabial sulcus, and the pogonion for the chin point (Fig. 10-1, *C*). Relating these points to the facial profile serves to point out abnormal anteroposterior displacements of the midfacial region, the maxillary and mandibular alveolar denture bases, and the chin. In general, these points lie harmoniously along the facial profile plane; any different relationship should alert the examiner to abnormalities of facial form. Any of the parts of the face represented by the four reference points may be deviated or displaced in an anteroposterior direction relative to the profile plane. The area of deviation may indicate to the examiner where the disharmony of dentofacial form exists; for example, a positive posterior displacement of the chin point suggests retrognathism, an anterior displacement suggests prognathism. One must bear in mind that the displacement of the mandible may be skeletal, dental, or functional in origin. Thus, the points of reference should be observed when the mandible is at rest position, when the mandible is in centric rela-

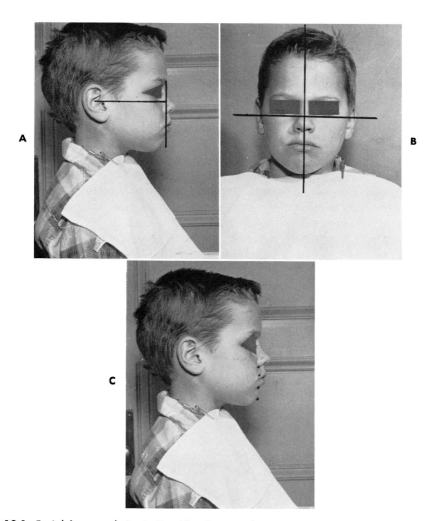

Fig. 10-1. *Facial form analysis.* **A,** Frankfort horizontal and anterior facial planes. **B,** Midsagittal plane. **C,** Displacement reference points; found by palpation. From top to bottom—subspinale, prostheon, infradentale, and pogonion.

tion, and when the teeth are in complete occlusion.

The relative size or mass of the maxilla and the mandible should be noted. This can be visualized as prominent, moderate, or reduced. The vertical proportions of the face should also be considered. Visual inspection of the space occupied by the nose, upper lip, lower lip, and chin while the lips are brought together lightly usually indicates that nasal height constitutes about 43 percent of the vertical height while the region below constitutes 57 percent (Dempster). Proportionate lengths of the body and ramus of the mandible should also be evaluated.

An estimate of the angles of the mandible, the angle between the maxillary occlusal and Frankfort planes, and the angle of inclination of the maxillary and mandibular teeth should be made. In children 8 to 12 years of age, the angle made by the base of the mandible and the ascending ramus should be an obtuse angle of about 140 degrees (McCoy). This is not a fixed value and only represents the average. Actual angular measurements need not be made; a general appraisal of the angle at the gonion is all that is necessary. Extreme variations are not difficult to observe. The inclination of the mandibular and maxillary anterior teeth should be approximately parallel with the median and facial profile planes. The angulation of the maxillary occlusal plane with reference to the Frankfort horizontal plane should be noted. Although this angle is generally in the region of 12 degrees, observations need only indicate that the angle is reduced, normal, or increased.

Asymmetries of the frontal facial form are best considered relative to the midsagittal plane. Although features tend to be associated with common patterns, the general proportions of the facial mass are symmetrical. A systematic comparison of definite areas should be carried out, for example, frontal bones, orbital regions, malar re-

gions, maxillary region, and mandibular region.

Some generalities of dentofacial form may alert the examiner to analyze the facial form. For instance, some facial features appear to be associated very frequently with certain types of malocclusion such as the adenoid facies associated with habitual mouth breathing. The typical adenoid facies is characterized by a thin face, pinched nose, high arched palate, and often retrognathia. The typical mouth breather shows a short upper lip and a lower lip that rests between the maxillary and the mandibular incisors. The maxillary incisors are frequently in labioversion and the mandibular incisors in linguoversion. In other instances, where the maxillary incisor teeth are in linguoversion to the mandibular incisors, the lower lip may be unusually prominent and the upper lip underdeveloped. The position and form of the lips are greatly influenced by the teeth and by breathing. It is also true that lip habits can produce changes in the position of the teeth and that abnormalities of occlusion can affect the position of the lips. One must remember that the position of the lips is directly related to the musculature and directly or indirectly related to the position of the teeth. In some instances the examiner may be alerted to the possibility of retrognathism by the presence of a rather pronounced mentolabial sulcus; this finding is not uncommon in this type of malocclusion. The presence of unusual facial forms generally referred to as hatchet face, flat face, mouse face, and dish face are obvoius indications for an analysis of the facial form.

It is not necessary to take cephalograms or photographs to generally appraise the form of the facial skeletal structures. The structures can be visualized in relation to the profile and midsagittal plane by holding up a piece of cardboard or other suitable material to the patient's face in approximate alignment with the reference landmarks (Fig. 10-2). The examiner should inspect the approximate placement of the chin point, the mandibular alveolar point, the maxillary alveolar point, and the midfacial region individually. Palpation of these bony landmarks may be necessary while the examiner holds the reference plane up to the face to determine their location. This is especially true if the lips,

nose, and soft tissues are large in relation to the skeletal structures. In general, these reference landmarks lie along the facial profile plane in the average face. The degree of anterior or posterior displacement of each area (midfacial, maxillary alveolar, mandibular alveolar, and the chin) should be noted. Generally, the examiner expresses

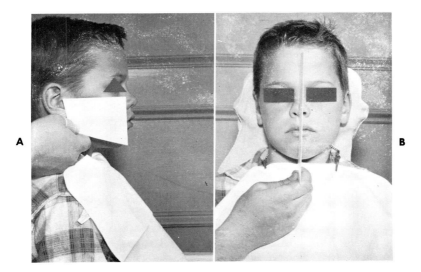

Fig. 10-2. *Facial form analysis.* **A,** Clinical method of determining the facial angle and alignment of the reference landmarks of the anterior facial plane. **B,** Checking symmetry by use of midsagittal plane.

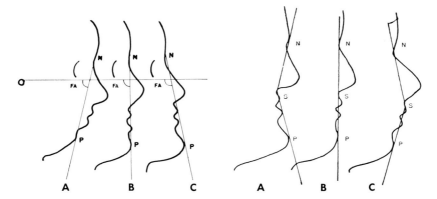

Fig. 10-3. *Facial form analysis.* **Left:** Variations in facial relationships by reference to the facial angle *(FA).* **A,** Retrognathic type of face. **B,** Straight or orthognathic face. **C,** Prognathic face, **Right:** Variations in facial relationships by reference to angle of convexity *(S).* **A,** Dish or concave face. **B,** Straight face. **C,** Hatchet or convex face. (After Downs.)

his findings of a variation in facial relationships by a reference to the facial angle and to the angle of convexity (Fig. 10-3). The facial angle is an expression of anteroposterior displacement of the chin. It is determined by a gross appraisal of the angle made by the Frankfort and facial planes. A facial angle of less than 90 degrees is suggestive of a retrognathic or Class II type of face; a right angle, an orthognathic or Class I type of face; an angle slightly greater than 90 degrees, a mesognathic face; and a wide obtuse angle, a prognathic or Class III type of face (Downs). The angle of convexity is formed by the intersection of a line drawn from the nasion to the nasospinale and a line drawn from the pogonion to the nasospinale. The angle formed by these two intersecting lines is a measure of the anteroposterior displacement of the maxillary part of the fact to the total profile. As indicated in Fig. 10-3, the angle made by these intersecting lines may be concave (dish face), straight, or convex (hatchet face).

The angular relationship of the occlusal and Frankfort planes is generally related to the facial angle. The cant of the occlusal plane is relatively steep in retrognathism and approaches parallelism in severe prognathism.

The inspection of the facial form for skeletal asymmetry may be accomplished by observation of both sides of the face when the piece of cardboard is placed in the midsagittal plane (Fig. 10-2). Palpation of the skeletal structures may be necessary to differentiate between soft tissue, muscle, and skeletal asymmetry. As previously mentioned, asymmetry may be muscular, soft tissue, or skeletal in nature, and these may be genetic, developmental, or pathologic in origin. The degree of asymmetry should be indicated in the same terms used previously—small, moderate, and wide. The examination of the facial form in the midsagittal planes should be made while the patient is closing his teeth together and

when the teeth are in occlusion. A deviation from the midline of the maxillary incisors may indicate a skeletal asymmetry or a malposition of the teeth in the arch. Asymmetry of the midline of the mandibular central incisors may indicate malposition of the incisors, asymmetry of the mandibular arch, or functional displacement of the mandible. It must also be remembered that an abnormal anteroposterior relationship of the mandible may be on a functional basis; for example, the mandible may be prevented from closing in the normal anteroposterior relationship because of premature contacts or occlusal interference. It is not uncommon to find what appears to be mandibular prognathism when the teeth are together yet find that the anteroposterior relationship is normal when the jaws are separated in centric relation.

Standardization of the relationships between facial structures cannot be dogmatized even with comprehensive methods of analysis. The evaluation of the findings of the type of facial form analysis presented here is based on the examiner's visual judgment and a sense of facial harmony. Thus, in most instances, the general practitioner is well equipped to detect moderate to severe abnormalities of the facial skeleton and relate them to malocclusion.

After the examiner has completed his analysis of the facial form, he will have some idea of the presence or absence of unfavorable or disharmonious bone growth and how it may relate to the development of the occlusion. In general his findings of disharmony will be those of skeletal displacement or asymmetry of the face. (Skeletal displacement is a term used to mean the malposition or maldevelopment of the arches.) Insufficient bony support for the size of the teeth may also be noted. It was previously stated that the development of malocclusion is related not only to skeletal development, but also to dental development. Therefore, to understand all the factors that may cause abnormal development of occlusion, the examiner needs to know something about the normal development of occlusion.

The development of occlusion is related to the harmonious development of the facial skeleton and to the functional harmony of the teeth, jaws, and musculature. Thus, while the development is in process, the examination of the patient for disturbances in this process must be related to the signs of disharmony or abnormality in all of the areas responsible for the development of the occlusion. The following presentation of the development of the occlusion is related to the position of the teeth in a more or less "ideal" arrangement for certain arbitrary set stages of occlusal development. These stages are related to the completion of the primary dentition, the mixed dentition, the occlusion of the permanent teeth in young adults, and a fourth stage, which takes into consideration the changes in occlusion that result from wear. The descriptions of so-called ideal or normal occlusions for any particular stage cannot be considered absolute. This arbitrary categorization is only of value when the examiner is able to visualize what variations of occlusion may exist and still be within the range of normal. Thus, the clinician should strive to use his knowledge of the development of occlusion and his knowledge of those factors that may alter the normal development of occlusion rather than to base his evaluation of occlusion on an ideal ararngement of the teeth.

Primary dentition analysis. The development of the primary occlusion is usually completed between the third and fifth year of life; it is generally considered to be more stable and to show fewer anomalies than either the mixed or permanent dentitions. It does, however, show a wide range of normal variation. Apparently there are no essential change in the occlusion once an interdigitation of the primary teeth has occurred. Growth in the height of the alveolar process and sagittal growth distal to the

dentition continues to occur. Most primary dentitions show a generalized spacing of the anterior teeth, and there may be wide spaces mesial to the maxillary cuspids and distal to the mandibular cuspids. Spacing is normal and does not change, that is, spaces do not close. An absence of spacing is normal, and spaces do no occur with advancing age.

The shape of the arch is usually ovoid. The length of the arch, from the distal surface of the second primary molar around to the distal surface of the opposite second primary molar, decreases after the eruption of the second primary molars. This decrease continues until the completion of the primary dentition and is caused by the mesial migration of the maxillary and mandibular second primary molars. The termination of the occlusion at the posterior surfaces of the second primary molars usually forms a straight terminal plane—vertical line tangent to the distal surfaces of second primary molars. Deformity of the facial skeleton, premature interproximal cavities, and sucking habits may cause the premature development of a terminal plane with a distal step. In other instances the anteroposterior occlusal relationship may be normal as manifested by a symmetrical midline and a satisfactory maxillary and mandibular cuspid position. However, a straight terminal plane is a more favorable condition for the establishment of the occlusal relationship of the first permanent molars. Occlusal irregularities of the primary dentition may result from severe sucking habits and from space closure associated with the premature loss of primary teeth.

In general, the primary dentition is characterized by a straight axial inclination of the incisors with an almost end-to-end relationship of these teeth. The mandibular teeth occlude one cusp anteriorly to the corresponding tooth in the maxilla. Deviations from this pattern are suggestive of malocclusion. In addition to an evaluation of the characteristics of the normal primary dentition, the examiner should search for all the local causes capable of bringing about irregularities of occlusion.

Due consideration should be given the prevention of malocclusion arising from neglect of the primary teeth and their early loss, from prolonged retention of the primary teeth, and from the presence of severe sucking and other oral habits. The premature loss of primary teeth from dental neglect and interproximal decay is quite likely to cause a loss of arch length with a consequent tendency for crowding of the permanent teeth. Retention of the primary teeth beyond their normal period of exfoliation may cause their permanent successors to erupt in an abnormal position. If a child persists in thumb sucking, an anterior open-bite usually results. In the presence of an abnormal anteroposterior relationship of the occlusion, severe malocclusion of the permanent dentition may result; however, where the anteroposterior relationship is normal, an open-bite of this type may be self-correcting, provided that the child ceases his severe sucking habit by the age of 4 years.

Mixed dentition analysis. The first permanent molars erupt at 6 to 7 years of age and represent the beginning of mixed dentition. The mandibular incisors usually follow the sixth-year molars and are frequently noted to be in a crowded and rotated position. At this age such crowding is not considered to be abnormal but may be abnormal in those instances where tooth eruption has preceded the growth of the jaw (dental age exceeds skeletal age). The crowding may be self-correcting because vertical growth of the alveolar processes up to the age of 9 or 10 years will usually allow for their proper positioning.

The first permanent molars may frequently erupt in a cusp-to-cusp relationship when there is no spacing in the primary arches and the terminal plane is straight. This molar relationship is of no significance, provided that the mandibular second pri-

mary molar is shed prior to the maxillary second primary molar so that a mesial shift shift (late mesial shift) of the lower permanent molar may take place (Baume). In the presence of generalized spacing of the primary arches the mandibular first permanent molar should erupt before the maxillary first molar to prevent the formation of unfavorable distal step in the terminal plane. If the maxillary first permanent molar erupts first, a distal step is established, and the mandibular first permanent molar may become locked in distal occlusion.

It has been shown by Lo and Moyers that a certain sequence of eruption is most favorable to the development of a normal occlusion. This sequence in the maxilla and mandible is shown in Fig. 10-4. In the maxillary arch the first molar (6) is the first to erupt, the central incisor (1) is second, the lateral incisor (2) is third, the first bicuspid (4) is fourth, the second bicuspid (5) is fifth, the cuspid (3) is sixth, and the second molar (7) is seventh. In the mandibular arch the first molar (6) is first to erupt, the central incisor (1) is second, the lateral incisor (2) is third, the cuspid (3) is fourth, the first bicuspid (4) is fifth, the second bicuspid (5) is sixth, and the second molar (7) is seventh.

Certain other sequences of eruption have

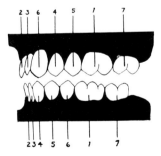

Fig. 10-4. *Mixed dentition analysis.* Most favorable sequence of eruption. Numbers indicate numerical order of sequence of eruption. (After Lo and Moyers.)

been found to be associated with an unfavorable development of the occlusion. In the maxilla the early eruption of the premolars or cuspid often results in Class II molar relationships. The most unfavorable sequence in the mandible is associated with the late eruption of the cuspid or the early eruption of the second molar. There appears to be a significant tendency for a Class II molar relationship to result when the maxillary molars erupt before the mandibular molars. Any clinical examination of the primary dentition cannot be considered complete without a radiographic study of the sequence of eruption. A study of radiographs will be of considerable aid in studying the sequence of eruption and anticipating the development of malocclusion. It should be noted, however, that a prediction of malocclusion based on the sequence of eruption without a consideration of such factors as endocrine disturbances, familial tendencies, density of bone, scar tissue, and keratinization of the epithelium may lead to an incorrect anticipation of occlusal irregularities.

Between the ages of 6 and 8, the incisors in the anterior segments of the mouth begin to erupt into occlusion. The lower central incisors erupt first and then the lower lateral. In the absence of retained primary incisors, these teeth move labially from the lingual aspect of the jaw. The primary incisors should be shed before the eruption of the permanent incisors so that the latter do not erupt lingual to the deciduous incisors. In general where there is no spacing in the primary dentition, the permanent mandibular lateral incisors tend to become crowded. Although there is some lateral displacement of the deciduous cuspids to compensate for simple crowding, there will be no displacement when the mandibular lateral incisors erupt lingually and are rotated. Excessive crowding of the lower central incisors can produce abnormal lateral displacement of the primary cuspids and cause them to be lost prematurely or produce a

functional retraction of the mandible with distal occlusion of the arches to utilize the increased intercanine width in the lower arch.

Careful attention should be given at this time to the premature loss of primary cuspids since their loss may prevent the normal rate of growth and development of the anterior segment of the jaw. The eruption of the maxillary central incisors occurs just after eruption of the mandibular central incisors. The permanent maxillary incisors erupt in a more labial inclination than the almost vertically positioned primary teeth. This inclination accompanied by spacing of the teeth is often considered by anxious parents to be a sign of serious malocclusion. However, this appearance is within the range of normal, and, if significant space is available, the teeth will erupt in their normal positions provided that no abnormal oral habits are present.

Not infrequently a diastema is seen between the maxillary central incisors, and the incisors will exhibit some distal inclination. This should not be considered abnormal unless the opening is extreme and interferes with the normal eruption of the lateral incisors. Closure of this space usually occurs in conjunction with the eruption of the permanent cuspids about the twelfth year. The maxillary lateral incisors may show some tendency for labioversion because of the approximation of the roots of the lateral incisors with the crowns of the erupting cuspids. However, as the cuspids erupt, their relationship with the lateral incisors changes and allows the latter to assume a more favorable position.

The development of the lateral segments of the mouth occurs between the ages of 9 and 12 years. At this time the sequence of eruption, the size of the teeth, and a normal retention of the primary cuspids and second molars are of considerable importance. As indicated previously, the most favorable sequence of eruption in the lateral segment of the mandible is cuspid, first bicuspid, second bicuspid, and then the second molar (provided that the sixth-year molars and the lateral and central incisors have already erupted). The eruption of the mandibular cuspids first tends to maintain a normal arch length and prevent a deep overbite, which is usually associated with the lingual collapse of the anterior segments. If the mandibular first bicuspid erupts before the cuspid, there is a tendency for the bicuspid to be tipped mesially, thereby preventing the cuspid from erupting normally. This occurs not infrequently when the primary cuspid is lost prematurely. If the mandibular second permanent molar erupts before the second bicuspid, there tends to be a loss of arch length and a mesial drift of the first molar, which blocks the second bicuspid out of its normal eruption position. This may also occur with the premature loss of the mandibular second primary molar although a certain amount of mesial drift is to be expected because of a favorable leeway space that usually exists as a result of the difference in tooth size between primary dentition and permanent dentition in this area. However, it is important that excessive mesial migration of the first permanent molar be prevented and sufficient space maintained to allow for the permanent successors. Thus, there must be sufficient space available for the size of the teeth that are to erupt; otherwise crowding and malocclusion will result.

Fortunately the examiner can predict the sum of the width of the cuspid, bicuspid, and second bicuspid within certain limits of probability by measuring the widths of the lower incisors. Thus, the sum of the widths of the four incisors is related to the sum of the widths of the teeth that are to erupt in the lateral segments of the jaw. This can be predicted with a certain level of confidence as indicated in Fig. 10-5 (Moyers). This chart may be used to predict, within certain limits of probability, the tooth size of the permanent cuspid and

the first and second premolars if the sum of the widths of the incisors is known. A prediction of the arch space available for these permanent teeth by such a probability chart is not clinically useful in all cases. However, a negative predicted value may be used as a basis for a referral to an orthodontist for consultation.

For example, in an 8-year-old child an end-to-end relationship of the first permanent molars and a predicted tooth size of 23.1 mm. for the mandibular cuspids and premolars suggest that the optimum space needed as measured from the distal aspect of the lateral incisors to the mesial aspect of the first permanent molar should be 24.8 mm. Crowding of the lower anterior teeth may be present, and the degree of crowding measured in millimeters has to be considered. In this example if 2 mm. of crowding exists in the four mandibular incisors, 1 mm. has to be added to the optimum space needed in each lateral segment of the arches. The figure 24.8 is derived by adding the mean increment of 1.7 mm. for the late mesial shift of the sixth-year molar to the predicted tooth size of the mandibular cuspids and premolars. A negtaive predicted value should alert the examiner to the probability of malocclusion because of a lack of arch space.

Many factors can influence tooth-to-tooth relationship, for example, shape of the dental arch, inclination of the teeth, loss of teeth, sequence of eruption, and environmental factors. From a practical standpoint the general practitioner may use this method of prediction of arch space reliably in a percentage of his cases. In fact, if the measurements are precise, there is a 95 percent probability that the predicted arch space will be correct within 2.5 mm. (Moyers). It is to be expected that a more precise evaluation will be undertaken by the orthodontist whenever a general practitioner has referred such cases because of a predicted negative mixed dentition value for the arch space.

The most favorable sequence of eruption of the teeth in the lateral segments of the maxilla is first bicuspid, second bicuspid, cuspid, and then second molar. Variations in this sequence in the first bicuspid and cuspid area are not so significant as those in the mandible. Mesial migration of the

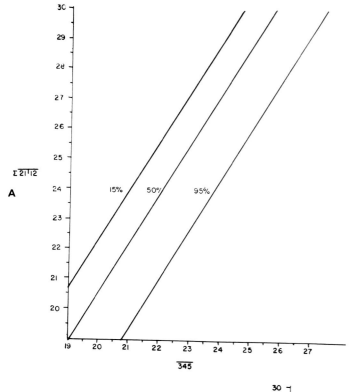

A

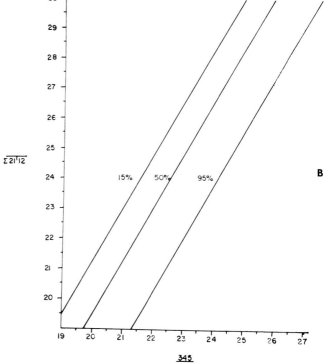

B

Fig. 10-5. *Mixed dentition analysis.* Percent probability of predicted tooth size of cuspids and premolars based on the sum of the widths of the mandibular incisors. If the sum of the widths in millimeters of the mandibular incisors is known (vertical axis), the sum of the widths of the cuspids and premolars can be predicted (horizontal axis) at the indicated probability (15%, 50%, 95%). **A,** Maxilla. **B,** Mandible. (From Moyers, R. E.: Handbook of orthodontics, Chicago, 1958, Year Book Publishers, Inc.)

maxillary first permanent molar from a premature loss of the primary second molar tends to allow a mesial drift of the first molar and the first and second bicuspids and often blocks out the normal eruption of the maxillary permanent cuspids. In some instances the second bicuspid is also crowded out of position. In general, the leeway in the maxilla is less than that in the mandible, and therefore less mesial migration of the first permanent molar can be tolerated. It can be seen that the most favorable sequence in the lateral segment of the arch occurs when the eruption of the mandibular teeth precedes the eruption of the maxillary teeth. Thus, the most favorable relationship between the upper and lower lateral segments of the arches is in lareg part dependent upon a favorable sequence of eruption of the teeth in this area.

Many of the problems that arise in the development of the occlusion arise from local factors that occur during the primary and mixed dentitions. Thus, the examiner should direct his attention not only to those factors affecting general facial and craniofacial development and imbalance of oral and facial musculature, but also to etiologic factors that can contribute to a loss of space. The premature loss of primary teeth, retention of primary teeth, congenital absence of teeth, dental anomalies, ectopic eruptions, and abnormal diastemas should be considered as important factors in the initiation and contribution to the development of an abnormal occlusion.

Functional as well as skeletal and dental factors are important for the development of a normal occlusion. Not only is the proper functioning of jaws and musculature important to the position of the teeth in the jaws, but also it is significant in its influence upon dentofacial growth. The importance of a harmonious balance between the oral and facial musculature and the teeth must not be minimized. Abnormal shifting of the mandible associated with occlusal interferences contributes to facial asymmetry, temporomandibular joint disturbances, and disturbances in the teeth and supporting structures. Malposed teeth, cross-bite, faulty restorations, and other occlusal interferences that produce unfavorable shifting of the mandible or of the teeth may affect the normal process of growth and development so that a more severe type of malocclusion results; for example, maxillary protrusion may be seen in association with hypotonicity of the upper lip, mouth breathing, or excessive lingual forces from abnormal tongue thrusting. A functional prognathic position of the mandible may be caused by muscle reflexes that are elicited to avoid occlusal interferences such as malposed teeth, faulty restorations, or occlusal anomalies. In these instances the lower jaw is habitually protruded to a point where the teeth can come together without interference. Lateral and other abnormal shifts of the mandible may be observed by the examiner when the patient is requested to occlude the teeth from the tonus or rest position of the mandible. Abnormal patterns of closure should be evaluated for the presence of malposed teeth, occlusal interferences; temporomandibular joint disturbances, and abnormal tonicity of the muscles.

• • •

In summary, the examination of the development of occlusion should consist of an adequate history, an analysis of the facial form, an analysis of the sequence of eruption, and the problems of space management, and an analysis of the function of the masticatory system.

Although judging malocclusion from a purely intraoral standpoint without regard for other dependent relationships has many shortcomings, a description or classification of the various types and forms of occluding teeth is a useful adjunct to occlusal deviations and terminology. However, two important considerations must be pointed out: a classification of malocclusion per se is never a diagnosis, and the determination of malocclusion simply on the basis of a description or classification of occlusal relationships is misleading and only a part of the total picture of malocclusion.

Angle introduced a system of classifying occlusal relationships into orthodontics in 1887. This classification was based on the assumption that the maxillary first permanent molar is always in the same position in the maxilla in relation to the base of the skull. He divided occlusal relationships into three classes according to the relationship of the maxillay and mandibular first permanent molars.

Class I comprises those arches that show a normal relationship of the maxillary and mandibular first permanent molars (mesiobuccal cusp of the maxillary molar fitting into the buccal groove of the mandibular first molar). This class also includes individual or groups of malposed teeth in which there is a normal molar relationship. Class II is comprised of those cases of malocclusion in which the mandibular first permanent molar is in distal relationship to the maxillary first permanent molar. This class is divided into two divisions. Division 1 includes protruding maxillary incisors and disocclusion of the lower molars and premolars in their relationship to the maxillary teeth. Mouth breathing, abnormal muscle pressure, and narrow maxillary arch are included. This division is subdivided to include unilateral distal molar relationships.

Division 2 includes bilateral distal molar relationships with retruding maxillary incisors; the maxillary arch is of normal width, and there is no mouth breathing or abnormal muscle pressure. This division is also subdivided to include unilateral cases. Class III includes all the cases of malocclusion in which there is mesial occlusion of both sides of the mandibular arch. The mesial occlusion must be one-half the width of the molar. Thus, the mesiobuccal cusp fits into the embrasure between the first and second mandibular molars. This classification of malocclusion based on molar relationship can be utilized even after extractions if the teeth are envisaged as replaced.

Although Angle's classification is simple and creates a framework for classifying malocclusion, it has many obvious shortcomings. The position of the maxillary first permanent molar is not constant in relation to the base of the skull; many factors may influence its position. For example, the signs of Class II, Division 1 or 2, may merely represent an exacerbation of a Class I and not the primary or essential changes underlying a true distal occlusion. Thus, a Class I occlusion may have the symptoms of a Class II, Division I, malocclusion, or the early loss of sixth-year molars may result in the mesial migration and tipping of the twelfth-year molars into a position that would simulate a Class I molar relationship when in reality there is a Class II relationship present.

Adult occlusion

An examination of the occlusion in the adult is necessarily concerned with those changes that occur with physiologic and pathologic processes. An occlusion that is considered normal at the age of 18 years cannot be considered normal for the same

individual at the age of 40 or 50 years. Even though the occlusion at 18 years of age may meet the criteria for ideal alignment and contact relation of the teeth, drifting, eruption, abrasion, extractions, loss of bone support, and prosthetic reconstructions continually alter the occlusion. These factors are of primary consideration in the continually changing pattern of occlusion and are difficult to separate from those changes that may be considered to be physiologic in nature. Therefore, it is difficult to state unequivocally what might be a normal occlusion for the adult. If it were possible to study the changes of occlusion over the years from adolescence to old age without the presence of pathologic disturbances, it might be considerably easier to establish a range of normal occlusion for an adult at any given age. The arrangement of the teeth and the occlusion of an adult are the results of changes that occur throughout life.

The occlusion of an adult at the time of examination cannot be assumed to have been constant over a long period of time. Other than extractions and replacement of teeth, attrition, extrusion, tipping, and migration appear to be the most obvious signs of occlusal changes in adult dentition. Attrition is a wearing away of the tooth surface from chewing foods that have a rough and gritty consistency. The condition progresses with advancing age. The pattern and degree of attrition are determined by the hardness of the teeth, the shape of the teeth, the amount of grit in the food, the age of the individual, the amount of force exerted on the teeth during the whole process of mastication, and the individual pattern of biting movements of the mandible. Attrition begins as soon as the teeth come into occlusal function. This is readily apparent in newly erupted incisors where the mamelons are soon worn down by incisal wear. Abnormal patterns of wear may be seen in localized areas where premature occlusion occurs or where abnormal occlusal surfaces are present. After second molars have erupted, there is little change in the width of the alveolar arches, but there is a slight increase in the length of the dental arches during the time that the third molars are erupting. It is impossible to tell exactly what the initial adult occlusion will be until all the permanent teeth have erupted.

In the United States the development of an edge-to-edge bite is not seen frequently either in the molar area of the primary dentition or in the incisor region of the adult dentition. As mentioned previously, characteristics of a normal primary dentition are the straight terminal plane and the almost end-to-end relationship of the maxillary and mandibular incisors. It is possible, however, for a step to develop in the terminal plane as a result of a forwarding shifting of the mandible associated with occlusal wear or because of a wide primary

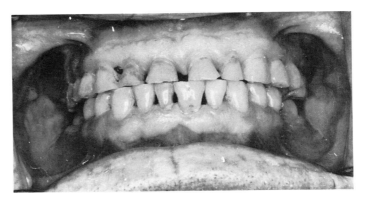

Fig. 10-6. *Occlusion.* Marked occlusal attrition sometimes associated with bruxism; note end-to-end relationship of anterior teeth and gemination of lower central incisor.

maxillary second molar. The edge-to-edge bite does not occur frequently in the United States because of our diet of soft and refined foods. In persons who eat a gritty diet, such as the Eskimos and aborigines, an edge-to-edge bite is common in the anterior teeth. Apparently the edge-to-edge bite is not manifest during the eruption of the permanent teeth and only occurs as a result of eating coarse and gritty foods (Fig. 10-6). Though there is a tendency for mesial shifting of the mandible in the primary dentition and the permanent dentition associated with attrition of the teeth, sufficient wearing of the teeth does not occur frequently enough for evaluation of the full manifestations of this type of occlusion.

Overjet and overbite relationship is related to the development of the occlusion and to function. Thus, a certain amount of overjet (horizontal overlap) and overbite (vertical overlap) must be considered normal. The degree of overbite must be related to the functional movements of the mandible, the presence or absence of extrusion of the maxillary and mandibular incisors, and the presence or absence of abnormal facial proportions. Abnormal horizontal overlap may be caused by maxillary protrusion, mandibular retrusion, labioversion of the maxillary incisors, or linguoversion of the mandibular incisors. Generally the maxillary incisors overhang the lower incisors about one-third of the length of their crowns. The degree of vertical overlap in the primary dentition is related to the amount of overbite in the mixed dentition; the overbite in the permanent dentition is influenced by the sequence of eruption of the permanent canines and premolars. A normal overbite usually results when the sequence of eruption is cuspid, first premolar, and second premolar in the mandibular arch and first premolar, cuspid, and second bicuspid in the maxillary arch.

From a practical standpoint the evaluation of the degree of overbite in the adult dentition should be related to the presence of impaired occlusal function, loss of vertical dimension in the posterior part of the mouth from extractions and loss of centric stops, extrusion of the maxillary and mandibular incisors associated with lack of centric stops, and impingement of the supporting structures by the maxillary and manibular anterior teeth. Thus, a deep overbite in itself cannot be considered pathologic without evidence of contributory signs of disease.

The form and localization of the occlusal changes associated with attrition apparently develop in accordance with the individual pattern of gliding movements. Thus, occlusal wear or attrition is related to the function of the masticatory system. Another important factor in the changes in occlusion in the adult dentition is a forward movement of the teeth by interproximal attrition. It is known that considerable interproximal wear of the teeth occurs and that a loss of up to 1 cm. from the length of the arch may be manifested in the older adult.

The significance of occlusal wear is directly related to the health of the supporting structures. Thus, in evaluating the relationship of attrition and the presence or absence of unfavorable stresses upon the supporting structure, one needs to consider the direction of the stresses transmitted to the supporting structures. In general, excessive attrition tends to produce oblique planes of wear that imply an increase in the horizontal stress on the teeth during mastication. If there is a general diminishing of cusp height and overbite, the teeth will receive a more favorable axially directed occlusal stress. Also, the smooth gliding movements of the mandible induced by this type of occlusal wear are more favorable to these supporting structures.

Another type of occlusal wear that has an unfavorable influence on the supporting structures can be observed when the incline planes of the cusps become steeper than usual and form plunger cusps. This pattern of wear seems to be seen most often when bilateral movements of the mandible predominate during mastication (Beyron). Other patterns of wear can be observed in association with restricted lateral movements of the mandible and when a patient chews only by moving his jaws up and down.

For some individuals protrusive movements seem to be most comfortable, and the occlusal changes brought on by these movements are primarily in the anterior teeth; these teeth frequently show considerable attrition, labial tipping of the maxillary incisors, and development of secondary spaces. In these instances there is a decrease in the incisor inclination and an increase in the cuspal inclination of the bicuspids and molars. The occlusal changes associated with unilateral and unilateral-diagonal movements during mastication and related to irregularities of the dentition, in-

cluding so-called unilateral cross-bite, are characterized by considerable attrition on the side used for mastication and a tendency for opening of the contacts of the anterior teeth (Beyron). Where unilateral movements predominate, the pattern of wear appears to be related to a combined lateral and up-and-down movement of the mandible. In unilateral-diagonal movements the patient is able to produce diagonal protrusive movements as well as lateral movements to one side, and the pattern of wear is related to these movements. Thus, more incisal wear may be observed in the unilateral-diagonal gliding movement than in the straight unilateral type of movements (Beyron). Extrusion and tipping of the most distal mandibular molars may result in a unilateral-diagonal restricted type of movement in which there is attrition of the bicuspids on a side of the extruded molar and extrusion of the maxil-

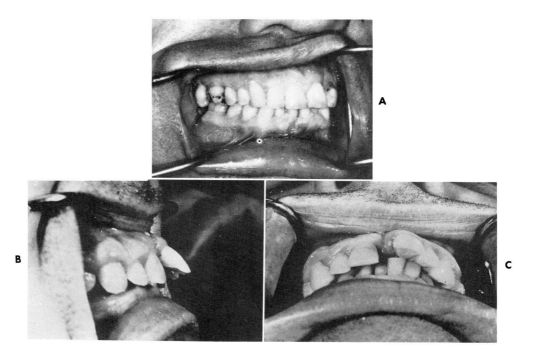

Fig. 10-7. *Occlusion.* **A,** Extruded upper right second molar in premature centric contact. **B** and **C,** Example of Thielemann's law.

lary anterior teeth diagonally opposite the extruded molar (Thielemann) (Fig. 10-7). Disturbances in the supporting structures in these types of movements appear to be related more to the lack of function than to the teeth that show the effects of attrition.

Functional analysis. The masticatory system has been described as a functional unit comprised of the teeth and their supporting structures, the jaws, the temporomandibular joints, the muscles attached to the mandible, the lips and tongue, and the vascular and nerve supply to these tissues. Thus, the so-called masticatory system constitutes groups of integrated parts capable of acting as a unit not only for the purpose of mastication, but also for the purpose of sucking, speaking, and any other function that reflects the behavior of the individual. It is impossible to adequately examine any one of the components of this system without consideration of the correlation that exists between the component parts.

Each component of the masticatory system may be examined individually, but the findings should be correlated by a functional analysis of the whole system. Thus, an analysis of the temporomandibular joint will not be adequate without an evaluation of the neuromuscular system, which makes the functional activities of the masticatory system possible. Furthermore, it is necessary to evaluate the physiologic adaptation of the masticatory system to functional wear and tear by compensatory eruption of the teeth, mesial drift, and changes in occlusal pattern. A practical approach to the analysis of disturbances of any of the components of the masticatory system demands that a clinical examination be made for the signs and symptoms of organic disease and that the findings be related to the functional or dysfunctional activities of each of the components and to the functional activities of the whole system. This means that each component part must be analyzed for organic disease, functional in-

capacitation, and production of disturbances in the rest of the system.

A functional analysis is a systematic examination of the anatomy and function of the masticatory system with special consideration given to functional disturbances and pathologic changes in the periodontium teeth, joints, and muscles of mastication. The analysis should consist of (1) a complete case history, including a review of the masticatory system for symptoms of dysfunction of the joints and muscles, psychic factors, fatigue, anxiety, and pain, (2) a clinical examination of the masticatory system, supplemented with (3) a radiographic examination of the teeth and periodontal structures and, where indicated, radiographs of the temporomandibular joint, and (4) an analysis of the occlusion with an articulator.

Occlusal trauma. A diagnosis of occlusal trauma must be made on the basis of an analysis of the occlusion during empty movements (such as lateral movements with the teeth in light contact), palpation for tooth mobility, and an evaluation of radiographs for signs of occlusal trauma (Fig. 10-8). Clinical observation should be directed toward the presence of predisposing factors such as occlusal habits, malocclusion, loss of teeth, loss of periodontal support, faulty restorations including bridges and partial dentures, occlusal interferences, and premature contacts in centric. Occlusal habits like clenching, biting on foreign objects, and bruxism should be considered in the analysis.

The most common clinical manifestation of occlusal trauma is abnormal tooth mobility. Changes in the supporting structures such as uneven width of the lamina dura, increased width of the periodontal membrane space (Fig. 10-8, *B*), and root resorption aid in making the diagnosis of occlusal trauma. Such manifestations should be related to the cause of abnormal tooth mobility. The relationship between cause and findings can be accomplished best dur-

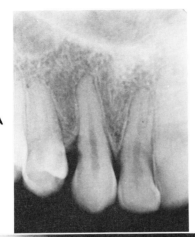

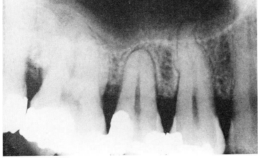

Fig. 10-8. *Occlusal trauma.* **A**, Changes in bone height, lamina dura, and periodontal membrane space. There was clinical evidence of bruxism, abnormal facets of wear, and increased mobility of the tooth. The lingual cusp of the tooth was an occlusal interference to lateral movement of the mandible. **B**, Occlusal trauma associated with periodontitis and bone loss. Note root resorption and increased width of periodontal membrane space.

ing the functional analysis of the masticatory system. Other important signs and symptoms of traumatic occlusion are included in the following list.

Increased tooth mobility
Migration of teeth
Root resorption
Pain (temporomandibular joint, pulpal, atypical facial, periodontal)
Alteration of lamina dura and periodontal membrane space
Atypical occlusal wear

Other reported manifestations of trauma from occlusion include periodontal abscesses, food impaction, internal resorption, osteosclerosis, pulpal calcification, periodontal pocket formation, gingival changes, and angular bony defects involving the alveolar crest (Fig. 10-8, *A*). Many reported relationships between occlusion and occlusal trauma have not been established. Except for acute trauma, often the symptoms of traumatic occlusion are not apparent to the patient.

Temporomandibular joint. Though the joints are considered briefly in a general examination (Chapter 6), a more detailed consideration of this area may be necessary during examination of the occlusion. The examination of the temporomandibular joint should begin by inspection and palpation of the tissues contiguous with the joint while it is at rest and during functional movements. Inspection for visible signs of swelling and ecchymosis, palpation for localized tenderness, and inquiry about pain on motion should be carried out in the region of the joint. Subjective complaints as described by the patient during the clinical history should serve to orient the examiner to a correlation of the symptoms of local manifestations of disease. Elevation of temperature, texture and induration of the overlying tissue, presence or absence of tenderness or fluctuation, and the characteristics of any enlargement are determined by palpation. Friction fremitus or joint crepitus can be detected as the joint is moved.

The muscles of mastication should be sufficiently relaxed to permit the patient to move the mandible comfortably through all functional movements. Movements may be restricted because of pain, joint disease, neuromuscular disease, or lack of muscle coordination. The range and freedom of active movements made by the patient should be evaluated in all excursions of the mandible, and, if indicated, the patient should be requested to bite on a piece of rubber or orangewood stick. Biting force per se probably has little significance to the

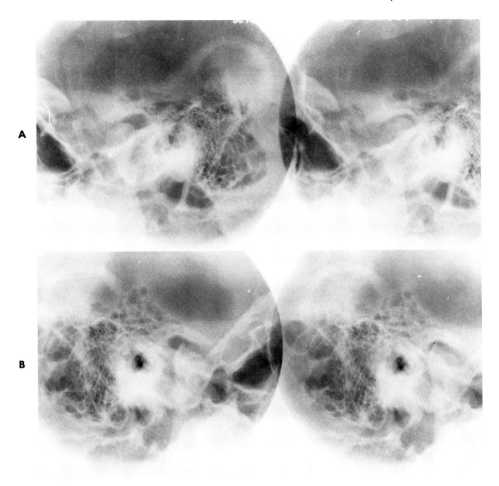

Fig. 10-9. *Radiograph of temporomandibular joints.* **A,** Right condyle in open and closed mandibular position with changes of traumatic arthritis. **B,** Left condyle with only slight changes of the articular surface.

natural dentition; however, biting down on something hard may produce symptoms that are not otherwise evident.

The temporomandibular joints are subject to luxation, subluxation, traumatic arthritis, acute suppurative arthritis, rheumatoid arthritis, and osteoarthritis associated with generalized degenerative joint disease involving all joints in the body (Fig. 10-9). Traumatic temporomandibular joint arthritis results from incomplete or complete dis-

location of the joint and from traumatic injury of the head of the condyle, the glenoid fossa, and the meniscus. If subluxation or traumatic injury is severe, the signs and symptoms are usually of an acute nature. Movements of the mandible are usually restricted by pain, and pain may be produced when the joints are palpated. On opening, the mandible may be deviated to one side because of unilateral pain involvement or because of immobilization of one side. Occasionally there is radiographic evidence of an increased joint space.

When traumatic injury to the joint is not sudden or severe but is of a low degree, chronic, or of a repeated nature, the history of onset will be vague and insidious. In these instances a disturbance in the other components of the masticatory system, such as occlusal disharmony, may be the factor responsible for trauma to the joints. The etiologic factors causing chronic traumatic arthritis may be present also in those patients exhibiting acute traumatic arthritis; they are not usually the cause of acute signs and symptoms unless they rather suddenly exceed the physiologic limits of the joint. The latter occurs not infrequently with occlusal disharmony. Dental procedures that require the mouth to be open for extended periods, high restorations, blows to the mandible, and extractions can be causes of traumatic injury to the joint. The signs and symptoms of such injury may be severe and of sudden onset, or the symptoms may be of a minor nature at first, only to give rise to severe symptoms later, either spontaneously or in association with another traumatic incident even of a minor nature.

The most common disturbance of the temporomandibular joint is chronic trauma and muscle pain related to psychic tension, muscle hypertonicity, and occlusal interferences. The initiating factor in chronic traumatic temporomandibular joint arthritis, TMJ-pain-dysfunction syndrome, may be an occlusal interference, psychic tension or both. In most instances neither the occlusal interference or the environmental factor causing psychic tension will be apparent to the patient. Whether or not disturbances occur in the components of the masticatory system will depend to a large degree on the adaptive capacity of the system.

The signs and symptoms of chronic temporomandibular joint arthritis may become very severe depending upon the duration of the cause and the environmental factors involved. During periods of severe psychic stress, clenching and bruxism may become exaggerated and lead to severe temporomandibular joint and muscle pain. Environmental factors include tensions of employment or occupation, marital problems, menopause, and fatigue. New restorations, drifting of teeth, dental procedures, and extractions may be the predisposing local factors. The most common manifestations of chronic temporomandibular joint arthritis and muscle pain are included in the following list.

> Pain in and around the joints
> Restriction of mandibular movements
> Tenderness of masticatory muscles
> Clicking noises in the joints

Palpation of the joint area will rarely uncover swelling or pain; however, jerky movements of the head of the condyle may be felt. Visual inspection will only rarely show signs of obvious deformity, but radiographic examination may show evidence of bone resorption or irregularity of the head of the condyle or anterior slope of the glenoid fossa.

An acute suppurative arthritis of the temporomandibular joint is usually a complication of gonorrheal urethritis or of other acute pyogenic joint involvement. Local manifestations consist of spasms of the masseter muscles, difficulty in opening the mouth, and the presence of the cardinal signs of inflammation in and around the affected temporomandibular joint. The systemic reaction consists of an elevation in temperature, leukocytosis, and general malaise. Radiographic examination of the joint will not reveal any change until rather extensive damage has taken place. Thus, it is necessary that early diagnosis and antibiotic treatment be instituted for the maintenance of a functional joint. The diagnosis of gonococcal arthritis can be confirmed by examination of fluid aspirated from the joint. The acute nature of the local and systemic signs and symptoms of disease should direct the examiner's attention to the possibility of an infective arthritis.

Etiologic factors responsible for disharmony of the masticatory system as well as for traumatic temporomandibular joint arthritis are discrepancy between centric relation and centric occlusion, abnormal tonicity of the masticatory muscles, local irritation associated with periodontal disease or dental caries, occlusal interference, psychic tension, loss of vertical dimension, neurologic disorders, abnormal habits of mastication and nonfunctional jaw positions, loss of teeth without replacement, faulty dental therapy, and bruxism.

Bruxism. Nonfunctional grinding of the teeth is an important predisposing factor in occlusal trauma and dysfunctional disturbances of the temporomandibular joint. Since most patients are not aware of the habit, the diagnosis is dependent upon the findings in the clinical examination (Figs. 10-10 and 10-11); however, a positive history may be obtained from the family or friends of the patient after the disturbance has been explained to the patient. The most common causes of bruxism include occlusal interferences, psychic tension, and periodontal disease. All those factors that lead to emotional or psychic stress can lead to the various forms of bruxism. In the presence of even minor occlusal discrepancies, a tendency for bruxism may occur when emotional stress is great. Occlusal habits related or unrelated to an individual's occupation may precipitate bruxism. It is important in making the diagnosis of bruxism to have a clear picture of the patient's emotional state as well as a knowledge of the signs of bruxism. The most

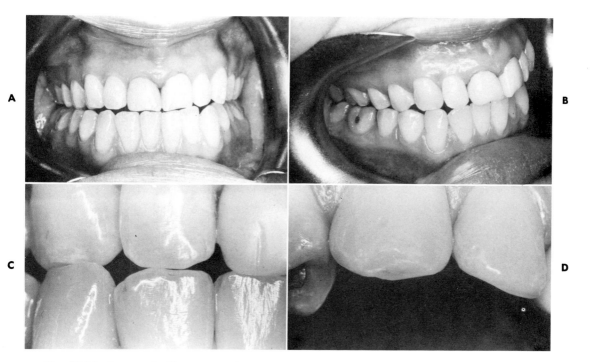

Fig. 10-10. *Bruxism.* **A,** The pattern of wear involving the anterior teeth is good evidence of a protrusive bruxing movement. **B,** Lateral protrusive contacts. **C** and **D,** Note facets of wear extending over onto the facial surface of the maxillary cuspid. Facets of wear in such nonfunctional positions are related to bruxism.

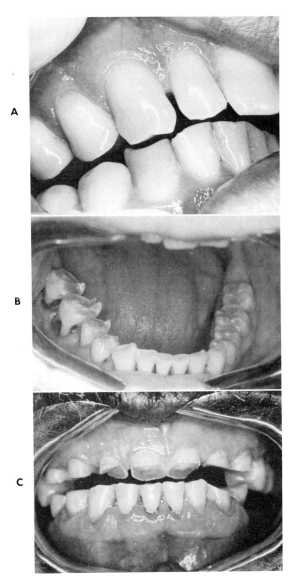

Fig. 10-11. *Facets of wear.* **A,** The type of wear illustrated is highly suggestive of bruxism. **B** and **C,** Extensive wear associated with bruxism.

important clinical manifestations of bruxism are included in the following list.

Nonfunctional facets of occlusal wear
Tenderness of masticatory muscles
Increased muscle tone and spasms
Hypertrophy of masticatory muscles
Temporomandibular joint stiffness and pain
Increased mobility of teeth

Examination for slide in centric. The examination of the masticatory system should include a search for a discrepancy between centric relation and centric occlusion. Centric relation is the most retruded position of the mandible from which lateral jaw movements can be made comfortably. Centric relation refers to a jaw-to-jaw relationship. The term "centric occlusion" refers to the position of the teeth when the jaws are closed and the teeth are at a maximum intercuspation. This is a tooth-to-tooth relationship.

When the mandible is closed in centric relation and there is no occlusal interference, the teeth should be in a position of maximum intercuspation without a sliding movement of the mandible. The sliding change from centric relation to centric occlusion is called a slide in centric. There may not be a slide in closing in centric relation; however, when premature contacts exist, the shift in the mandible will occur. The intial contact in centric relation that causes the slide is referred to as a premature contact or a centric interference (Fig. 10-12). Premature contacts represent a potential source of tissue injury and are significant etiologic factors in temporomandibular joint arthritis and bruxism.

The most likely position for premature contacts on the mandibular molars in "normal" occlusions (supporting cusps make contact with fossae and marginal ridges in centric occlusion) are the distal slopes of the triangular ridges and the cusp ridges. The most common areas for premature contacts for the maxillary molars and premolars are the mesial inclines of the cusp ridges of the lingual cusps and the mesial inclines of the oblique ridges of the maxillary molars (Fig. 10-13, *A*). On the mandibular premolars the premature contacts occur most frequently on the distal slopes of the triangular ridges of the lingual cusps (Fig. 10-13, *B*).

The success in determining the presence of a slide in centric occlusion is determined

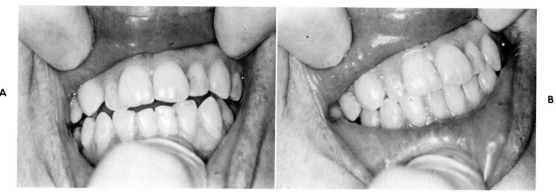

Fig. 10-12. *Premature contact.* **A,** Premature contact in centric relation caused by lingual version of the maxillary lateral incisor. **B,** Relationship of contacts of the lateral incisors in centric occlusion.

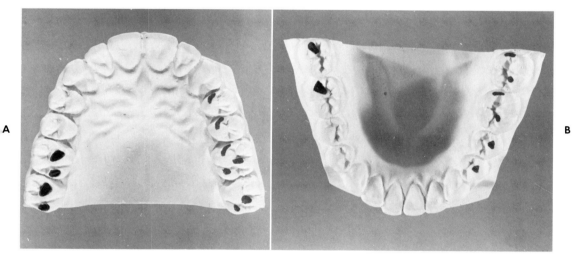

Fig. 10-13. *Areas of premature contacts and balancing interferences.* **A,** Maxillary arch showing most likely areas for premature contacts—mesial inclines of lingual cusp ridges and oblique ridges. Balancing interferences involve buccal inclines of lingual cusps. **B,** Mandibular arch showing potential areas for premature contacts—distal inclines of triangular and cusp ridges of lingual cusps. Balancing interferences most frequently involve the triangular ridges and cusps tips of the distal buccal and distal cusps of the molars.

by the ability of the examiner to manipulate the mandible about its hinge axis. This maneuver may be complicated by temporomandibular joint dysfunction and by abnormal tonus of the muscles of mastication. The initial objective of the examiner should be to get the patient to assume a relaxed, unstrained retruded position of the mandible without exerting unnecessary pressure. When there is hypertonicity of the muscles, the patient may require considerable training in relaxation of these muscles.

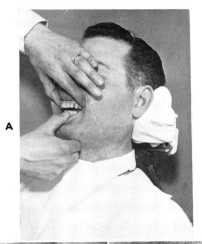

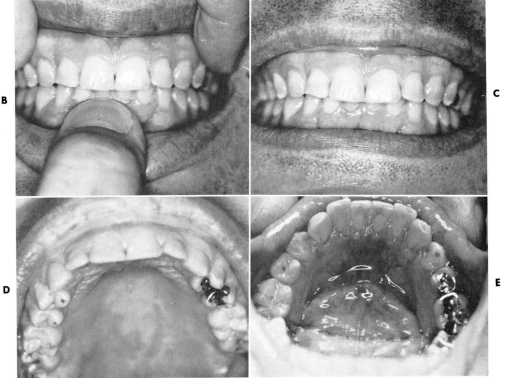

Fig. 10-14. *Occlusion.* **A,** Examination for premature centric contact. **B,** Centric relation. **C,** Centric occlusion. **D** and **E,** Carbon marks indicating points of premature contact; note marks on mesial aspects of the lingual cusps of the maxillary first bicuspid; this is a common location of premature contacts.

The use of relaxant drugs such as Robaxin may be of assistance in such cases. The chin should be held between the index finger and thumb (Fig. 10-14), and the mandible should be moved up and down in small arcs. Initially it may be necessary to ask the patient to assist in making these movements. As the jaw is manipulated, the mandible should be directed passively posteriorly and upward to decrease the inner occlusal distance. When the muscles are completely relaxed and the mandible is in the retruded position and the teeth are in close approximation, the examiner should have a sense of rotary or hinge axis movement. Further slight closure will serve to establish the first occlusal contact. If premature contacts are present, the mandible will be displaced anteriorly on closure. Where no slide in centric occlusion is present, a maximum number of teeth will contact simultaneously. During the hinge axis closure, the examiner may palpate for the tooth exhibiting the first premature contact, for percussion vibrations, and for movements of the teeth.

The areas of premature contact may be marked with articulating paper or 28-gauge wax (Fig. 10-15). The process should be repeated until the patient is aware of what is being done and until the muscles are completely relaxed. It may take some time to train the patient in centric relation closure. This may require considerable patience on the part of the examiner as well as the patient. The determination of centric relation should be carried out several times so that the examiner may feel sure that the hinge axis movement is being made without benefit of the patient's muscle effort. In general, the examiner will find that the most retruded position of the mandible becomes more apparent after several manipulations of the mandible. The patient may be requested to stop his centric closure just as he first comes into occlusal contact; at this point visual inspection of the teeth may reveal the position of the premature contact. After this is noted, the patient should be requested to press his teeth together; the path of closure is noted. In some instances it may be difficult to determine the exact

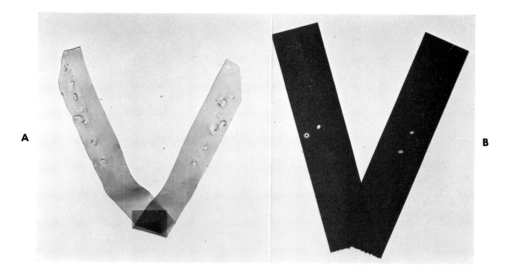

Fig. 10-15. *Occlusion.* **A,** Premature contacts identified by perforations in 28-gauge Kerr green wax. **B,** Premature contacts identified by perforation in carbon paper; this method also marks the teeth.

position of a premature contact. Various methods are used to determine a position of the premature contacts, depending upon the ability and success of their use by the operator. The examiner should always question the patient regarding his location of a tooth contact, for in many individuals the sense of location is very highly developed; in others misleading information will be given. The sound of the teeth coming together may indicate where the premature contact is located; however, it is only of limited value to most operators. The presence of worn facets on the teeth is suggestive of premature contacts. Polished gold restorations present some difficulty in marking with articulating paper. In these instances especially, the use of 28-gauge green wax may be helpful. In some instances where there is hypermobility of the teeth, the initial occlusal interference will tend to move a tooth in a lateral direction. This movement can be easily felt by the examiner.

Mandibular movements. The relation of the teeth to mandibular movements should be observed in working, balancing, and protrusive positions (Fig. 10-16). In working position the buccal cusps of the mandibular teeth may contact the lingual inclines of the buccal cusps of the maxillary teeth (group function). However the cuspids may provide all or most of the guidance in lateral movements. Both group function and cuspid guidance, or cuspid guidance only, may be normal. The examiner should determine whether or not selective grinding will provide for smooth lateral working excursions.

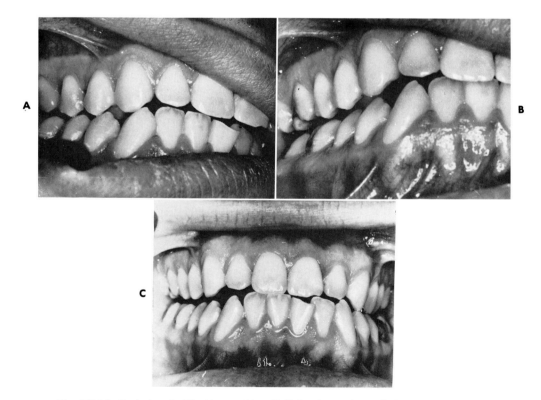

Fig. 10-16. *Occlusion.* **A,** Working position. **B,** Balancing position. **C,** Protrusive position.

The extent of grinding will depend on the working interferences present and the need to distribute occlusal forces.

Balancing interferences most often involve the buccal inclines of the lingual cusps of the maxillary molars, and the lingual inclines of the buccal cusps of the mandibular molars (Fig. 10-13). Balancing contacts may be observed when lateral excursions are being made by the patient. The examiner should guide the jaw with the teeth in contact on the working side. Balancing side contacts may be light but are not necessary in the natural dentition (Fig. 10-17). Having the patient move in lateral and lateral protrusive movements with the teeth in contact (called "empty movements") are not necessarily those movements encountered in chewing or bruxism. Avoidance patterns may be established so that interferences are difficult to detect. Abnormal, jerky, and restricted movements may be caused by interferences on the balancing side. Balancing interferences, especially related to new restorations, are significant factors in the etiology of bruxism, traumatic occlusion, temporomandibular joint dysfunction, and muscle pain.

Movements that result from balancing interferences prevent maximum efficiency on the working side, tend to place undue lateral stress on the teeth on the balancing side, and predispose to temporomandibular joint arthritis because of movements of the mandible to avoid the interferences.

Protrusive movements should be observed for abnormal patterns of movements. The teeth should be in occlusion when the excursions are performed so that jerky, eccentric, and deviated protrusive movements caused by undesirable posterior contacts can be observed (Fig. 10-18). Quite frequently cuspal interferences will prevent the mandible from performing smooth gliding protrusive movements.

The mandibular movements should be repeated while the teeth are out of contact (Fig. 10-19). In many instance the patient will be able to perform these excursions better than when the teeth are in contact because of the occlusal interferences present that restrict excursions of the mandible when the teeth are in contact. In other instances the patient will not be able to perform the movements adequately because of forced inactivity of some of the usual patterns of muscle activity caused by restricted movements resulting from occlusal interferences. Less frequently, muscle spasms, tenderness, or paralysis will prevent certain of the mandibular movements.

Cases of prognathism should be observed for the possibility of an occlusal interfer-

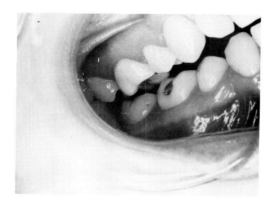

Fig. 10-17. Balancing side interference causing loss of contact on the working side in "empty movement" and the development of an avoidance pattern in voluntary, unguided lateral movement.

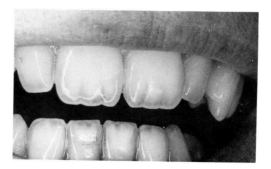

Fig. 10-18. Posterior contacts causing functional anterior open bite. Note absence of wear on maxillary incisors.

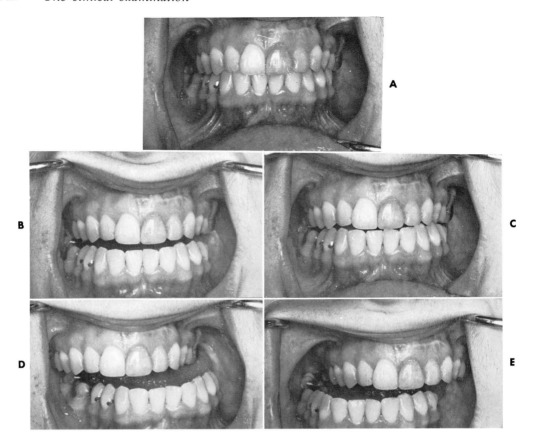

Fig. 10-19. *Mandibular movements.* Observation of mandibular movements. **A,** Centric occlusion. **B,** Protrusive movement without occlusal contact. **C,** Protrusive movement with occlusal contact. **D** and **E,** Lateral excursions without occlusal contact. The movements shown in **B** through **E** are called border movements.

ence preventing the closure of the mandible in centric relation. This functional type of prognathism can be determined easily by having the patient close in centric relation and then in his convenience centric occlusion. In centric relation a functional prognathism will disappear (Fig. 10-20).

Tonus or rest position of the mandible. The involuntary maintenance of the position of the mandible in an individual who is awake and in an upright position is determined by the tonus of the masticatory and functionally related muscles. The reflex contraction of the muscles that results from a pull such as gravity is called the stretch or myotatic reflex. A steady reflex contraction as seen in the muscles that are concerned with posture and gravity is called tonus. Factors such as learning, pain, fear, fatigue, mental relaxation, and the positions of the patient will affect tonus. Occlusal irregularities and periodontal disease may also alter normal tonus position of the mandible.

The tonus or rest position is of clinical importance because of its relationship to the interocclusal space (freeway space) that is usually present between the occlusal surfaces of the maxillary and mandibular teeth. The width of this space varies considerably but most generally is from 2 to 5

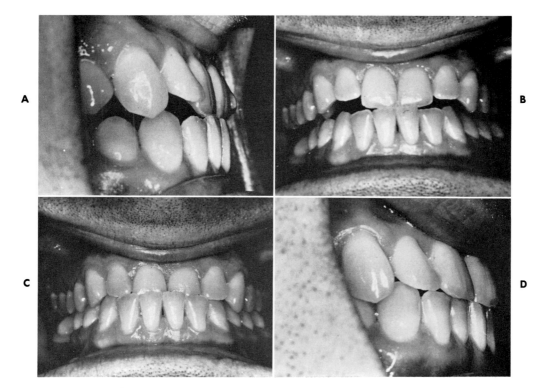

Fig. 10-20. *Mandibular positions.* Functional Class III relationship of mandible caused by malposed maxillary incisors. **A** and **B**, Mandible in centric relation. **C**, Teeth in acquired centric occlusion producing prognathism. **D**, True centric occlusion following labial movement of incisors.

mm. in the anterior portion of the mouth. The exact amount of freeway space should be determined independently in each individual.

To obtain a reasonable recording of the rest position, it is necessary to eliminate factors that can disturb the tonus. Relaxing procedures, such as repeated swallowing, the use of phonetics or word sounds to be repeated by the patient such as *m* or *o* or word syllables such as *O-hi-o* or *Miss-i-ssipp-i*, and training in muscle relaxation are of help in obtaining an acceptable rest position of the mandible. Such maneuvers will give fairly good results provided that there are no disturbing factors such as occlusal interference, periodontal disease, tongue and lip habits, fear apprehension, and pain. A radiographic registration is

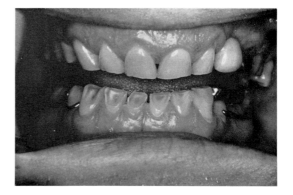

Fig. 10-21. *Dysfunctional occlusion.* Attrition of anterior teeth caused by deep overbite and loss of posterior teeth; note presence of bite-raising appliance in the mandibular arch.

probably more accurate than other methods for registration of the rest position of the mandible; however, this method does not lend itself readily to most clinical procedures. Under normal conditions the rest position is considered to be constant, except for minor changes with age.

Vertical dimension is the vertical height of the face as determined by muscle relationships and the rest position of the mandible. Its determination is of importance when the examiner seeks to evaluate the possibility of an increase in the freeway space (so-called closed-bite) (Fig. 10-21).

Inasmuch as vertical dimension is related to the position of rest of the mandible and this rest position is stable, changes in the interocclusal space (freeway space) can be related to the vertical dimension of the face. An increase in the space results occasionally from excessive attrition of the teeth without compensatory eruption. Encroachment on the space may result from extrusion of teeth; this is usually limited to localized areas of the arches where teeth or centric stops have been lost. Sometimes, encroachment on the freeway space will result from misguided bite-raising procedures. When there has been encroachment upon the space by some bite-raising procedure, there will be a constant undue stimulus to the stretch reflex of the muscles of mastication that will promote undue muscle contractions and produce pathologic sequelae. An increase in the freeway space is not of direct significance for muscle tonus and rest position, but it may directly influence the tonus and other functional relations of the masticatory system by associated abnormal or strained occlusal relations.

The diagnosis of an abnormally wide freeway space or loss of vertical dimension should not be made simply on the basis of altered facial expression, for many factors can produce changes in facial expression. Wrinkles caused by age and the disappearance of fat pads with a loss of tissue contour cannot be considered as signs of loss of vertical dimension. A deep overbite in itself is not a sign of lost vertical dimension. Excessive attrition of the teeth is not necessarily an indication that the patient has a loss of vertical dimension or an abnormally wide freeway space, since a loss of tooth structure may be compensated for by eruption of the teeth and increase in the height of the alveolar process. Where an older individual has what appears to be a closed-bite and an abnormally wide freeway space but does not have untoward signs or symptoms of this condition, the clinician should be very cautious about attempting to greatly reduce the freeway space without an effort to determine the actual status of the vertical dimension and freeway space.

Usually an attempt to restore vertical dimension will result in failure because the appearance of the freeway space is not related to the actual status of the vertical dimension. When extensive reconstruction is planned, it is necessary that the clinician give due consideration to the measurement of vertical dimension. Though the vertical dimension may be determined by its relationship to the rest position of the mandible, it has been pointed out that the procedure for obtaining the exact location of the rest position is not precise. A temporary splint may be used as a diagnostic aid for the evaluation of a vertical dimension that is considered to be the right one for the patient. If the patient tolerates the appliance well, the derived freeway space is probably correct. In general, it is better to underdiagnose cases of a loss of vertical dimension than to overdiagnose them. All too frequently a diagnosis is made of a loss, and treatment for the loss results in an encroachment upon the freeway space.

When a patient with a deep overbite complains of soreness of the palatal tissue around the incisive papilla, the clinician should not necessarily consider this evidence of a closed-bite or loss of vertical dimension unless additional facts justify the diagnosis. Many individuals have a deep overbite that is within the range of normal for them. However, if a patient complains of an incisive papilla being painful because of traumatization from the lower incisors, the clinician should determine whether there is a loss of centric stops on these teeth, whether there is extrusion of these teeth, or whether there is hyperplasia of the gingival tissues and incisive papilla.

Quite frequently the inclination and the anatomy of the maxillary central incisors do not present adequate centric stops for the lower incisor teeth. This may be accompanied by an extrusion of the lower incisors with impingement upon the incisive papilla, causing an inflammatory reaction. Although this may be considered an anterior closed-bite or an encroachment upon the freeway space, it is not satisfactory evidence of a generalized change in the vertical dimension. In the majority of these cases there is no change in the posterior vertical dimension. Unfortunately many of these cases are diagnosed as having loss of vertical dimension, and attempts are made to intrude the anterior teeth and cause eruption of the posterior teeth. Such a diagnosis and treatment plan are based on lack of understanding of the rest position of the mandible and the freeway space. The difference in the occlusal plane between the anterior portion of the mouth and the posterior teeth in such cases does not represent a lack of development of the alveolar process and eruption of the posterior teeth but reflects the lack of centric stops on the maxillary teeth by an extrusion of the mandibular or maxillary central incisors. Thus, the treatment should not be based upon a loss of vertical dimension but upon a correction of the factors responsible for it. In this particular instance a diagnosis is directed toward the extrusion of teeth in the absence of adequate centric stops. Therefore, the treatment plan should be based upon the establishment of centric stops either by orthodontic movements of the

teeth or restoration to provide centric stops for the lower incisors. In either event, some occlusal adjustment will be necessary for the correction of the height of the lower incisors and in some instances for the correction of the length of the maxillary incisors. A more detailed study of the occlusion may be necessary, and the examiner may desire to mount the models of the patient's teeth on an articulator. This is accomplished by a face-bow registration, a centric relation wax bite, and a protrusive relation wax bite. Casts of the teeth to be studied may be mounted on an adjustable articulator. Articulation of the models is an important aid in the functional analysis of occlusal relations and is of significant value many times in diagnosis and treatment planning (see Chapter 15).

REFERENCES

Anderson, G. M.: Practical orthodontics, St. Louis, 1948, The C. V. Mosby Co.
Baume, L. J.: Physiological tooth migration and its significance for the development of occlusion, J. Dent. Res. 1950:
   I. Biogenetic course of deciduous dentition, **29**:123-132.
   II. Biogenesis of accessional dentition, **29**:331-337.
   III. Biogenesis of the successional dentition, **29**:338-348.
   IV. The biogenesis of overbite, **29**:440-447.
Beyron, H.: Occlusal changes in the adult dentition, Sven. Tandlak. Tidskr. **45**:119-169, 1952.
Downs, W. B.: Variations in facial relationships: their significance in treatment and prognoses, Amer. J. Orthodont. **34**:812-840, 1948.
Friel, S.: The development of ideal occlusion of the gum pads and teeth, Amer. J. Orthdont. **40**:196-227, 1954.
Greene, C. S.: A survey of current professional concepts and opinions about the myofossal pain-dysfunction (MPD) syndrome, J.A.D.A. **86**:128, 1973.
Ingervall, B.: Range of movement of mandible in children, Scand. J. Dent. Res. **78**:311, 1970.
Kawamura, Y.: Neurophysiologic background of occlusion, J. Amer. Soc. Periodont. **5**:175-183, 1967.
Lo, R. T., and Moyers, R. E.: Studies in the etiology and prevention of malocclusion, Amer. J. Orthodont. **39**:460-467, 1953.
Lupton, D. E.: Psychological aspects of temporomandibular joint dysfunction, J.A.D.A. **79**:131, 1969.
McCall, C. M., Szmyd, L., and Rotter, R. M.:

Personality characteristics in patients with temporomandibular joint symptoms, J.A.D.A. **62:** 694, 1961.

Møller, E.: Clinical electromyography in dentistry, Int. Dent. J. **19:**250, 1969.

Moyers, R. E.: Handbook of orthodontics, Chicago, 1958, Year Book Medical Publishers, Inc.

Moyers, R. E.: Development of occlusion, Dent. Clin. N. Amer. **13:**523, July, 1969.

Ramfjord, S. P., and Ash, M. M.: Occlusion, Philadelphia, 1971, W. B. Saunders Co.

Ramfjord, S. P., Kerr, D. A., and Ash, M. M. (editors): World workshop in periodontics, Ann Arbor, Mich., 1966, The University of Michigan Press.

Schwartz, L. L., and Chayes, C. M.: Facial pain and mandibular dysfunction, Philadelphia, 1969, W. B. Saunders Co.

Sheppard, I. M., and Sheppard, S. M.: Maximal incisal opening, a diagnostic index, J. Dent. Med. **20:**13, 1965.

Thielemann, K.: Biomechanik der Paradentose, Leipzig, 1938, Herman Meusser.

11

Examination of the edentulous and partially edentulous mouth

The examination of the edentulous patient should include all the components of a complete and thorough examination except for those parts concerned with the evaluation of the natural dentition. The examination of the patient in preparation for the construction of dentures differs only slightly from that of the patient already wearing dentures. The main difference lies in analysis. The analysis of the areas to receive dentures relates to effective impressions for adequate construction of denture bases, whereas the analysis of denture-bearing areas relates to dentures already in use.

Periodic examination of denture-bearing areas and artificial dentures is as important as the periodic examination of the natural dentition. It should serve to outline the denture-bearing areas, to determine structures or areas that may require relief, to ascertain what anatomic features can be found in the impression, to evaluate the hard and soft structures that are used for the denture base, and to evaluate dentures already being worn.

The preparation of the mouth for dentures may require the removal of bony spines, unerupted teeth, retained roots, hyperplastic tissue, tori, and protuberant localized areas of the alveolar ridges that would prevent proper placement of dentures because of lack of intermaxillary space. Occasionally it may be necessary to push back the frenula and deepen the mucobuccal fold. These factors should be taken into consideration before denture construction is started. Although dentists are quite adept at compensating for many defects of the denture-bearing areas, alveolectomies and other surgical procedures many times provide a more favorable denture base than can be obtained by compensatory procedures.

The anatomic features that should be considered prior to taking an impression are those hard- and soft-tissue landmarks that must be identified in the impression and those tissues that may, because of their consistency and contour, interfere with the taking of an impression. It is very necessary that the examiner determine what soft tissue displacements must be considered before taking the impression. Inspection and palpation of the structures of the denture-bearing areas and periphery will enable the clinician to interpret these structures in the impression. It will also enable him to determine what areas are to bear the dentures and what areas must be relieved to prevent interference with function, movement, retention, and placement of the dentures.

Inspection and palpation of the edentulous areas should be systematic and should follow a routine procedure so that no feature will be overlooked (Figs. 11-1 and 11-2). The following characteristics of the ridges should be noted: roughness, sharpness, flatness, height, and relation to the opposing arches; relation to the anterior nasal spine, zygomatic process of the maxilla, hamulus, mental foramen, mental trigone, buccal shelf, retromolar trigone, genial tubercles, and mylohyoid line; and relation to position of the tongue and the floor of the mouth.

Inspection and palpation of the maxillary arch can begin at the midline. The prominence of the anterior nasal spine and its relationship to the alveolar ridges can be noted by pressing a finger lightly over the midline above the attached gingiva. By palpating laterally, the examiner can feel the slight concavity of the canine fossa just anterior to the canine eminence. The alveolar ridge should be palpated in these areas for evidence of sharp bony spicules. Then, by palpating posteriorly, the examiner can feel the maxillary buttress of the zygomatic arch and should note its relation to the alveolar ridge. Its obliqueness and promi-

nence should be related to the position of the periphery of the denture. The position and prominence of labial and buccal frenula should be noted; when the attachment is high on the ridge, special consideration may be necessary. The superior buccal fornix should be considered in relation to its depth and position of the buccal flange of the denture. The maxillary tuberosity should be inspected and palpated for hyperplastic tissue and nearness to the opposing alveolar ridge. Occasionally the tuberosity extends to the mandibular ridge and makes recontouring necessary.

The relation of the pterygoid hamulus to the hamular notch should be noted. The position of the posterior palatal seal must be accurately determined to avoid interference with the action of the tensor veli palatini muscle. The location of the distal posterior

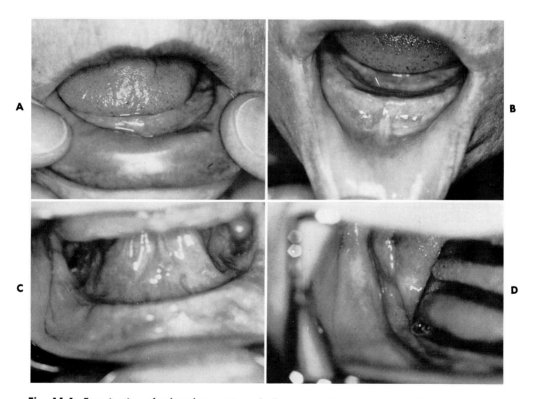

Fig. 11-1. *Examination of edentulous patient.* **A,** Tongue position. **B,** Position of labial frenulum. **C,** Position of lingual attachment of soft tissue. **D,** Retromolar pad and lateral throat form.

palatal seal must be visualized at the junction of the hard and soft palates (vibrating line). The junction can be seen clearly when the patient says "aah." The tissue over the greater palatine foramen should be palpated for texture and softness. Not infrequently these tissues are soft, fluctuant, and easily compressed by impression materials. The tissues of the palate and alveolar ridges should be palpated and the compressibility of these areas compared. This comparison should extend from the midline to the alveolar ridges and from the juction of the hard and soft palates to the incisive papilla. Obviously, the degree of compressibility is of considerable importance in recording an accurate impression.

The presence of a palatine torus can present denture problems (Fig. 2-6, *A*). The incisive papilla may lie on a level with the alveolar ridge, and, if it is soft and hyperplastic, relief of this area may be necessary. This is especially true if the patient complains of tenderness when this area is palpated.

The position of the palatine foveas is often used as a landmark for the establishment of the posterior border of the upper denture (Fig. 11-2). However, because of considerable variation and difficulty in seeing these depressions, these foveas cannot be relied upon as landmarks for the peripheral posterior border of the denture.

The mandibular buccal fornix and the

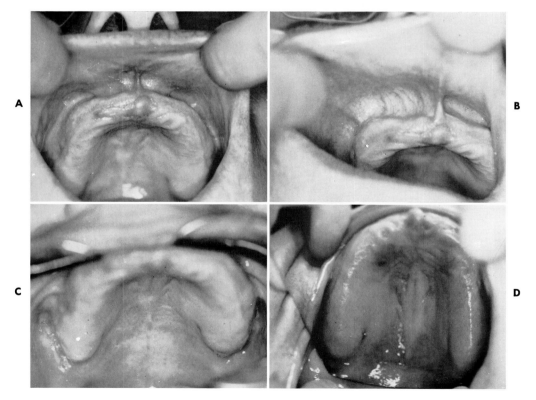

Fig. 11-2. *Examination of edentulous patient.* **A,** Labial frenulum. **B,** Buccal frenulum. **C,** Vibrating line (junction of hard and soft palate). **D,** Tuberosity and midsagittal suture; note relationship of pterygomandibular raphe to palate.

buccal shelf should be palpated in the molar region to determine the direction of the slant of the surface of the shelf and the relationship to the attachment of the buccinator muscle fibers. It is necessary to determine these anatomic landmarks since the buccal flange or periphery of the lower denture is related to the usable surface presented here. Palpation will also facilitate the determination of the periphery of the impression tray. The buccal fornix is also frequently involved in overextension of the buccal flange of dentures and should be inspected for signs and symptoms of this condition.

The anterior border of the ramus of the mandible should be palpated at rest and during movements of the mandible. The relationship between the alveolar ridge, retromolar pad, pterygomandibular raphe, and buccinator muscle should be evaluated. The pterygomandibular ligament passes by the lateral posterior palatal seal area and frequently impinges on the junction of the alveolar ridge and the palate (Fig. 11-2,

D). The attachment of the pterygomandibular ligament must not impinge upon the periphery of the denture. Dislodgement of the denture may result when the mouth is opened wide if this area of attachment is not considered.

The anteroposterior ridge relationship is of considerable importance in the placement and arrangement of the teeth. The mandibular alveolar ridge may be in distal or mesial relation to the maxillary ridge and occasionally presents difficulties in the placement of teeth and the retention of the dentures. The lateral ridge relationship is also of similar importance to the stability of the dentures.

Vertical dimension should be established during the initial phases of the examination and more accurately during the construction of the denture. Some change in the rest position of the mandible may occur with older age. This fact must be considered when vertical dimension is evaluated. The external features of the face should be noted from frontal and profile

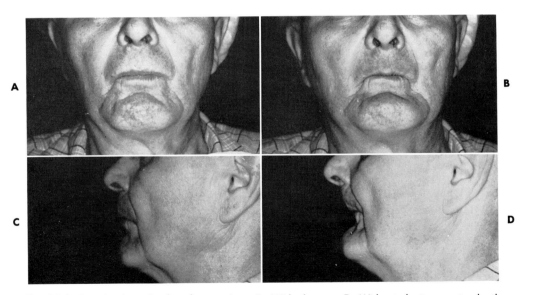

Fig. 11-3. *Examination of edentulous patient.* **A,** With denture. **B,** Without denture; note depth of labial folds and loss of support for cheeks. **C** and **D,** Examination of profile with and without dentures.

aspects (Fig. 11-3). Loss of tissue tone does not in itself indicate a loss of vertical dimension.

The tissues that are to bear the dentures should be evaluated for their ability to support dentures. Thin, atrophic, and spongy tissues are easily traumatized, and special consideration may be necessary to prepare them for dentures. Older patients, especially women past the menopause, may require massage of the tissues, small posterior teeth, and a special soft lining over the surfaces of knifelike alveolar ridges. It may also be necessary for these patients to alternately leave out one of their dentures at night.

The periphery of the buccal posterior border of the lower denture can be estimated by palpation during functional movements of the mandible and later can be fully evaluated by a functional impression. The lingual tubercle (the mandibular eminence below and medial to the most distal lower molar) and the postmylohyoid fossa of the mandible should be palpated to determine the undercut that this eminence and fossa present so the examiner can get some idea of the extent of the lingual flange of the lower denture. It is important in the selection of an impression tray since an over extended flange of an impression tray can injure the bony tissue and also prevent an adequate impression. The position of the attachment of the lingual frenulum is of significance in establishing the periphery of the denture. If the alveolar ridge height is minimal and the attachment high, there may be difficulty in establishing a proper lingual flange in this region. This area is also of significance in the placement of lingual bars of partial dentures.

The alveololingual sulcus should be palpated, since the floor of the mouth and the prominent structures that lie in it may be raised during the impression taking and may obliterate a portion of the ridge in the impression. This is especially true if there are prominent glands in the floor of the mouth together with extensive resorption of the molar area of the mandibular alveolar ridge. When this arrangement of structures is known, the examiner can prevent them from affecting the impression by modifying the impression tray.

The examiner should observe and palpate the lingual aspects of the mandible in the region of the bicuspids for the presence of mandibular tori since these structures occasionally prevent the proper placing of dentures and of necessity have to be removed surgically. The location of the mylohyoid ridge should be determined by palpation, especially in cases of extreme absorption of the alveolar ridge; the effect that the position of the mylohyoid ridge will have on the periphery of the lingual flange of the lower denture should be visualized.

The examination of the patient with dentures should consist of an evaluation of the response of the tissues to the dentures, the patient's adjustment to the dentures, and an analysis of the function of the dentures. The response of the tissues may be that of physiologic adaptation or pathologic regression. Although most patients adjust esthetically, functionally, and emotionally to the dentures, some patients refuse to wear dentures because of a lack of adjustment in any one or all of these areas. A patient may be completely satisfied with his dentures, yet an analysis of their function may reveal many shortcomings that prevent their maximum efficiency. It is not uncommon in such instances for pathologic factors to be present that the patient has unknowingly tolerated. Some patients with a high degree of tolerance believe that soreness, looseness, and poor chewing ability are inherent qualities of all dentures. At the other extreme are those who refuse to adjust to any denture regardless of its perfection. The emotional aspects of complete denture service and the adjustment of the patient make it imperative that the examination of dentures and denture-bearing areas for determination of proper function and the presence of disease be thorough and complete.

The diagnosis of complaints regarding complete dentures may present serious difficulty (Fig. 11-4). The separation of complaints of organic origin from those caused by lack of adjustment often taxes the skill and patience of the examiner. A well-taken history is often of significant value in making the differentiation. Proper preparation of the mouth and proper psychologic preparation of the patient are important considerations in the avoidance of denture problems.

The patient's complaints are usually directed toward soreness of the tissues after insertion of the dentures. Another common complaint during the adjustment period is lack of stability of the dentures. It must be pointed out that patients must learn to wear dentures, and the importance of this fact is sometimes completely overlooked by the patient. From the dentist's standpoint, many complaints may arise from a lack of adjustment of the patient to the dentures.

A complaint of soreness should be evaluated in terms of an overextension or overpressure of the denture, faulty occlusion, excessive vertical dimension, and a lack of patient adjustment. Localized areas of soreness may be manifested by a break in the mucosa or by areas of tenderness that can be determined by palpation. Ulceration of the tissues may arise because of overpressure from the denture or because of bony spicules beneath the mucosa. The exact location of the area of overpressure may be localized on the denture by using soft wax. This is painted on the mucosal surface of the denture in the general location of the offending area. Replacement of the dentures and functional movements of the mandible will displace the wax if overpressure or extension is present.

Generalized soreness of the alveolar crest may be related to excessive vertical dimension, encroachment on the freeway space, locked occlusion, lack of accommodation for Bennett's movement, or the presence of tissues that are not capable of denture support (Kingery). Denture-sore mouth is commonly caused by lack of denture stability, rarely by a sensitivity to the denture material itself. The stability of the dentures is related to occlusal balance, peripheral seal, vertical dimension, and the freeway space. Constant rocking and displacement result in chronic irritation of the underlying soft tissues.

Soreness at the periphery of the denture in the mucobuccal fold is usually caused by an overextension or overpressure of the buccal or lingual flange. The soreness is related to abrasion or ulceration of the mucosa. Soreness in the anterior part of the mouth can result from an overextension of the lingual flange, excessive pressure caused by a slide in centric occlusion, or overextension of the buccal flange in the molar region. Soreness on the lingual aspect of the denture flange may be caused by overextension on the labial or buccal side, occlusal interference on the same or opposite side, or warpage of the denture (Kingery).

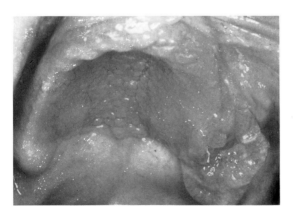

Fig. 11-4. *Examination of edentulous patient.* Lesion detected in patient who has worn same denture for 35 years. There is palatal papillomatosis and large fungating carcinoma with central necrosis involving left tuberosity. This lesion almost hidden by the denture was undetected through three periods of hospitalization for cataract removal.

Soreness in the posterior part of the mouth may result from occlusal interference or overextension of the labial flange in the anterior part of the mouth.

Looseness of dentures is another complaint that the examiner may encounter either shortly after the denture has been delivered to the patient or after it has been worn for a considerable length of time. The patient may complain of the maxillary denture dropping each time the mouth is opened or only occasionally. The causes may be multiple, and the occlusion, posterior seal, and overextension of the denture should be evaluated. Not infrequently a patient will complain that the upper denture drops when he talks or sings; this may be caused by overextension of the periphery of the denture or overactivity of the soft palate.

If the denture becomes loose on one side while the patient chews on the other side, the occlusion should be checked for teeth set too wide on the denture, inadequate overject, and entrapment of food because of the inclination of the buccal cusps. Cheek chewing may result from inadequate overjet of the maxillary molars both buccally and distally. A denture may come loose after being worn for only a few hours; this is frequently caused by accumulation of thick mucinous saliva under it. Having the patient wash the denture off occasionally will usually indicate whether this is the cause.

The stability of the lower denture is related, among other things, to the position of the bicuspids and the thickness of the periphery of the denture. The buccal aspect of the first bicuspid should not be more prominent buccally than the buccal flange of the denture. The peripheral flange should be thin in the region of frenula, lips, and molar region.

Partially edentulous mouth

Examination of the partially edentulous mouth includes a thorough examination of the whole mouth, the remaining teeth, and the denture-bearing areas (Fig. 11-5). The examination may be given for the purpose of considering the mouth preparatory to partial dentures, for evaluating dentures that are already in use, or for appraising the response of the tissues to the dentures. Whatever the reason for the examination, the mouth should be completely examined for the presence of disease or potentially harmful conditions.

It goes without saying that a complete examination of the mouth is necessary prior to the preparation for partial dentures. The prerequisite of a complete examination has been discussed previously. The condition of the teeth and their supporting structures must be known prior to the construction of partial dentures. It is only after these structures have been evaluated that the dentist can know what elements of the partial denture prosthesis have to be considered. Whether or not a tooth and its supporting structure is a suitable abutment can be determined only by an examination of these structures. Thus, periodontal disease, carious lesions, devital teeth, poor root form, malposed teeth, teeth with abnormal anatomic crowns, unerupted teeth, root fragments, soft tissue lesions, and systemic disease are factors that have an important bearing on the placement of partial dentures; each must be evaluated by history and examination.

It is not the purpose of this book to dwell on the indications and contraindications for partial dentures or to justify the use of fixed or removable appliances. Both forms of appliances have common aims: to increase the function of mastication; to prevent extrusion, drifting, and hyperfunction of the remaining teeth; and to improve esthetic and phonetic qualities of the mouth.

The examination of the partially edentulous mouth should consider the following items: (1) vitality of the teeth, caries, attrition, (2) condition of the supporting tis-

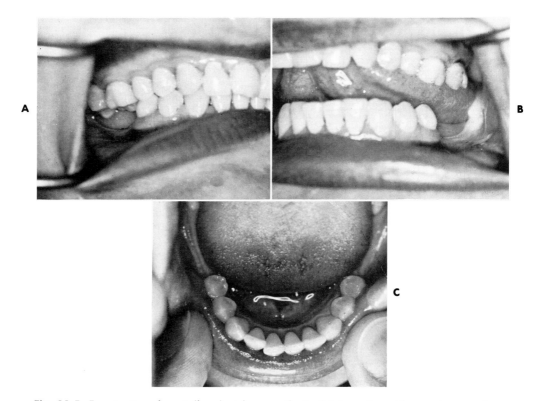

Fig. 11-5. *Examination of partially edentulous mouth.* **A,** Relation of maxillary molars to edentulous area. **B,** Position of sublingual tissue to edentulous area. **C,** Clinical survey regarding planes of insertion of an appliance.

sues of the teeth, (3) status of the edentulous areas, (4) arrangement and position of the remaining teeth, (5) occlusal relationships, (6) intermaxillary space and vertical dimension, (7) oral hygiene, (8) form of roots and crowns of the teeth to be used as abutments, (9) relationship of the alveolar ridge to frenula, soft tissues, and bony eminences, (10) relationship of free gingival margin to placement of the appliance, (11) anteroposterior and lateral relationship of opposing arches, and (12) ability of the tissues of the edentulous areas to act as a denture-bearing area. These are the basic principles of the examination necessary for the restoration of any edentulous space, whether it be with a fixed or removable appliance.

The examination of the appliance already placed should involve all of the preceding factors plus an evaluation of the adjustment of both the tissues and the patient to the appliance. These factors should be brought out and elaborated upon in the history and examination of the patient. A periodic examination of appliances as well as the structures of the masticatory system should be a part of an efficient dental practice.

The consideration and selection of abutment teeth for a fixed or removable appliance must follow the needs and dictates of each case, and consideration must be given to the status of the pulp, the form and length of the root, the stability of the tooth, and the condition of the supporting tissues. Irrespective of the type of appliance, the ability of the tooth to be used and retained as an abutment must receive due consideration. Thus, the first step in an examination of the teeth and arches for a prosthetic appliance should be the determination of the status of the teeth and supporting structures.

The vitality of any tooth to be used or that has been used as an abutment should be routinely tested. Retrograde pulp changes may not be obvious to the patient or to the examiner until the extra load on an abutment tooth causes a rapid deterioration of the pulp. Although pulp testing may not completely appraise minor pulp abnormalities, a sufficient number of abnormal teeth may be discovered by routine testing to make the effort well worth while. The location and extent of carious lesions should be determined. Such a determination may require removal of all the decay before a final evaluation can be made.

The condition of the supporting structures of the teeth also has to be evaluated before proceeding with the construction of an appliance. If periodontal disease is present, extensive treatment may be required to prepare the mouth for an appliance. In many instances, teeth that appear superficially to be good abutments have to be extracted because of bifurcation and trifurcation involvement.

Edentulous areas should be examined clinically and radiographically for the presence of lesions, unerupted teeth, retained root tips, and foreign objects such as amalgam.

The arrangement and position of the teeth are directly related to the design of an appliance. Malposed teeth present problems in the final placement of fixed appliances, preparation of the teeth for retainers, and interocclusal harmony. They also present problems in the design of clasps, line of insertion, and line of draw for removable appliances. These factors can best be evaluated by the use of a surveyor.

The location of edentulous areas is of importance in determining whether an appliance is to be fixed or removable. The use of a classification system to describe the type of partial edentulism present facilitates the discussion of a case without resorting to the cumbersome task of naming all the teeth present in the arch. Such a classification as advocated by Kennedy is an aid to the terminology used in oral diagnosis and has practical application in partial denture design. It must be remembered that such a classification is never a diagnosis. The designation Class I is given to those cases in which bilateral edentulous areas are located posterior to the remaining teeth; Class II, to those cases in which a unilateral edentulous area is located posterior to the remaining teeth; Class III, to those cases in which there is a unilateral edentulous space with teeth remaining posterior and anterior to it; and Class IV, to those cases in which a unilateral edentulous space is present involving the midline.

Occlusal relationships are important to the stability, retention, and maintenance of appliances as well as to trauma of the remaining teeth when occlusal disharmony exists. Extruded and drifted teeth should be analyzed in their functional relations and in relation to the appliance that is to be placed (Fig. 11-6). Equilibration of the natural dentition may be necessary for the preparation of the mouth. This must be considered before construction of the appliance begins. Working, balancing, and protrusive relationships should be evaluated. An alteration of the form of the remaining teeth should be considered in relation to improving the function of the occlusion. Not infrequently an appliance is constructed without first considering what modification of the teeth can be accomplished to improve the number of harmonious contacts in lateral excursion. Unfortunately in many such instances the working bite will consist of only one or two teeth being in contact in lateral movements of the jaw. In a large number of instances judicious grinding will result in bringing more of the remaining teeth into contact in the working bite. It will also allow the replacement of the missing teeth in the appliance in a functional position for lateral movements.

The intermaxillary space should be evaluated, since in many instances little space may be present for the placement of teeth or the ideal placement of the metal framework, connectors, and occlusal rests (Fig. 10-25). Frequently a patient will have lost all of the lower molars, with the result that the upper molars have drifted and encroached upon the denture area of the

lower arch (Fig. 11-6). This is a significant finding and has an important bearing on the preparation of the mouth for an appliance and on the design of the appliance.

Oral hygiene is an important factor in the maintenance of any appliance. Establishing good oral hygiene and teaching the patient to maintain it are important factors in the health of the supporting structures. This phase of treatment should be considered prior to the placement of an appliance. Any type of appliance requires that the patient take additional care of the mouth to prevent the accumulation of debris in abutment areas. Poor oral hygiene in itself

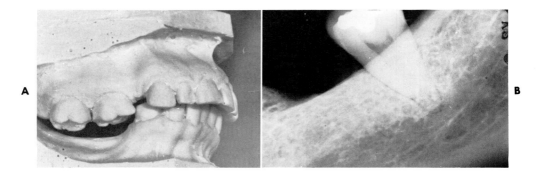

Fig. 11-6. *Examination of partially edentulous mouth.* **A,** Cast showing relationship of teeth to edentulous area. **B,** Root form unfavorable for an abutment tooth.

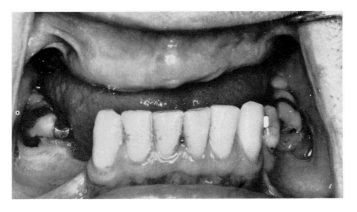

Fig. 11-7. *Examination of partially edentulous mouth.* Relationship of remaining teeth to edentulous arch.

may be a strong contraindication for many or all appliances.

The form of the roots of teeth that are to be used as support for an appliance is of considerable importance. Short conical roots may preclude the use of a tooth for an abutment (Fig. 11-6, *B*). The form of the crown is important to the type of retainer that may be used and to the placement of clasps if the appliance is of the removable type. The presence and location of undercuts in the anatomic crown of an abutment tooth are directly related to the position and design of the retaining parts of the appliance. In some instances, the crown of a tooth may have to be completely altered either by grinding or by full crown restorations in order to have a line of draw or retention areas for clasps.

The relationship of the alveolar crest to frenula, soft tissues, and bony eminences should be determined (Fig. 11-7). Lingual bars of lower partial dentures may encroach upon the lingual frenulum when its attachment is high or when the alveolar process has been resorbed. When this occurs, frenula attachments may have to be altered, or the design of the partial denture may have to be altered to the point that the lingual bar does not rest on soft tissue but on the teeth. The presence of undercuts in the alveolar ridge and adjacent tissues may of necessity require that the line of draw be altered or the undercut removed. Such conditions should be evaluated during the examination of the mouth; in some instances such an evaluation may determine what type of appliance, if any, can be constructed for the patient. The use of casts and a surveyor will be of significant benefit in evaluation of the undercut areas. The presence of large bony eminences like palatine and mandibular tori directly affects the design and position of palatal and lingual bars if not removed. These protuberances should be noted in the examination and considered in the treatment plan.

The location of the gingival margin should be considered in relation to the design and placement of the framework of partial dentures. Also of importance is the relationship of the gingival margin to the placement of a retainer. In some instances its position may also affect the placement of clasps. Hyperplastic papillae on the mesial or distal aspects of an abutment tooth are a potential source of trouble and can also interfere with the design of an appliance. This tissue with its relationship to the appliance and abutment predisposes to the development of deep crevices or even periodontal pockets. Removal of the tissue should be considered in the examination and related to the preparation of the mouth for the appliance. Lingual bars and connectors of partial dentures have to be designed in order to avoid encroachment on the free gingival margin.

The anteroposterior and lateral relationships of the opposing arches should be noted and evaluated. As in the construction of full dentures, the proper relationship of the teeth to the arches is an important consideration. The anteroposterior relationship of the maxillary and mandibular arches should be determined in centric relation as well as in centric occlusion. Premature contacts may result in a false anterior displacement of the mandible.

The state of the soft and hard tissues that are to bear the prosthetic appliance is an important factor in the successful wearing of the appliance. Thin, atrophic, or soft and hyperplastic tissue is not a good base for partial dentures; the examiner should evaluate all such areas that are to be used for supporting the denture. Older patients may frequently have thin and atrophic tissue that cannot stand the trauma of an appliance. Patients with Plummer-Vinson syndrome frequently complain of the inability to wear any type of tissue-borne appliance. When the examination reveals that tissue is soft and atrophic in those areas to be used as a denture base, careful consideration must be given to the design of the appliance and to the possibility of removal of redundant tissue.

Complaints relative to partial dentures already being worn are similar to those relative to full dentures. In addition, complaints concerning sore teeth may be found. Sore teeth may result from occlusal trauma, especially associated with occlusal test being "high," from constant displacement of the teeth during the insertion of the appliance. Complaints concerning fixed appliances are usually related to occlusal trauma, balancing interferences, and heavy loading of an abutment tooth not accustomed to its increased function.

REFERENCES

Atwood, D. A., and Coy, W. A.: Clinical, cephalometric, and densitometric study of reduction of residual ridges, J. Prosth. Dent. 26:280, 1971.

Boitel, R. H.: Problems of old age in dental prosthetics and restorative procedures, J. Prosth. Dent. 26:350, 1971.

Brill, N., Scübeler, S., and Tryde, G.: Aspects of occlusal sense in natural and artificial teeth, J. Prosth. Dent. 12:123, 1962.

Carlsson, G. E., and Persson, D.: Morphologic changes of the mandible after extraction and wearing of dentures: a longitudinal, clinical, and x-ray cephalometric study covering 5 years, Odont. Revy 18:27, 1967.

Kingery, R. H.: Lectures on complete dentures, Ann Arbor, Mich., 1958, The University of Michigan, School of Dentistry.

Tallgren, A.: The effect of denture wearing on facial morphology, Acta Odont. Scand. 25:563, 1967.

Wright, C. R., Muyskens, J. H., Strong, L. H., et al.: A study of the tongue and its relation to denture stability, J.A.D.A. 39:269, 1949.

SECTION III

RADIOGRAPHIC AND SUPPLEMENTARY EXAMINATIONS

Dental radiographs, when correlated with the case history and clinical examination, are among the most important diagnostic supplements in oral diagnosis. Well-taken radiographs examined under the proper conditions may reveal evidence of disease that cannot be discovered by any other method. There are numerous pathologic situations that cannot be detected clinically until a large amount of normal tissue is involved; yet, a radiograph may reveal such a situation while it is still incipient. This can be said of such entities as odontogenic cysts and tumors, neoplasms of bone, reaction of bone to devital teeth, and many others. If the dentist neglects to use an adequate number of radiographs at regular intervals, he ignores an extremely valuable diagnostic procedure. Misuse of radiographs by using them only for the detection of dental caries encourages neglect of other major dental problems.

There has been much discussion among dental radiologists relative to the most desirable method or technic for obtaining radiographs. Regardless of the preference for a particular technic, the final product is, of course, of the utmost importance. The technic used should be mastered so that all of the features that a diagnostician desires in a radiograph are present. The requirements of any good radiograph, regardless of technic, are (1) a clear sharp image of the anatomic area involved, (2) inclusion of a sufficient normal area surrounding the pathologic area being examined, (3) proper contrast between tissues of varying densities, and (4) minimal distortion.

It is important that radiographs be examined under proper lighting conditions. Properly exposed radiographs will show varying amounts of detail, depending upon the intensity of the light used to view them. Quite frequently detail is not seen in a radiograph because the viewing light is too dim; in many instances, a bright light will bring out detail that is not seen under ordinary lighting conditions.

In addition to an adequate history, physical examination, and radiographic examination, supplementary diagnostic aids may be necessary to complete the examination of a patient. Such aids include bacteriologic studies, blood studies, serologic tests, urine studies, contact sensitivity tests, biopsy, pulp vitality tests, the articulation and surveying of study casts, and the use of disclosing solution. Clinical laboratory studies of occasional value to the dentist are bacteriologic tests, screening blood studies, and urinalysis.

Laboratory tests should not be considered routine examination procedures; they should be done only when indicated. In many instances too much emphasis is placed on the information expected from a battery of such tests. In reality there can be no substitute for a carefully taken and weighed history and the examination and observation of the patient by a competent clinician. Without these procedures, diagnostic laboratory aids cannot be intelli-

259

gently utilized; in fact, a complete examination in most instances makes them unnecessary. Laboratory tests and radiographic observations are often important in confirming and establishing a diagnosis; however, they are not always employed with judgment. Of primary importance is the proper recognition of the need for laboratory studies; at no time should they become a substitute for an adequate history and examination of the patient. Dependence on laboratory aids and neglect and misinterpretation of the history and clinical findings often reveal a lack of understanding of the true value of laboratory studies. Such an approach is often conducive to errors in diagnosis and is an unnecessary expense to the patient. The examiner should not rely upon any one method of examination in his diagnostic procedure. Reliance should not be placed primarily on laboratory studies since, more often than not, a correct diagnosis can be more adequately determined by subjective and objective clinical symptoms alone than by laboratory studies alone.

OUTLINE FOR RADIOGRAPHIC EXAMINATION
Complete mouth radiographs

1. Lamina dura associated with teeth and the cortical bone associated with denture-bearing areas—continuity and thickness
2. Periodontal spaces—variations in width
3. Level of the alveolar crest in relation to cementoenamel junction
4. Periapical radiolucency
5. Pathologic conditions of the teeth
6. Pathologic conditions of the jaws—osseous radiolucencies and osseous radiopacities
7. Other dental findings

Posterior bite-wing radiographs

1. Lamina dura continuity at the alveolar crest
2. Alveolar crest level in relation to the cementoenamel junction

3. Tooth crown shape and formative defects of the tooth crown
4. Pulp size and degree of pulpal calcification
5. Existing restorations
6. Location of calculus
7. Location of carious lesions

OUTLINE OF SUPPLEMENTARY EXAMINATIONS
Bacteriologic studies

Antibiotic sensitivity tests
Wound, abscess, lesions, and surgical incision cultures
Caries activity tests
Root canal cultures
Fresh moist preparations and smears

Blood studies

Hematologic diagnosis associated with anemia and polycythemia
    Red cell count
    Hemoglobin determination
    Hematocrit determination
Hematologic diagnosis associated with bleeding
    Bleeding time
    Coagulation or clotting time
    Partial thromboplastin time
    Clot retraction
    Tourniquet test
    Platelet count
    Prothrombin time
Hematologic diagnosis associated with infections
    White cell count
    Differential white cell count
Hematologic diagnosis associated with lymph node enlargement
Hematologic diagnosis associated with leukemias
Serologic tests
    Complement-fixation test
    Flocculation test
    Alkaline phosphatase, calcium, phosphorus, and serum protein determinations

Urine studies
Biochemical profiles
Contact sensitivity tests
Biopsy
Exfoliative cytology and aspiration
Pulp vitality tests
Study casts
Stomatomicroscope
Disclosing solution

12
Radiographic examination

The most common mistake made in radiographic examinations is that of omission. It is not an uncommon practice in dentistry to include posterior bite-wing radiographs and periapical radiographs of the anterior teeth only in the initial radiographic examination and then to repeat only the posterior bite-wing radiographs in subsequent examinations at 6-month or yearly intervals. In instance after instance it can be shown that posterior bite-wing radiographs without periapical radiographs of the complete mouth are far from sufficient (Fig. 12-1). Too frequently, pathologic areas involving the apices and radicular portions of teeth are missed because an insufficient number of radiographs are taken. The minimum to be taken in the initial examination of any patient, dentulous or edentulous, should include radiographs of the complete mouth as well as posterior bite-wing radiographs if the posterior teeth are present.

It is a common practice to charge a separate fee for radiographs. This makes it seem as though the dentist is offering a product for that fee. It is far more desirable to charge one fee for the service of conducting a thorough and efficient examination, including interpretation of the radiographs. The radiographs in themselves are of no value to the patient—it is the ability of the dentist to interpret those radiographs accurately for which the patient pays the fee.

INTERPRETATION OF NORMAL RADIOGRAPHS

The basic prerequisite for radiographic interpretation is an understanding of what constitutes normal. The normal architecture of the hard tissues as seen radiographically, as well as the normal landmarks, must be recognized by the examiner and distinguished from pathologic conditions. One must remember that the radiographic image seen on the x-ray film is a "shadow" of hard tissues that do not permit the complete passage of x-rays through them. The varying degrees of density or calcification of bone and teeth permit varying amounts of x-rays to reach the x-ray film. The areas occupied by the denser structures such as teeth and bone appear lighter (radiopaque) on x-ray film, since a large portion of the x-rays is stopped and therefore not permitted to reach and expose the x-ray film. Areas occupied by the soft tissues or by air allow the passage of almost all of the x-rays and appear black (radiolucent) on film. What one actually sees when he examines a radiograph is a two-dimensional shadow of the structure radiographed. The fact that the radiograph is only two dimensional permits superimposition of one structure upon another in the radiograph. When the diagnostician examines a radiograph, he must always keep in mind that what he sees is merely variations in density of hard tissues and that he also sees a shadow of all of the tissue that occupied the space between the x-ray film and the source of the x-rays.

Normal landmarks— periapical radiographs

There are several normal anatomic landmarks that can be recognized on radiographs taken in different parts of the mouth. These landmarks vary in position, size, and clarity from one individual to another, and

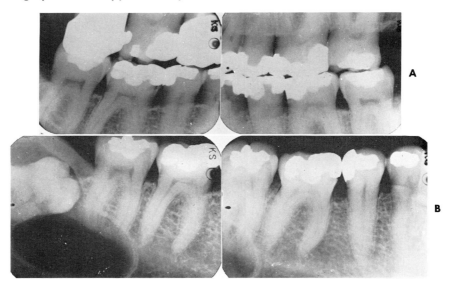

Fig. 12-1. *Radiographic examination.* **A,** Posterior bite-wing radiographs. **B,** Periapical radiographs. **B** shows that posterior bite-wing radiographs are inadequate to demonstrate findings other than those associated with the crowns of the teeth; note that dentigerous cyst and impacted molar are not seen in posterior bite-wing radiographs.

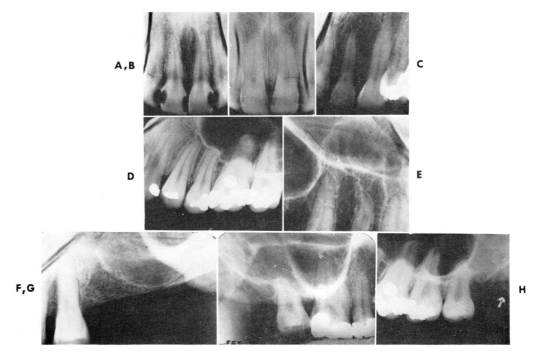

Fig. 12-2. *Radiographic examination—landmarks.* **A,** Incisive canal. **B,** Nasal septum. **C,** Incisive fossa. **D,** Maxillary sinus. **E,** Antral Y. **F,** Molar bone. **G,** Coronoid process. **H,** Hamular process.

they correspond to normal anatomic structures that are seen by every dental student in anatomy dissections.

The maxilla (Fig. 12-2). The following landmarks are recognizable in radiographs of the maxilla.

Incisive foramen. The incisive foramen is visible in the anterior midline of the maxilla between the roots of the maxillary incisor teeth. The foramen usually appears as an oval-shaped, somewhat radiolucent area surrounded by a relatively dense layer of bone.

Nasal septum. The nasal septum is visible as a vertical radiopaque band well above the apices of the central incisors and is centrally located in the radiograph.

Incisive fossa. Between the roots of the cuspid and central incisor teeth and over the apex of the lateral incisor tooth is an area that appears to be less dense than the surrounding tissue. This corresponds to the incisive fossa and is in fact an anatomic area that contains less thickness of bone than the areas lateral to it.

Maxillary sinus. The maxillary sinus produces a large radiolucent area usually extending from the bicuspid area posteriorly to the second molar region. Sinus septa can be seen as radiopaque lines running through the maxillary sinus, and an important landmark, the so-called antral Y, marks the separation of the anterior portion of the maxillary sinus from the nasal cavity. The antral Y is seen in the radiograph of the cuspid region. In young persons the maxillary sinus is confined to an area near the apices of the teeth, whereas in older persons this sinus extends well down toward the alveolar crest, and it may appear as though the roots of the maxillary bicuspid and molar teeth actually project into the maxillary sinus.

Malar bone. This appears radiographically as a U-shaped radiopaque band at the maxillary first molar area and is frequently superimposed on the roots of the maxillary first molar.

Coronoid process. Quite frequently when the second molar region is radiographed, a fingerlike projection can be seen in the inferior and posterior corner of the film. This bony structure represents the coronoid process of the mandible.

Hamulus. A small projection of bone may be seen just posterior to the maxillary tuberosity in many radiographs of the second molar region. This represents the hamular process of the medial pterygoid plate.

• • •

The maxillary radiographic landmarks that are likely to cause confusion are the maxillary sinus, which is often confused with a cystic area by the inexperienced examiner; the incisive fossa, which may give the impression of a rarefied area about the lateral incisor root apex; and the incisive foramen, which, when rather large, may suggest the presence of an incisive canal cyst or an area of bone rarefaction over the central incisor if superimposed on the apex of the central incisor (Fig. 12-3).

The mandible (Fig. 12-4). The following landmarks are recognizable in radiographs of the mandible.

Lingual foramen. In the anterior midline of the mandible inferior to the apices of the central incisor teeth is the lingual foramen. This is not seen on all mandibular in-

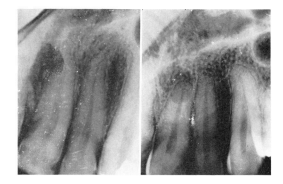

Fig. 12-3. *Radiographic examination—landmarks.* Incisive foramen superimposed on apex of central incisor.

cisor radiographs. However, when visualized, it is a circumscribed radiopaque area with a center that is radiolucent and about 0.5 mm. in diameter.

Genial tubercles. The genial tubercles can be seen only when the base of the mandible is visible in the mandibular central incisor radiograph. They appear as sharp radiopaque projections from the lingual cortical plate of bone.

Mental foramen. The mental foramen is located near the apices of bicuspid teeth

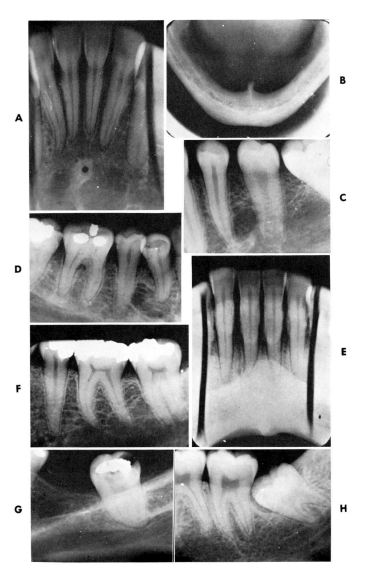

Fig. 12-4. *Radiographic examination—landmarks.* **A,** Lingual foramen. **B,** Genial tubercle. **C** and **D,** Mental foramen. **E,** Mental ridge. **F,** Submaxillary fossa. **G,** Mandibular canal, mylohyoid, and external oblique line moving from inferior to superior. **H,** Projection of impacted third molar roots into inferior alveolar canal.

in the mandible. In the greatest percentage of human jaws the mental foramen is seen radiographically between the two bicuspid teeth. However, its position may vary from a position anterior to the first bicuspid to one that is posterior to the second bicuspid. Multiple mental foramens do occur.

Mental ridge. Because of the heavy cortical plate of bone in certain areas of the mandible, there are definite linear structures that produce normal radiographic landmarks. The mental ridge is one of these structures. It appears as an inverted V-shaped radiopaque structure and may be superimposed on the incisor roots.

Submaxillary fossa. Another normal radiographic finding on the mandible is that of the depression beneath the mandibular molar roots that is occupied by the submaxillary salivary gland. This area of the mandible is somewhat thinner than the surrounding bone and therefore may lack trabecular pattern and may appear comparatively radiolucent.

Mandibular canal. In the area beneath the first, second, and third molar roots the mandibular canal appears as a horizontal linear radiolucent band bordered by two radiopaque lines.

External oblique line. Immediately superior to the mandibular canal is another radiopaque linear structure that represents the external oblique line.

• • •

The areas in the mandible that produce confusion in interpretation of radiographs for the inexperienced examiner are the mental foramen, particularly when it is superimposed over the apex of one of the bicuspid teeth, and the submaxillary gland fossa, which sometimes appears an an area of bone rarefaction.

General landmarks (Fig. 12-5). The general landmarks recognizable in radiographs include the alevolar process, alveolar bone, and periodontal space.

Alveolar process. The alveolar process is that bone which is trabecular in pattern and surrounds the roots of the teeth. The bony architecture of the alveolar process varies from one area to another, particularly in the size of the trabeculae and the size of the marrow spaces. Patterns of trabeculae also vary from one person to another. One particularly characteristic variation in pattern is that of the "stepladder" trabecular arrangement that is frequently seen between the roots of the mandibular incisor teeth.

Alveolar bone. The alveolar bone is the cortical bone that immediately surrounds the teeth and therefore lines the alveolus of the tooth. It is often referred to radiographically as the lamina dura, and under normal circumstances is a radiopaque line of relatively uniform thickness that is continuous around the entire root of the tooth. The term lamina dura also includes the cortical bone that extends over the alveolar crest and gives the impression that the lamina dura is a continuous line from one alveolus to another. The most coronal portion of the alvoelar process, as well as the lamina dura, which occupies the space between two adjacent teeth, is referred to as the alveolar crest. The crest is normally within 1 to 1.5 mm. of the cementoenemal junction of the adjacent tooth.

Periodontal space. The radiolucent line

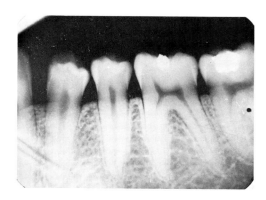

Fig. 12-5. *Radiographic examination—landmarks.* Alveolar process and alveolar bone.

between the root of the tooth and the alveolar bone represents the space occupied by the periodontal membrane. Normally the periodontal space is of nearly uniform width around the entire root of the tooth.

METHOD OF RADIOGRAPHIC EXAMINATION

As previously stated, the minimum dental radiographic examination should include radiographs of the complete mouth (14 periapical films) and posterior bitewing radiographs (No. 1 and No. 2 size films to allow two views with different horizontal angulations in order to reduce overlap areas) if enough posterior teeth are present to warrant them. Auxiliary radiographs may be used wherever indicated and will be discussed later.

Well-organized, methodic examination of the radiograph is imperative if the dentist is to make complete use of this valuable diagnostic aid. Whenever possible, correlation between clinical and radiographic findings is extremely important to minimize the interpretation of an artifact in the radiograph as a disease process. The organization of the radiograph viewing procedure minimizes the possibility of overlooking important details. A methodic approach to radiographic viewing develops the habit of examining all radiographs in the same sequence, thereby increasing the accuracy of the viewing procedure.

RADIOGRAPHS OF THE COMPLETE MOUTH
Lamina dura—continuity and thickness

The lamina dura normally forms a continuous line around the roots of the teeth and over the alveolar crest between the teeth. It should be examined in the same numerical sequence as the teeth are examined to preclude the possibility of missing any area. Periapical films provide the means for examining the lamina dura in most areas, although the bite-wing films are often helpful in determining its continuity

over the alveolar crest in the posterior part of the dental arch.

A lack of continuity of alveolar crest lamina dura is indicative of active periodontal disease (Fig. 12-6). This very important finding, if overlooked, can cause the examiner to miss the diagnosis of incipient periodontal disease, since resorption of the alveolar crest lamina dura is the initial bone loss that occurs in periodontitis. The success of periodontal treatment can be evaluated radiographically in many cases since the lamina dura will reappear when the gingival inflammatory process is eliminated.

A break in continuity of lamina dura at the apical area of the tooth occurs as the result of inflammatory reaction of the periapical tissue to a devital pulp (Fig. 12-7). The break will occur in either an acute or chronic periapical inflammation and the extent of the lack of continuity is dependent

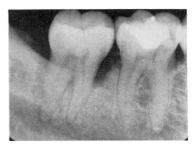

Fig. 12-6. *Absence of lamina dura at alveolar crest and lateral surface of root.*

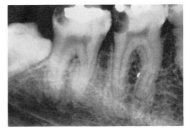

Fig. 12-7. *Absence of lamina dura at apex of mesial root of first molar caused by devital pulp.*

on the extent of the inflammatory process. An acute periapical inflammatory process can always be correlated with the clinical findings of a tooth that is painful to percussion or biting pressures, and the presence of swelling or abscess formation, depending on how severe the inflammatory response is and how far it has progressed. A chronic inflammatory process will show varying degrees of involvement of the lamina dura and usually will be asymptomatic.

Interruption of the lamina dura associated with the lateral aspect of the root of a tooth is usually caused by the extension of periodontal disease. In acute periodontal abscess the resorption of the lamina dura

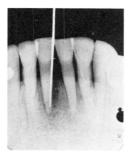

Fig. 12-8. *Absence of lamina dura* from lateral root surface associated with periodontal abscess. Note probe in the area of abscess.

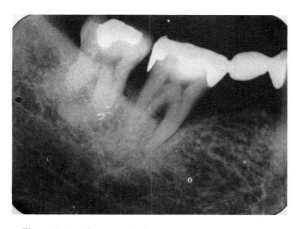

Fig. 12-9. *Absence of lamina dura* in bifurcation area of mandibular second molar.

occurs very rapidly and is accompanied by clinical signs and symptoms of abscess formation (Fig. 12-8). A periodontal pocket that is progressing rapidly also shows interruption of the lamina dura and can be demonstrated clinically, although it may be asymptomatic. When no periodontal pocket or abscess formation can be demonstated clinically in relation to the disappearance of the lamina dura from the lateral root surface, then the possibilities of trauma, lateral root cyst formation, or neoplasm should be considered. Other radiographic evidence of lateral root cyst or neoplasm usually accompanies the disappearance of lamina dura.

In radiographs that show considerable periodontal disease, examination for continuity of the lamina dura in the trifurcation area of maxillary molars and the bifurcation area of mandibular molars is very important (Fig. 12-9). A disappearance of lamina dura in these areas indicates that the periodontal destruction has advanced to the area of root division and the degree of destruction becomes very important in the consideration of retention of teeth so involved.

The cortical bone is continuous in edentulous arches under normal conditions. It should appear as a regular unbroken line at the crest of the well-healed edentulous ridge (Fig. 12-10). The cortical bone in edenulous areas is susceptible to the same resorptive changes as the lamina dura about functioning teeth. Pressure and inflammation are capable of disrupting the cortical bone at the crest of the edentulous ridge. By far the most common resorptive change in cortical bone over the edentulous ridge occurs in the situation in which a maxillary denture is worn opposing natural mandibular anterior teeth and without posterior support. When a mandibular partial denture that needs rebasing is worn and does not support the posterior part of the maxillary complete denture, anterior resorption will occur in the maxilla. This

A

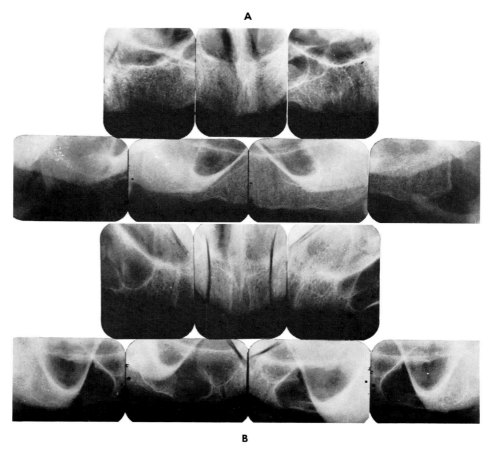

B

Fig. 12-10. *Continuity of cortical layer of bone in edentulous arch.* **A,** Lack of continuity in left cuspid region. **B,** Lack of continuity in right and left cuspid regions.

type of resorption is evident radiographically from bicuspid to bicuspid region of the anterior portion of the edentulous maxillary arch. The resorption can be correlated with the clinical finding of a flabby ridge and in many instances with an accompanying inflammatory reaction in the overlying tissue. The patient in such instances complains of looseness of the maxillary denture or uses denture adhesive constantly to provide denture stability.

The thickness of the lamina dura about the roots of teeth is, in general, uniform. There are minor degrees of variation from one area of the mouth to another but the radiographic interpreter should be alerted by variations of thickness of lamina dura on the same tooth. The changes that occur in traumatic occlusion are evidenced by a compensatory widening of lamina dura associated with the portion of the tooth where tension is applied to the periodontal membrane as the tooth is traumatized (Fig. 12-11). A clinical appraisal of occlusal function will usually substantiate the radiographic findings.

Periodontal spaces—variations in width

Uniformity of the width of the periodontal space is evident about teeth that are

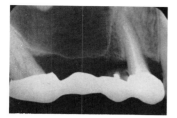

Fig. 12-11. *Increased width of lamina dura and widened periodontal space caused by occlusal trauma.*

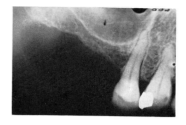

Fig. 12-12. *Widened periodontal space, calculus on distal aspect of second bicuspid and loss of alveolar bone.*

functioning normally. The space averages from 0.18 to 0.25 mm. in width (Kronfeld). The minor variations in width depend on the level of the periodontal membrane under consideration. Physiologic movement of a tooth results in slightly wider periodontal membrane at the apical and cervical regions as a result of movement around a fulcrum point near the midpoint of the root of the tooth. Nonfunctional teeth show narrowing of the periodontal space. A tooth in traumatic occlusion shows characteristic excessive widening of the periodontal space near the alveolar crest (Fig. 12-12). Excessive widening of the periodontal space is often visible near the apical portion of the root on the contralateral side of the traumatized tooth. The horizontal angulation of the radiograph sometimes masks one or both of these changes because the variation of breadth of periodontal space that is parallel to the x-ray at different horizontal angulations and because the involved surface of the tooth may be buccal or lingual and therefore not visualized. Widening of the periodontal space in the bifurcation and trifurcation areas of molars may be suggestive of either advance of periodontal disease to these areas or traumatic occlusion (Fig. 12-9). Widened periodontal spaces may be confirmed by clinical examination of the traumatized tooth, which frequently shows increased mobility and produces a dull percussion note.

Initial periapical reactions to devital pulps are manifest radiographically as widened periodontal spaces at the apices of involved teeth. Recognition of this incipient finding may prevent extensive periapical involvement or severe pain and possibly severe infection. Confusion in diagnosis may arise when the periapical periodontal membrane is widened as a result of vertical occlusal trauma to the affected tooth. The suspicion of a devital tooth in the course of the radiographic examination should always be confirmed by the appropriate plup tests.

Level of the alveolar crest in relation to the cementoenamel junction

The normal level of the alveolar crest is from 1 to 1.5 mm. apical to the cementoenamel junction (Fig. 12-13). Reduction of the level is indicative of the extent of periodontal disease but not always indicative of active periodontal disease; however, when the alveolar crest is seen at a reduced level without the lamina dura intact over it, the examiner can assume that the periodontal disease is active.

There may be confusion in judging the level of the alveolar crest in the maxillary molar region because of the vertical angulation at which this area is radiographed and the buccolingual width of the crest. The vertical angulation results in a projection of the buccal portion of the alveolar crest coronally (Fig. 12-14). The "long cone" technic is capable of producing a

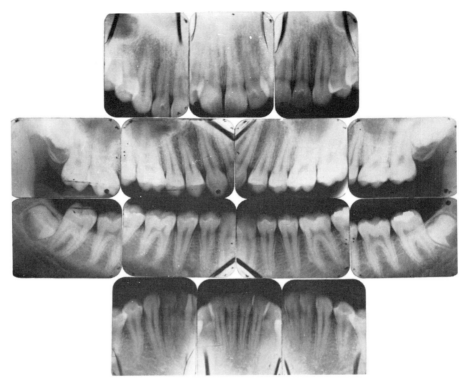

Fig. 12-13. *Normal complete mouth radiograph.*

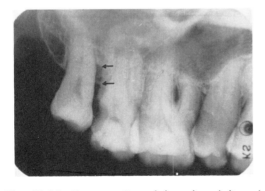

Fig. 12-14. *Demonstration of buccal and lingual bone levels. Note trifurcation involvement of first molar and deep caries on mesial aspect of second bicuspid and distal aspect of second molar.*

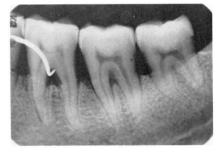

Fig. 12-15. *Horizontal loss of alveolar bone and alveolar process. Note bifurcation involvement on first and second molars.*

truer radiographic reproduction of this area.

The level of the alveolar crest is a very important consideration in the selection of teeth to be retained in periodontal treatment and in the selection of abutment teeth for prosthetic appliances. No rule of thumb will hold for the acceptable level of the

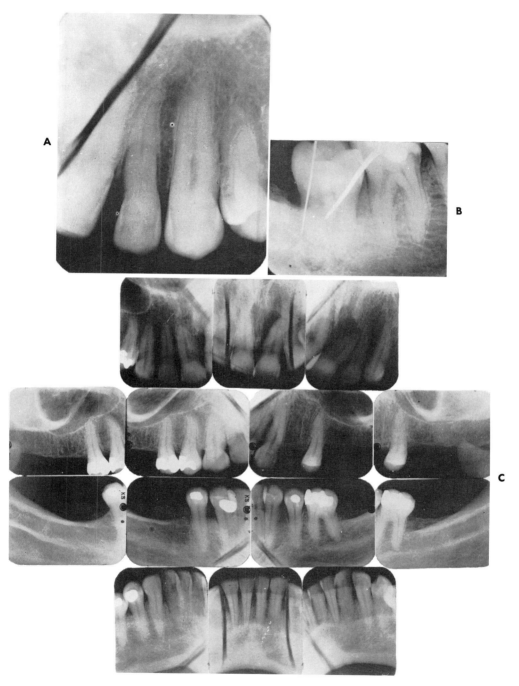

Fig. 12-16. *Vertical loss of alveolar bone.* **A,** Lingual aspect of lateral incisor. **B,** Distal and lingual aspect of second molar. **C,** Single area of involvement on mesial aspect of maxillary right central incisor.

alveolar crest because of the variation in root form and root size. However, when a tooth has less than half its original periodontal support, it is usually not able to withstand the additional load of a prosthesis.

The terms horizontal and vertical bone loss have been applied loosely to the two different patterns of reduction in height of the alveolar crest. The term horizontal bone loss applies to a more or less uniform reduction of the alveolar crest that is associated with periodontal disease on the basis of a uniform inflammatory process (Fig. 12-15). The inflammatory process results mainly from plaque, calculus, and poorly adapted cervical margins of restorations. Vertical bone loss, on the other hand, refers to localized reduction in height of the alveolar crest, in which case one or several teeth will show supporting bone destruction while adjacent teeth show little or none (Fig. 12-16). Vertical bone loss can sometimes be related to occlusal trauma, food impaction, and a periodontal abscess, but is generally a sign of periodontitis.

Examination of the level of the alveolar crest is particularly important in relation to molar teeth when the level of the crest is lowered to the bifurcation or trifurcation area. As a result of the angulation of maxillary molar radiographs, the involvement of root trifurcation is difficult to determine. The difficulty arises because, as stated before, the buccal level of alveolar crest is projected more to the occlusal than to the lingual level. Careful examination in the maxillary molar region will reveal the lingual level of the alveolar crest as an indistinct line apical to the buccal level. The lingual level is a more accurate level since it is the anatomic portion of the jaw in that area that is closest to the film and, therefore, less subject to distortions of angulation. It is not always possible, on clinical examination, to determine the involvement of trifurcation areas in periodontal disease, but a radiographic finding suggestive of

trifurcation involvement should prompt specific clinical examination procedures for confirmation.

Periapical radiolucency

Periapical radiolucency usually indicates a devital tooth. The exceptions to this are frequent enough, however, to warrant clinical confirmation by pulp test of any tooth suspected of being devital on the basis of radiographic findings (Fig. 12-17).

Periapical radiolucencies may be the result of a variety of causes such as chronic periapical granuloma, radicular cyst, periapical abscess, and neoplasms. The most common causes are periapical granuloma and periapical abscess. Neoplasms are infrequently responsible for periapical rarefaction of bone, but when neoplasia is the cause, this finding may be of grave importance. The odontogenic neoplasm, cemen-

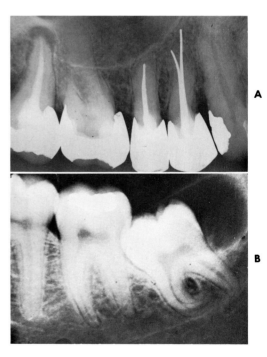

Fig. 12-17. A, Radiolucency of apex of second molar. **B,** Radiolucency caused by lateral dentigerous cyst on distal aspect of third molar.

toma, in its osteolytic stage may be the cause of periapical radiolucency.

Acute periapical abscess in its initial stages may produce very little periapical change in radiodensity of bone, but as it becomes recurrent or long standing, the area of apical bone destruction becomes obvious. Usually there is sufficient clinical evidence of acute periapical inflammation to confirm early bone rarefaction at the apex of the tooth.

Chronic periapical granuloma is a chronic inflammatory process that represents reaction to a devital pulp. The area of bone involved varies considerably, depending on the period of time the tooth has been devital and on the individual human defense mechanism. There is a variation in relative radiolucency of granulomas that makes one easily discernible and another difficult to detect radiographically. There is seldom any clinical symptom to indicate that a tooth has a chronic periapical radiolucency.

Radicular cysts are always associated with devital teeth (Fig. 12-18). In their initial stages they cannot be distinguished with any accuracy from chronic periapical granuloma. When large, they have the characteristics of any bony cyst. A large radicular cyst is a radiolucent area surrounded by a thin layer of compact bone appearing radiographically similar to lamina dura. Radicular cysts are products of proliferation of the epithelial rests of Malassez in a chronic periapical granuloma. Such cysts are not accompanied by clinical symptoms unless secondarily infected, but, if they are large enough, they may produce local swelling and looseness of teeth.

Multiple cementoma is an odontogenic tumor that, at different stages of its development, produces both periapical radiolucency and radiopacity. The most common area of involvement is the mandibular anterior region. The initial stage is the osteolytic stage in which one or more teeth are involved; this stage presents a radiographic picture identical to that of chronic periapical granuloma. Pulp testing will show the involved teeth to be vital.

Traumatic devitalization of teeth occurs readily in the mandibular anterior region. Teeth devitalized by trauma are often free of caries; therefore, a radiolucent zone at the apex of a mandibular anterior tooth that is free of caries may lead to confusion between periapical granuloma and cementoma. Vitality tests by reliable means provide the diagnosis.

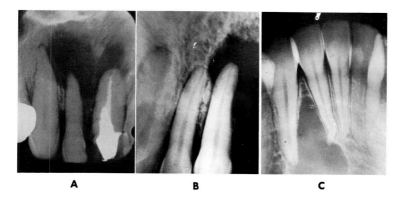

A   **B**   **C**

Fig. 12-18. *Periapical radiolucency.* **A,** Radicular cyst associated with devital central incisor. Lateral incisor and cuspid are vital. **B,** Radiolucency around cuspid caused by metastatic neoplasm. **C,** Radiolucent area between and below the apices of cuspid and lateral incisor is a traumatic bone cyst.

Pathologic conditions of the teeth

Calcification of the pulp. Complete calcification of the pulp occurs for the most part in the incisor and cuspid teeth. In most cases of complete calcification, a history of trauma to the involved tooth can be obtained. Although complete calcification does occur after trauma, it is not unusual for only part of the pulp to become calcified. Quite frequently the entire coronal portion of the pulp calcifies in a relatively short period of time after acute trauma to the tooth. In most instances teeth that show an increased degree of calcification of the pulp are vital, and clinically they will show changes in color when compared to the adjacent teeth.

Minor degrees of calcification are seen in the dental pulp shortly after the tooth has reached occlusal contact and has received a functional load. Secondary dentin is laid down at a rate that varies with many factors such as occlusal attrition, dental caries, and the size of restorations and their proximity to the pulp (Fig. 12-19). Calcification of the pulp is a continuous process that is seen to a minor degree in the teeth of young persons and to a greater extent in older individuals.

Pulp stones are frequently seen in various places in the pulp. They occur in the chamber and in the canals. Radiographically they appear as radiopaque, regular, round areas of calcification and may be isolated in the center of the pulp chamber or apparently attached to one of the walls of the chamber (Fig. 12-20). Pulp stones, as well as the amount of secondary dentin that can be seen radiographically in the pulp canals, are of particular importance when a tooth is being evaluated for root canal therapy.

Caries. Dental caries is by far the most common pathologic change that will be seen radiographically in the teeth (Fig. 12-21). It is necessary that radiographs have proper contrast in order to show dental caries in all of the areas of the tooth in which decay occurs. Radiographs should be examined for caries in the same sequence each time. The carious lesions should be listed in numerical order as they are discovered on the radiograph. The list may be supplemented during the clinical examination, and, at the same time, lesions found radiographically can be verified clinically.

Initially, the carious process will appear as a V-shaped radiolucent zone in the enamel, with the apex of the V toward the dentoenamel junction when it occurs at the contract point of the tooth. When an initial carious area is in an occlusal developmental fissure, the process involving enamel is not easily detected, so that occlusal caries involves dentin before it is dis-

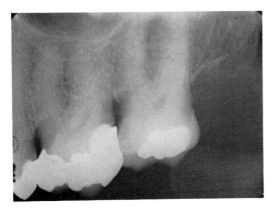

Fig. 12-19. *Secondary dentin formation associated with deep restoration on distal aspect of first molar.*

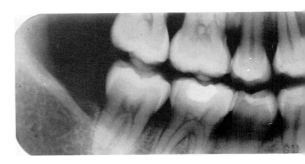

Fig. 12-20. *Pulp stones.*

covered radiographically. As the carious process involves the dentin, a wider radiolucent zone can be seen extending well beyond the apex of the lesion in the enamel along the junction between the enamel and dentin. In advanced dental caries the radiolucency will appear as a large dished-out area. When dental caries is advanced, it is quite simple to interpret radiographically. However, initial incipient caries involving occlusal fissures requires close examination of the radiographic film. It is important to confirm clinically the radiographic findings of dental caries whenever possible. Clinical confirmation of caries is particularly important in the anterior part of the mouth where silicate restorations are placed, since silicate restorations are radiolucent and

may resemble caries radiographically. Silicate or plastic restorations are sometimes placed in bicuspid teeth in an attempt to preserve esthetics, and these also appear radiolucent and may be mistaken for carious lesions radiographically.

One of the most difficult of carious lesions to interpret on the dental radiograph is that of recurrent caries at the margins of existing restorations. Recurrent caries is particularly difficult to interpret in radiographs where steep vertical angulations have been used. Recurrent caries is virtually impossible to detect radiographically when it occurs beneath a buccal or lingual restoration. The most common picture of recurrent marginal caries is that of a radiolucent zone extending inward from the cer-

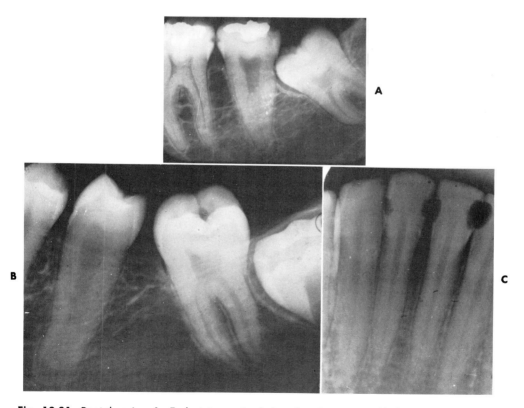

Fig. 12-21. *Dental caries.* **A,** Early interproximal dental caries on mandibular first and second molars; recurrent caries beneath and distal to occlusal restoration of second molar. **B,** Occlusal caries. **C,** Interproximal caries in mandibular anterior teeth.

vical margin of interproximal restorations. Another location in which recurrent dental caries is somewhat difficult to detect radiographically is under existing silicate filings in the anterior part of the mouth. A loss of the sharp outline of the cavity preparation may be the only radiographic evidence of recurrent carries under a silicate restoration.

Attrition. Occlusal attrition is an obvious clinical finding that may be confused radiographically with extensive occlusal caries. Of course, clinical confirmation of attrition is readily made; even so, attrition and dental caries are occasionally coexistent.

Calculus. Certain types of calculus can be seen radiographically on careful inspection of the x-ray film (Fig. 12-22). Calculus may appear as a spurlike projection near the proximocervical aspect of the tooth or as a linear radiopaque line running from mesial to distal aspects of the tooth, representing calculus on the buccal or lingual aspect of the tooth. Calculus that has been altered in contour with a scaler but incompletely removed will lose its angular appearance radiographically and will appear as a somewhat rounded elevation along the root surface of the tooth. The fine flat type of calculus that is tenaciously adherent to the root surface of the tooth is virtually impossible to detect radiographically, and therefore clinical examination is always important in spite of a lack of radiographic evidence of calculus.

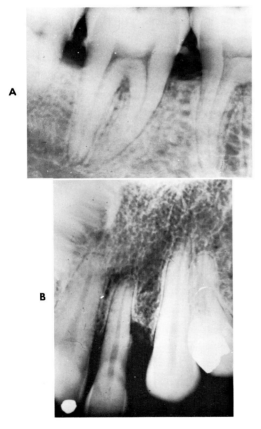

Fig. 12-22. *Calculus.* **A,** Spurs of calculus of all molars. **B,** Flat mass of calculus at bottom of deep periodontal pocket of distal lateral incisor.

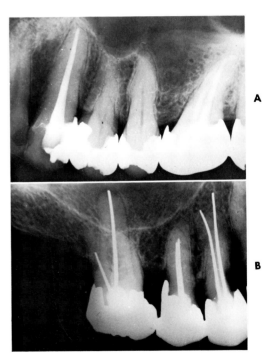

Fig. 12-23. A, Overhanging fillings on distal of cuspid and mesial of first molar. Note recurrent caries under restoration on the distal of first molar. **B,** Overhanging restorations on all teeth. Note caries under restoration on distal of cuspid and calculus below restoration on distal of first bicuspid.

Conditions caused by overhanging restorations. Overhanging restorations at the proximocervical margin are rather easy to detect when the filling material is radiopaque in nature (Fig. 12-23). Overhanging margins of restorations on the buccal and lingual aspects of interproximal restorations or on buccal or lingual restorations are difficult to detect radiographically. However, careful clinical examination of the buccal and lingual areas will reveal any existing overhanging margins and the gingival inflammation that they produce.

Resorption. Root resorption is not an uncommon radiographic finding and may be described as external and internal (Fig. 12-24). External root resorption may occur anywhere along the root of the tooth. Areas of root resorption give a radiographic picture of a noticeable irregularity in the contour of the root surface of the tooth. When resorption has occurred to a somewhat advanced degree at the apex, it may give the impression that the apical portion of the tooth has been cut off. Root resorption that occurs in an area where the periodontal membrane is intact is almost without exception caused by trauma of some type. Types of trauma to be considered are traumatic occlusion, orthodontic movement, and prosthetic abutment overload. When external root resorption occurs opposite a radiolucent zone and the lamina dura and periodontal space are not intact, it should be a matter for serious consideration since neoplasms occurring about the roots of teeth have the ability to erode through the lamina dura and produce resorption of the root.

Internal resorption is a less frequent finding than external resorption and always occurs somewhere along the pulp canal or adjacent to the pulp chamber. Radiographically it will appear as an indistinct and irregular zone of radiolucency and may be confused with dental caries when the coronal pulp is involved. Where there has been extensive buccal recession of the gingiva, allowing the occurrence of carious lesions on the buccal or lingual root surface of the tooth, the carious lesion may give a radiographic impression of internal resorption.

Hypercementosis. Hypercementosis, or excessive cementum deposition on the roots of the teeth, varies in degree from a situation that is barely discernible to one in which a rather massive amount of cementum has been laid down. The radiographic picture of hypercementosis shows an increase in the bulk of the root, and usually the portion of the root involved is easily detected radiographically since there is

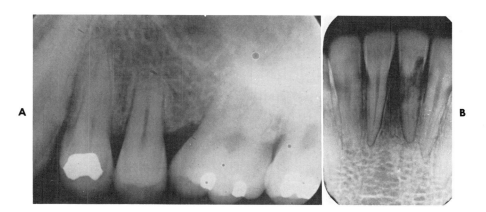

Fig. 12-24. *Root resorption.* **A,** External resorption associated with occlusal trauma. **B,** Internal resorption.

some change from expected contour of the root surface (Fig. 12-25).

Dilaceration. Dilaceration, or pronounced angular curvature of the root, is readily detected on periapical radiographs (Fig. 12-26). It occurs in varying degrees and may involve the root at any level. A very common area in which minimal dilaceration is seen is at the apical one-third of the maxillary lateral incisors. Dilaceration is an important consideration in the diagnosis of teeth that require endodontic treatment or extraction, since there is a limit to the root curvature that will permit passage of a root canal file and that will permit simple extraction without fracture of the root. Occasionally dilaceration is a factor in the selection of abutment teeth for bridges and partial dentures.

Abnormalities of root form. Root form and length, the number of roots on teeth, and the portion of root supported by bone are important considerations in the selection of abutment teeth for dental prosthesis and are readily discernible on properly taken periapical x-ray films. It is especially important to minimize distortion of root length in obtaining periapical radiographs of possible abutments.

The degree of calcification of the radicular (root) portion of the pulp canal, the degree of curvature of the pulp canals, and the number of pulp canals present are important considerations in endodontic treatment. No arbitrary limits on the degree of curvature that can be negotiated by a root canal instrument are in existence, so the radiograph and the amount of root curvature will be regarded differently, depending on the ability of the individual dentist.

Formative defects. Formative defects (see Chapter 9) of enamel may be localized or generalized. Radiographically, localized areas of hypoplastic enamel appear similar to dental caries. Localized areas of hyperplasia are frequently multiple, round radio-

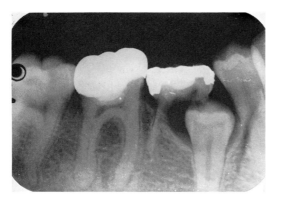

Fig. 12-25. *Hypercementosis* of first molar roots.

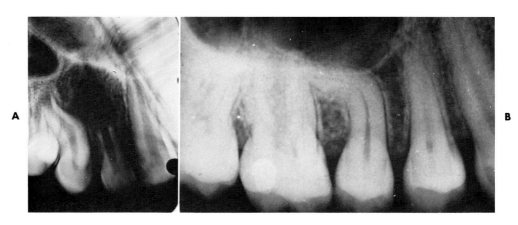

Fig. 12-26. *Dilaceration.* **A,** Cuspid root; periapical granuloma on lateral incisor. **B,** Second bicuspid.

lucent zones. It is not unusual to see hypoplastic pits with associated underlying carious areas.

There are several different types of generalized defects of enamel, all of which have a hereditary etiology. Radiographically the finding in all the types are similar because of the tendency for the enamel to be thin and to abrade or fracture easily. The teeth tend to appear small radiographically because of the thinness of enamel. Attrition varies in degree with the age of the affected individual. Absence of pieces of enamel may be seen radiographically if fractures have occurred.

Turner's teeth show a deformity of the crown of the tooth, which may involve only the incisal or occlusal portion of the enamel. Hutchinson's incisors have a screwdriver shape radiographically, with the cervical width of the tooth being greater than the incisal width. They may also show a notched incisal edge. Mulberry molars have the radiographic appearance of a constricted occlusal surface without the normal cuspal pattern.

Defects of dentin are hereditary in etiology. Two important hereditary entities are dentinogenesis imperfecta and dentin dysplasia. Dentinogenesis imperfecta, or hereditary opalescent dentin, produces a radiographic picture of attrition, absence or near absence of root canals and pulps, and inconstant periapical radiolucency. Dentin dysplasia i s characterized radiographically by absent or poorly developed roots, absence of root canals and pulp chambers, and presence of periapical radiolucencies on all teeth.

Other minor formative defects of teeth such as dens in dente, gemination, fusion, and concrescence are well described in oral pathology textbooks.

Pathologic conditions of the jaws

At this point in the radiographic examination the parts of the radiograph that have not received specific attention are inspected. There are numerous pathologic processes that might be cited under each of the subheadings; however, it is not the purpose of this book to present specific pathologic entities other than as examples to illustrate general principles.

Because of the wide variety of pathologic conditions that could be included, it is necessary to organize the possible findings into large general groups that have some common characteristics. Radiographic characteristics of osseous lesions listed in the following outline can serve as a guide to the examiner and lead him to a tentative diagnosis.

I. Osseous radiolucencies
  A. Osteolytic lesions
    1. Cysts (other than radicular)
    2. Neoplasms
      a. Benign
        (1) Odontogenic
        (2) Nonodontogenic
      b. Malignant
        (1) Primary
        (2) Secondary
    3. Endocrinopathic bone dysplasia
  B. Systemic disease
  C. Osteomyelitis
  D. Residual postoperative osseous defect
II. Osseous radiopacities
  A. Tumors
    1. Odontogenic
    2. Nonodontogenic
  B. Foreign bodies
  C. Bone dysplasias
III. Combination of osseous radiolucency and radiopacity
  A. Neoplasms
    1. Benign
      a. Odontogenic
      b. Nonodontogenic
    2. Malignant—primary
  B. Bone dysplasias
  C. Osteomyelitis
  D. Foreign bodies
IV. Other dental findings—impacted teeth, supernumerary teeth, root canal fillings

Osseous radiolucencies

When a radiolucent area is discovered in radiographs of the complete mouth, the examiner should evaluate the lesion in a specific way. There is no justification for an examiner merely "feeling" a diagnosis; a diagnosis should be based on sound principles. Because of the great variation possible in each type of radiolucent lesion, in examining a pathologic area specific attention must be given to certain details and characteristics of the lesion. In evaluating radiolucent areas, the following should be considered: (1) location and extent of the radiolucency in reference to teeth, normal landmarks, and anatomic region, (2) relative degree of radiolucency, (3) presence or absence of any radiopaque areas or lines in the substance of the lesion, (4) nature of the borders of the lesion, (5) apparent effect of the process that is producing the radiolucency on the teeth and anatomic landmarks, and (6) possible origin of the lesion.

The location and extent of the radiolucency in reference to teeth, normal landmarks, and anatomic region reveal important information about the degree of involvement and the nature of a lesion of the bone. It is important to note whether a radiolucent zone is associated with an area from which teeth have been extracted or are congenitally absent. Certain pathologic conditions of the jaws have a tendency to occur in a certain area of either jaw or in one jaw in particular. In many pathologic conditions, location does not aid in the diagnosis. The amount of involvement is extremely variable in different radiolucent lesions; nevertheless, more extensive involvement may be expected of certain diseases. The extension and location are extremely important in considering the type of treatment and the prognosis.

The relative degree of radiolucency of different lesions is quite variable, depending on the nature of the pathologic process. Some processes produce tissue that is less radiolucent than that produced by other pathologic entities. A cystic process is generally more radiolucent than a process that is producing soft tissue. The amount of normal bone superimposed on a radiolucent area will alter the degree of radiolucency.

The presence or absence of radiopaque areas in the substance of a radiolucent lesion will reveal evidence of ossification centers or sequestra in the lesion. Radiopaque lines may show a tendency toward formation of compartments within a zone of osseous destruction. Although loculation is not characteristic of a specific pathologic process, it is a radiographic feature that characterizes certain processes.

The nature of the borders of a radiolucency relates to some degree the growth characteristics of certain lesions of the jaws. Infiltrative, invasive lesions are not well demarcated by a sharp line of contrast between the normal and the radiolucent area. Lesions that grow rather slowly and are not invasive tend to be well outlined, and in many instances slow-growing lesions are surrounded by a definite layer of compact bone. Certain pathologic processes tend to invade surrounding bone in a locular or budding pattern and therefore present a rather characteristic border between the lesion and normal tissue.

The apparent effect of the pathologic process that is producing the radiolucency on the teeth and anatomic landmarks may help the examiner further characterize a radiolucent zone. There are a number of pathologic processes that produce resorption of the roots of the teeth adjacent to, or involved in, the process. Root resorption is by no means diagnostic of a particular lesion, but it should call several possible causes to the examiner's mind. Root resorption associated with a radiolucent zone should always be regarded seriously, since it is seen in association with infiltrative neoplasms. Effects on landmarks such as obliteration of normal detail or expansion of normal boundaries of the jaws must also be considered as evidence of a pathologic process of an extensive and serious nature.

Possible origin of the lesion may be derived from its location and general characteristics. If the other considerations for examining radiolucent zones are carefully evaluated, the examiner should have at least one or several possible diagnoses in mind. He should consider the possibility of origin from tissues normally present in the jaws, from direct extension from outside the jaws such as from the maxillary sinus or oral mucosa, or from some distant tissue by indirect extension or metastasis.

The summary of the six general considerations for radiolucent zones should channel the possible diagnoses into the general areas listed previously.

Osteolytic lesions. Osteolytic lesions visible as radiolucent lesions include cysts, benign and malignant neoplasms, and endocrinopathic bone dysplasia.

Cysts. Cysts are osteolytic in that they destroy bone by expansion. Because of their lack of clinical symptoms (unless very large or secondarily infected), they are usually discovered radiographically. They vary considerably in size, depending on the length of time they have been actively enlarging. Cysts adjacent to the maxillary sinus have been known to increase in size until the sinus is replaced by cystic structure.

In general, cysts are very radiolucent. As a result of their expansion in all directions and the limited buccolingual spaces in the jaws, there is usually little or no normal trabecular pattern superimposed on the cyst. The central portion may show signs of septal separation of locules or compartments. The borders are usually distinct because of a tendency for a thin cortical layer of bone to be maintained at the walls of the cyst. The borders appear similar to lamina dura. The presence of a radiopaque cyst wall is not a constant criterion for radio-

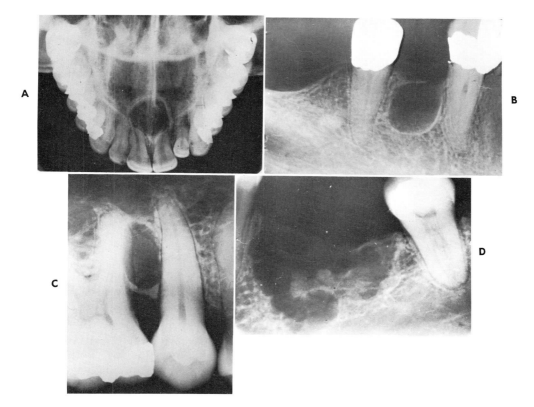

Fig. 12-27. *Osseous radiolucencies.* **A,** Nasopalatine cyst. **B,** Residual cyst. **C,** Lateral root cyst. **D,** Fibrosarcoma.

graphic diagnosis, since it does not always occur and because other lesions may form a similar boundary pattern.

The effects on structures surrounding a cyst are mainly the result of pressure from expansion of the cyst. Spreading of teeth, expansion of the normal buccal or lingual plate of the maxilla or mandible, and obliteration of normal radiographic landmarks are radiographic changes that may be caused by a cyst (Fig. 12-27).

Cysts, other than radicular, may arise from residual epithelium in lines of fusion of the jaws and are known as fissural cysts. Cysts may arise from primordial or residual odontogenic tissue in the jaws from the development of the dentition or from periodontal epithelial debris residual after the extraction of the teeth. The location of a cyst is suggestive of the origin of the lesion. Fissural cysts are seen in the midline of the maxilla or between the maxillary cuspid and lateral incisors or rarely at the symphysis of the mandible. Fissural cysts, particularly the globulomaxillary (arising between the maxillary cuspid and lateral incisor), may extend to involve the apices of adjacent teeth. When this occurs, it is difficult to differentiate between a fissural and a radicular cyst radiographically. When the apices of teeth are involved, the vitality of the teeth must be established to rule out radicular cyst. This distinction is important since the treatment of a fissural cyst differs from treatment of a radicular cyst.

Benign neoplasms. Benign neoplasms visible as radiolucent zones may be divided into odontogenic and nonodontogenic.

Odontogenic neoplasms. Neoplasms arising from odontogenic tissue that produce radiolucent areas in the radiograph are those that do not have the ability to form calcified structures. Since this group of odontogenic neoplasms includes ameloblastomas, there is a considerable variation in the extent of involvement of the jaws in this group of lesions. In general, "soft" or radiolucent odontogenic neoplasms may

arise in any area where there is or has been odontogenic tissue. In particular, ameloblastomas show a singular tendency to arise in the mandibular third molar area and, depending upon the time at which they are discovered, may involve small to very large areas of the jaw.

The relative degree of radiolucency varies according to the type of neoplasm. The ameloblastoma shows a great deal of variation from one type to another, since it may be solid or cystic. Cystic ameloblastomas may be a single cystic mass or multilocular in character. The single cystic mass shows the high degree of radiolucency that characterizes most cysts, whereas the bony septa of the multilocular cystic ameloblastoma results in less penetration of x-rays; therefore, the cyst is less radiolucent. Other soft odontogenic neoplasms, such as soft mixed odontogenic tumors and odontogenic myxomas, shows a relative radiolucency similar to that of any soft tissue in an area of bone destruction.

Radiopaque lines and areas are frequently seen in soft odontogenic neoplasms. A multilocular cystic ameloblastoma shows multiple trabeculae that represent the thin bony walls of the multiple compartments of the cyst. The mixed odontogenic neoplasm that has some potential for forming enamel, cementum, or dentin may show small areas of radiopacity within the substance of the radiolucent mass.

The borders of odontogenic neoplasms in general are not clearly defined. Even the cystic ameloblastoma tends to grow in a budding, invasive pattern, thereby producing an indistinct boundary compared to the relatively distinct border of cysts that are increasing in size by expansion only. Solid ameloblastomas also are invasive in growth character and offer no distinct radiographic boundary. Other soft odontogenic tumors are less invasive in character and therefore show more distinct radiographic delimitation.

Teeth and anatomic structure approximating a soft odontogenic neoplasm may show minimal to sharp change radiographically as the result of pressure or expansion of the neoplastic mass. Disappearance of the lamina dura about the roots of teeth encroached upon by the mass is a common finding. Ameloblastomas are well known for their ability to produce external resorption of the roots that they involve. When large enough, any of the soft odontogenic tumors may produce expansion of the cortical plate.

The origin of soft odontogenic tumors is, of course, from the dental anlage. The degree of differentiation, when the tissue becomes neoplastic, and the tissue involved determine the type of tumor. None of the tumors can be classified positively by radiographic means alone.

Nonodontogenic neoplasms. Benign neoplasms of the jaws are difficult to characterize because of the variety of radiographic patterns they may produce and because of their rarity. Their general characteristics may be similar to those attributed to a multilocular cystic lesion or a soft odontogenic tumor. The variation in pattern should impress the examiner with the need for establishing a diagnosis by means of biopsy.

Benign neoplasms may arise from any connective tissues elements present in the jaws; therefore, they include myxomas, fibromas, chondromas, neurofibromas, or salivary gland adenomas.

Malignant neoplasms. Malignant neoplasms visible as radiolucent zones may be either primary or secondary.

Primary malignant neoplasms. Different types of malignant neoplasms will show different patterns of radiolucency depending upon the origin of the neoplastic cells. These neoplasms are characterized by their rapid growth and their ability to invade surrounding tissue and become widespread in their involvement. If discovered on routine radiographic examination, they are likely to be small, but in many instances

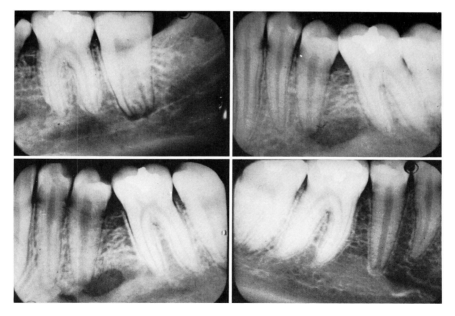

Fig. 12-28. *Osseous radiolucency.* Neurogenic sarcoma involving mental foramen and extending along the inferior alveolar canal to the retromolar area; note innocent appearance of this lesion on routine radiographic examination.

they rapidly involve a large area (Fig. 12-28).

The primary malignant neoplasms of the jaws arise from connective tissue. Only on rare occasions is a primary intraosseous malignant neoplasm of epithelial origin. Epithelial neoplasms usually involve the jaws secondarily by local invasion or by metastasis. The primary radiolucent lesions include fibrosarcoma and multiple myeloma for the most part.

Fibrosarcoma gives a radiographic picture of widespread, diffuse involvement, whereas multiple myeloma tends to produce round radiolucent zones that are often referred to as "punched out" in character. In multiple myeloma, complete skeletal radiographs usually reveal involvement of other bones. Fibrosarcoma has no distinct radiolucent character nor characteristic border; rather, it is the aggressive nature of the process that impresses the examiner. The tentative radiographic diagnosis of any malignant intraosseous neoplasm requires prompt action in obtaining the positive diagnosis by means of biopsy so that therapeutic measures can be undertaken as soon as possible.

Secondary malignant neoplasms. Malignant neoplasms may involve the jaws secondarily by local invasion or by metastasis. For the most part these lesions are epithelial in origin. Squamous cell carcinoma of the alveolar ridge and others areas of the mouth adjacent to bone may invade the underlying osseous structures. Radiographic findings are supported by clinical evidence or history of carcinoma. On rare occasions the first evidence of a carcinoma originating in the oral mucosa may be that of diffuse radiolucency beneath the mucosal origin of the lesion. Osseous involvement by a carcinoma is more likely to occur in the endophytic type rather than in the exophytic type of carcinoma.

Metastatic involvement of the jaws by carcinoma is relatively rare. Certain types of carcinoma, namely thyroid, breast, and prostatic, and hypernephroma have a pronounced tendency to metastasize to bone. No distinct radiographic characteristic can be stated for metastatic lesions in the jaws. They appear as nonspecific areas of radiolucency in any location. By the time there is radiographic evidence of metastasis to the jaws, the primary lesion usually has been discovered.

Endocrinopathic bone dysplasia. Radiolucency seen in endocrine dysfunction is the result of hyperparathyroidism. The involvement may be more extensive, but otherwise the process is indistinguishable from central giant cell tumor. The histologic findings must be supported by proper blood studies to establish the diagnosis (see Chapter 13).

Systemic disease. Systemic diseases producing an osseous radiolucency include such entities as eosinophilic granuloma and Hand-Schüller-Christian disease. Both of these diseases may produce destruction of the alveolar process in a somewhat generalized pattern. Eosinophilic granuloma may produce solitary or multiple lesions. The radiolucency produced is distinct, and the borders of the lesions are not well defined. The radiolucent zone is not trabeculated and may show some angularity of outline in eosinophilic granuloma. Often the teeth are involved and appear radiographically to have lost all of their bony support. Hand-Schüller-Christian disease may involve developing teeth, resulting in destruction of the follicle or malformation.

Osteomyelitis. Osteomyelitis, a suppurative inflammatory process, is accompanied by radiographic changes in radiolucency in its earlier stages while bone is being destroyed. The bone appears to be "moth-eaten," and zones of radiolucency surround islands of necrotic bone or sequestra.

The margins of the radiolucency are ill defined. Later stages of the process show new bone formation with areas of destruction. Clinical manifestions of osteomyeli-

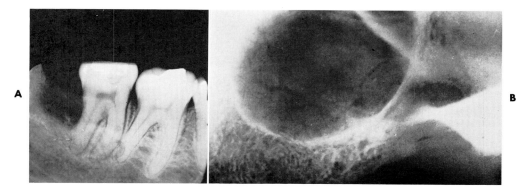

Fig. 12-29. *Osseous radiolucencies.* **A,** Postoperative defect after removal of third molar. **B,** Oro-antral fistula.

tis should be correlated with radiographic findings.

Residual postoperative defects. Postoperative defects are seen after extraction of mandibular third molars (Fig. 12-29, *A*). Incomplete repair of an osseous defect in the maxilla usually results in a round radiolucent area that is well defined and surrounded by normal bone. Occasionally a cyst may be suspected, but the history of a surgical procedure will aid considerably in establishing a diagnosis. An oro-antral fistula may be detected as a radiolucent zone between the floor of the sinus and the alveolar crest (Fig. 12-29, *B*).

Osseous radiopacities

Radiopacities in general do not have the grave significance that is attendant to radiolucencies. Nevertheless, in evaluating radiopacities, one must make a diagnosis because of the potential destructive processes associated with some of them. The following should be considered in evaluating radiopacities: (1) location and extent, (2) relative degree of radiopacity, (3) variations in radiopacity within the radiopaque lesion, (4) nature of the area immediately surrounding the radiopacity, and (5) possible origin of the lesion.

The location and extent often suggest a specific process. For example, torus mandibularis will usually appear as a radiopacity superimposed on the roots of the mandibular bicuspids. The extent of radiopacities, whether they are generalized or localized, offers much information toward a diagnosis. The extent of localized radiopacities may be an important consideration in the surgical attack of such a lesion.

The relative degree of radiopacity is helpful in determining whether the lesion is made up of bone, tooth tissue, or a metallic foreign object. Bone is generally less radiopaque than tooth structure, and both bone and tooth allow passage of more x-rays than metallic objects and are less radiopaque than metal.

Variations in radiopacities within a radiopaque area and the architecture produced by the variations are helpful in establishing the type of calcified tissue being visualized. For example, close inspection of a suspected retained root tip usually reveals evidence of pulp canal in the long axis of the radiopaque area.

The nature of the area immediately surrounding a radiopaque zone may be suggestive of a tooth follicle or periodontal space, thereby narrowing the possible diagnosis to a lesion of odontogenic origin. Osseous structures producing radiopacities are usually less well demarcated radiographically than are odontogenic lesions.

Consideration of the foregoing factors will lead the examiner to a determination of the origin of the lesion. The possible origin of a radiopacity is much more limited and usually more easily determined than is the origin of a radiolucency. The possible origin of a radiopacity is limited by the types of tissue in the body that are calcified. The origin of metallic foreign bodies is usually determined readily by the history.

Tumors. Tumors visible as radiopacities include odontogenic and nonodontogenic.

Odontogenic tumors. Odontogenic neoplasms that produce an opaque image radiographically are the hard odontomas. The radiopacity is produced by a calcified mass made up of combinations of enamel, dentin, and cementum (Fig. 12-30, *A*).

The relative degree of radiopacity is vari-able throughout the mass in mixed odontomas as a result of the variation in radiopacity of the constituent calcified tissues. The enamel in the mass will be recorded as more radiopaque than either dentin or cementum.

The degree of involvement varies from masses of about 1 cm. to several centimeters in diameter. Odontomas do not seem to favor any particular location of the jaws. When they occur in close association with teeth, the result is usually failure of one or more teeth to erupt. Although the outline or margins of an odontoma are generally irregular, the margins are distinct. Frequently there is evidence of a follicle associated with the periphery of an odontoma, and there may also be evidence of a periodontal space.

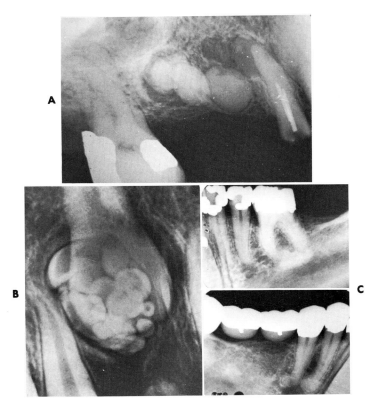

Fig. 12-30. *Osseous radiopacities.* **A,** Complex odontoma. **B,** Compound odontoma. **C,** Hypercementosis.

Enamel pearl. Enamel pearls are misplaced spherical masses of enamel that appear at the cervical areas of teeth especially in the trifurcation and bifurcation areas of molar teeth. The pearls are of the same degree of radiopacity as the enamel on the crown of the tooth; however, they are rather distinct in outline because of their association with the root portion of teeth and their relatively greater opacity in comparison with dentin and cementum.

Cementoma. Multiple cementoma has been discussed previously under periapical radiolucency. In its final stage of development the cementoma is an irregular radiopaque mass involving the apex of one or more teeth.

Nonodontogenic tumors. The following nonodontogenic tumors are visible as radiopaque zones.

Bone whorls. Islands of compact bone, sometimes referred to as sclerotic bone or bone scars, are seen on routine periapical radiographs. Radiopacities of this general nature may occur without apparent cause or as the sequela of an inflammatory process such as a periapical abscess. Bone whorls are irregular in outline and are without clear-cut margins. They are of no significance as a radiographic entity, but areas of sclerotic bone are sometimes confused with odontomas or with root tips.

Enostoses and exostoses. Enostoses are inward growths of bone that appear radiographically similar to bone whorls and have the same significance as bone whorls. Exostoses are outward overgrowths of bone and include the tori of the maxilla and mandible. The most common exostosis seen radiographically is the torus mandibularis and appears as a well-circumscribed area of increased radiopacity superimposed on the roots of the mandibular bicuspids. A radiographic findings of exostosis bears little significance but should be confirmed during the clinical examination. Exostoses that occur on the buccal aspect of the alveolar processes do not show any remarkable radiographic change. Hyperostosis may produce a generalized radiopacity (Fig. 12-30, *B*).

Foreign bodies. Metallic objects and root tips are the most common foreign bodies seen in the periapical radiograph. Root tips are usually recognized rather easily as a result of their almost constant association with an edentulous area. Root tips that are well tolerated by the body may or may not

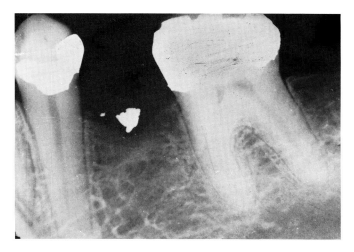

Fig. 12-31. *Osseous radiopacities. Amalgam fragment in tissue of extraction site.*

be surrounded by a thin radiolucent line comparable to the periodontal space. When an inflammatory reaction occurs around a retained root tip, the surrounding area may show radiolucent changes; root tips seen with a surrounding radiolucent zone are discussed below under the subject of osseous radiolucency and radiopacity.

In periapical radiographs of the complete mouth, metallic foreign bodies are a frequent finding in association with edentulous areas as a result of the frequent accidental deposition of amalgam in an extraction socket. In the extraction procedure the forceps fracture off varying sizes of amalgam particles from the restoration of the tooth being extracted. The silver amalgam fragments may appear as small granular radiopaque deposits or as large angular pieces. Silver amalgam is well tolerated by the body; so the fragments are usually an isolated, incidental radiographic finding (Fig. 12-31). Amalgam in the tissue is frequently confirmed clinically by an area of bluish pigmentation of the oral mucosa at the extraction site.

Other metallic fragments may be observed as the result of accidental inclusion of metal in the soft tissues of the face and mouth. Shot residual from shotgun wounds, steel fragments, and a variety of other metallic objects may be seen radiographically and the diagnosis usually can be made on the basis of information about the event that caused the deposition of metal. Frequently metallic foreign bodies are super-imposed radiographically on bone when in actuality the object is embedded in soft tissue. When foreign bodies are visualized radiographically, clinical examination should include inspection for scars and palpation of the involved soft tissue. Occasionally radiopaque areas that are the result of retained contrast media in sinus cavities or in the mouth are recorded on dental radiographs. A history of an examination requiring the use of radiopaque contrast media is sufficient to identify the foreign radiopacity.

Bone dysplasias. Dysplasias visible as radiopacities include, among others, leontiasis ossea and osteopetrosis.

Generalized radiopacity of the jaws. Generalized obliteration of narrow spaces by osteosclerosis should suggest to the examiner that he is confronted with a generalized bone dysplasia such as leontiasis ossea or osteopetrosis. Confirmation of the existence of these processes requires the aid of a medical radiologist.

Combination of osseous radiolucency and radiopacity

The following factors must be considered when periapical radiographic examination reveals an area or areas of combined radiolucency and radiopacity: (1) location and extent of the area in question, (2) relative degree of radiolucency, (3) relative degree of radiopacity, (4) variations in radiopacity within the radiopaque part of the area in question, (5) nature of the

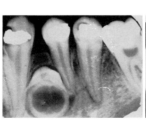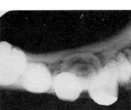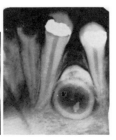

Fig. 12-32. *Combined radiolucency and radiopacity. Dilated odontoma.*

borders of the area in question, (6) apparent effect of the lesion on teeth and anatomic landmarks, and (7) possible origin of the lesion. These have been discussed under osseous radiolucencies and osseous radiopacities.

Neoplasms. Benign and primary malignant neoplasms may produce a combination of radiolucency and radiopacity.

Benign neoplasms. Benign neoplasms include odontogenic and nonodontogenic.

Odontogenic   neoplasms.   Calcifying mixed odontogenic tumors show a varying degree of calcification in a radiolucent zone. The calcified portion is generally a mixture of enamel, dentin, and cementum that produces a variation in the radiopacity of the calcified portion of the lesion while the noncalcified portion results in an ill-defined margin. Mixed odontogenic tumors do not favor a particular location in the jaws and are marked by variation in degree of involvement and degree of calcification (Fig. 12-32).

Hard mixed odontomas may produce a combined radiolucency and radiopacity if the follicular epithelium associated with an odontoma undergoes cystic degeneration. When cystic change is associated with an odontoma, the combined radiographic features of both a cyst and an odontoma are evident.

The proliferative stage of multiple cementoma, as described previously, shows a combined radiolucent and radiopaque lesion (Fig. 12-33).

Nonodontogenic neoplasm. An ossifying fibroma has the same radiographic characteristics as a fibroma with the additional finding of ossification occurring in the radiolucent zone in varying amounts, depending upon the stage of maturity of the neoplasm.

Primary malignant neoplasms. One neoplasm, osteogenic sarcoma, is outstanding in the category. Osteoblastic osteogenic sarcoma is characterized by rapid growth and bone production. Radiographically the area of involvement is usually extensive with no definite border. Radiopaque areas are visualized that show a "sunray" effect produced by divergent spicules of neoplastic bone. The "sunray" radiographic feature should suggest osteogenic sarcoma, although it may be seen in other neoplasms.

Bone dysplasias. Bone dysplasias that cause a combination of radiolucency and radiopacity are frequently generalized processes in the involved bone; however, single isolated lesions may occur.

Paget's disease, or osteitis deformans, is a generalized process that may affect the maxilla in its involvement of bones of the head. The radiographic appearance of bone

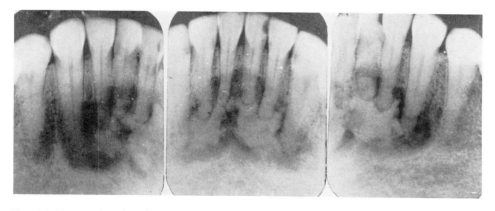

Fig. 12-33. *Combined radiolucency and radiopacity.* Periapical osteofibrosis or multiple cementoma.

that is produced in Paget's disease is frequently described as "cotton wool." Maxillary bone enlargement and hypercementosis or resorption of the teeth are seen when the maxilla is involved.

Fibrous dysplasia may be characterized radiographically only by a change in trabecular pattern. Single or multiple lesions may be seen, and the dysplasia may be confused with osteogenic sarcoma both radiographically and histologically by an inexperienced examiner.

Bone dysplasias that suggest a generalized process are not within the scope of dental treatment. Medical consultation should be sought for patients whose dental radiographic examination suggests that a generalized process is being manifested in the maxilla or mandible.

Osteomyelitis. Chronic osteomyelitis is a productive infection. Areas of radiopacity representing bone production are seen in relation to radiolucent areas in long-standing osteomyelitis. Clinical manifestations suggest bone infection and confirm radiographic findings.

Foreign bodies. Root tips that are not tolerated by the body may be associated with radiolucent zones suggestive of a cyst or ganulation tissue such as that seen at the apex of a devital tooth.

Other dental findings

Radiographs of the complete mouth are valuable in the evaluation of impacted teeth, the presence and position of supernumerary teeth, the tolerance of periapical bone to root canal fillings, and the presence of root irregularities; they are also of value in planning extractions and in planning for bridge and partial denture abutments.

Unerupted or impacted teeth are easily recognized radiographically. The radiograph is of value in planning the surgical approach to an impacted tooth (Fig. 12-34).

Supernumerary teeth are normal-appear-

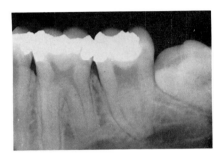

Fig. 12-34. *Other dental findings.* Impacted third molar; note that radiograph is inadequate for complete appraisal of root form.

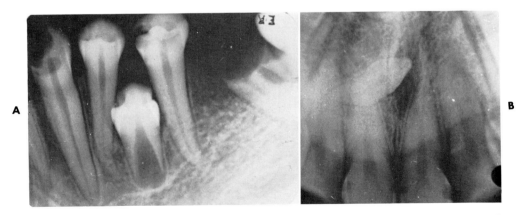

Fig. 12-35. *Other dental findings.* **A,** Supernumerary mandibular bicuspid. **B,** Supernumerary tooth in anterior midline of maxilla.

ing teeth in excess of the normal number of teeth in the mouth (Fig. 12-35). The most common location for supernumerary teeth is in the maxillary anterior region (Stafne, 1932). Occasionally a supernumerary tooth will be visualized radiographically parallel to the long axis of the x-ray film; this results in a confusing radiograph. Supplemental radiographs can be used to provide visualization of the long axis of the tooth. Supernumerary teeth are associated with a follicle that may undergo cystic change and produce a dentigerous cyst or, rarely, an ameloblastoma.

Careful evaluation of root canal fillings and periapical reaction to them are always included in the radiographic interpretation procedure. Newly placed as well as long-standing root canal fillings should be evaluated. Adaptation of the filling material to the walls of the root canal should be noted. Fillings that do not reach the apex of the tooth are of significance because of the frequent periapical radiolucency that is produced or that remains persistent at the apices when the root canal is incompletely filled. Overextension of the fillings into the periapical area is not uncommon. Such fillings are generally well tolerated by the periapical tissue of the tooth, but they may incite an inflammatory response.

POSTERIOR BITE-WING RADIOGRAPHS

The posterior bite-wing radiograph supplements radiographs of the complete mouth. It has limited use and should never be used as the only means of radiographic examination for a new patient nor for one who is returning for an examination and has not had radiographs of the complete mouth taken during the preceding 1 or 2 years.

Posterior bite-wing radiographs are used (1) to determine lamina dura continuity at the alveolar crest, (2) to estimate alveolar crest level in relation to the cementoenamel junction, (3) to evaluate tooth crown shape and formative defects of the tooth crown, (4) to determine pulp size and degree of pulpal calcification, (5) to evaluate existing restorations, (6) to locate calculus, and (7) to locate carious lesions.

Lamina dura continuity

Determining continuity of alveolar crest lamina dura may be less difficult in posterior bite-wing radiographs than in periapical radiographs that have been taken at steep vertical angulations in the posterior part of the mouth. The 8-degree vertical angulation used to obtain the bite-wing radiograph reduces the amount of superimposition of buccal alveolar crest image in a coronal direction that occurs in the periapical radiograph. Recognition of early periodontal disease is aided by careful inspection of the lamina dura for continuity. Interruptions of continuity can often be related to other findings in the interproximal area such as presence of calculus, overhanging margins, and open contacts (Fig. 12-36).

The width of the periodontal space associated with the cervical area of the tooth may be evaluated by means of posterior bite-wing radiographs; however, the evaluation is incomplete since the entire periodontal space must be evaluated by means of periapical radiographs.

Alveolar crest level

Within the limits of the coverage of posterior bite-wing radiographs, the level of the alveolar crest in relation to the cementoenamel junction can be determined accurately. Resorption of the crest to the point of bifurcation and trifurcation involvement of molar teeth is not always visualized in posterior bit-wing radiographs because of the limited amount of root that is included on the film (Fig. 12-36).

Crown shape and formative defects

In planning restorations of carious teeth, the shape of the crowns of the teeth to be restored is often important in determining the best type of restoration and the best

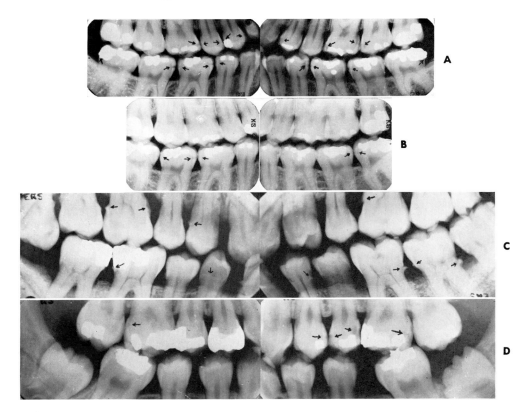

Fig. 12-36. *Posterior bite-wing examination.* **A,** Caries, overhanging restoration, normal bone level, and continuity of lamina dura over alveolar crest; interproximal caries indicated by arrows; overhanging restorations on lower second molars; and recurrent caries under restoration on distal aspect of lower right third molar. **B,** Auxiliary films to eliminate overlapping in molar area for visualization of interproximal caries. **C,** Loss of continuity of lamina dura at alveolar crest, caries, calculus, spacing of teeth, extrusion of maxillary third molar, and reduction of pulp size; calculus indicated by arrows; occlusal caries on upper and lower right first molars; and incipient interproximal caries on distal upper right second bicuspid. **D,** Pulp size, interproximal caries, spacing, and impaction; caries indicated by arrows.

means of preparing a tooth to receive a restoration. The characteristics of the contact areas are easily determined in the bite-wing radiograph if the contact overlap areas have been eliminated by supplemental films at different horizontal angulations. The level of the contact point and the vertical length of the interproximal contact of adjacent teeth or the lack of a contact between two adjacent posterior teeth should be determined.

Local formative defects such as hypoplastic pits and alteration of crown form can be seen readily in posterior bite-wing radiographs. More generalized formative defects such as amelogenesis imperfecta, dentinogenesis imperfecta, and dentin dysplasia can also be recognized by the crown characteristics described under radiographs of the complete mouth.

Pulp size and pulpal calcification

Cavity preparation is performed with less possibility of pulp exposure if bite-wing radiographs are examined carefully to determine the size of the pulp of the tooth to be prepared. The degree of pulpal calcification represents the response of the pulp to occlusal function, restorations, and dental caries. The pulp size may be a determining factor in the type of restoration that can be placed in a tooth. Teeth of young individuals have large pulps and require more conservative types of preparation for restoration, whereas pulps that have undergone considerable calcification allow more room for extensive or radical restorations (Fig. 12-36).

Existing restorations

Marginal fit, recurrence of dental caries, adequacy of contact points, and depth of involvement are important factors in examining restorations by means of posterior bite-wing radiographs. The reasons for replacing restorations are usually unsatisfactory function or recurrent caries, which are determined by radiographic examination and confirmed wherever possible by clinical findings. Open and overhanging cervical margins of otherwise satisfactory restorations are important to recognize as contributory to periodontal disease. The effects of faulty restorations can usually be seen at the alveolar crest as resorption of the lamina dura (Fig. 12-36).

Location of calculus

Interproximal subgingival calculus is quite well visualized on posterior bite-wing radiographs. It usually appears as a spur-like projection on the proximal surface of a tooth. Incompletely removed calculus after dental prophylaxis may present a rounded or flattened appearance on the bite-wing radiograph. Calculus occurring on the buccal or lingual surface of a tooth has the same linear appearance as it does in the periapical film (Fig. 12-36). Not all calculus can be seen radiographically; therefore, the bite-wing radiograph serves only to supplement thorough clinical exploration.

Location of carious lesions

Posterior bite-wing radiographs, together with radiographs of the complete mouth and clinical exploration, provide the complete procedure for location of carious lesions. Carious areas evident on bite-wing radiographs should be recorded numerically, and the combined findings by all three methods should be analyzed to produce a final list (see Chapter 9).

Interproximal carious lesions are well visualized in carefully taken posterior bite-wing radiographs when the lesions have progressed through the enamel and have involved the dentoenamel junction. Initial incipient carious lesions that have not entirely penetrated the enamel may be less easy to detect.

Carious lesions occurring in teeth without periodontal involvement are seen most commonly at the contact point or under the occlusal enamel at the apex of a developmental fissure. When periodontal disease is evident, the involvement of teeth by dental caries is frequently in the area of the cementoenamel junction.

Recurrent dental caries may be detected more readily in posterior bite-wing radiographs than in periapical radiographs because of the more favorable vertical angulation used for bite-wing radiographs.

Careful inspection for recurernt dental caries should be directed to the interproximal cervical margins of restorations and to the occlusal floor under the restoration. Recurrent caries are frequently indistinct and may present a poorly defined radiolucent line or zone at a restoration margin or wall.

The inspection of a bite-wing radiograph for carious lesions should be done in a routine manner so that all areas of the radiograph receive the same attention. All of the maxillary teeth should be inspected in sequence followed by the same procedure for the mandibular teeth (Fig. 12-36).

SUPPLEMENTAL RADIOGRAPHS

Radiographs of the complete mouth and posterior bite-wing radiographs are ordinarily sufficient to render a satisfactory diagnosis and treatment program for a patient. However, occasions arise when additional radiographs are extremely helpful. No special equipment or special training is required either in taking or interpreting supplemental radiographs. Types of supplemental radiographs are given in the following list.

1. Occlusal radiographs (Fig. 12-37)
   a. Maxillary and mandibular topographic occlusal views
   b. Maxillary and mandibular anterior occlusal views
   c. Maxillary posterior occlusal views
2. Lateral views of the body of the mandible (Fig. 12-38)
3. Lateral views of the condyle
4. Temporomandibular joint radiographs (Fig. 12-39)
5. Panographic radiographs (Fig. 12-40)

The selection of proper supplemental radiographs depends on the area that needs further radiographic investigation and the pathologic condition suspected by the examiner.

Supplemental radiographs are indicated (1) when a bone fracture is suspected, (2) when a salivary calculus is suspected, (3) when the extent of a radiographic lesion cannot be determined by means of periapical radiographs, (4) when the exact location of a radiographic lesion, foreign body, or tooth cannot be determined by periapical radiographs, (5) when the patient is unable to tolerate intraoral films, and (6) when there is suspicion of temporomandibular joint changes.

The location of fractures by the general practitioner of dentistry is limited to the mandible. Maxillary fractures require special radiographic technics that are best done in hospitals at the request of an oral surgeon.

Fractures tend to occur in specific areas of the mandible such as the symphysis, the angle, or the head of the condyle. Lateral views of the body of the mandible, lateral views of the condyle, and occlusal radiographs may all be used to establish the presence or absence of a fracture.

Salivary calculi in Wharton's duct and Stensen's duct can usually be visualized

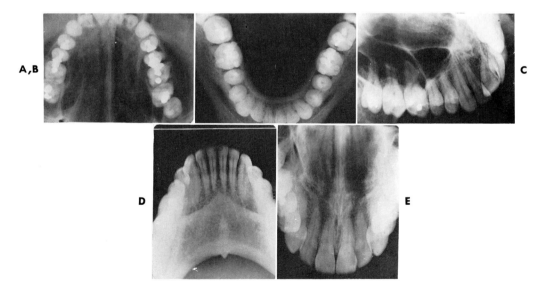

Fig. 12-37. *Supplemental radiographic examination.* **A,** Maxillary topographic occlusal view. **B,** Mandibular topographic occlusal view. **C,** Maxillary posterior occlusal view. **D,** Mandibular anterior occlusal view. **E,** Maxillary anterior occlusal view.

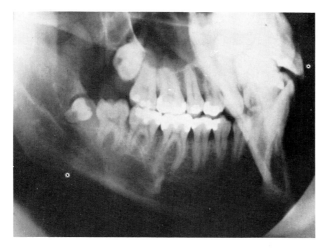

Fig. 12-38. *Supplemental radiographic examination.* Lateral view of body of mandible.

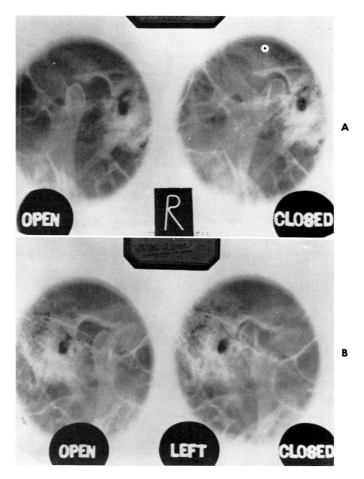

Fig. 12-39. *Supplemental radiographic examination.* Temporomandibular joint open and closed. **A,** Right. **B,** Left.

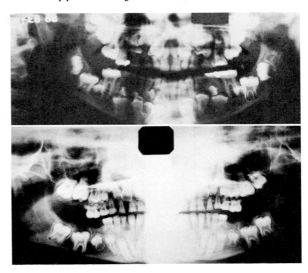

Fig. 12-40. *Panographic radiographs.*

radiographically. Calculi in Wharton's duct are best seen on mandibular topographic occlusal radiographs. Lateral films of the jaw are useful when a Stensen's duct calculus is suspected.

The limited area covered by periapical radiographs often does not provide a complete view of a pathologic process. Lateral films of the jaw or occlusal radiographs are usually large enough to provide a complete picture of most pathologic processes that occur in the jaws.

The exact location of pathologic areas, impacted teeth, or foreign bodies is simplified by utilization of the proper supplemental radiograph. Buccolingual relations of objects are easily determined by occlusal radiographs. Lateral views of the jaw are helpful in location of foreign bodies such as broken injection needles embedded in soft tissues; the insertion of landmark needles helps localize foreign objects on the radiograph.

Situations that prevent the use of intraoral x-ray film may be intense gag reflex, infection and swelling, or an extremely sore mouth. The selection of supplemental (or, in these patients, substitution) radiographs is limited to lateral films of the jaw

and perhaps anterior occlusal views of the maxilla and mandible. The detail of the teeth is not as clear in the lateral view of the jaw as it is in the periapical radiograph, but the lateral film is sufficient to be used for diagnostic purposes in most cases where intraoral films are not obtainable.

Radiographs of the temporomandibular joint are of limited value since it is difficult to obtain a clear radiograph of the joint area and because seldom is anything of diagnostic importance recorded on the radiograph. Neoplastic involvement or bony ankylosis of the temporomandibular joint produces radiographic changes, and occasionally osteoarthritic changes with the osteophyte formation are seen in the temporomandibular joint area. The majority of temporomandibular joint problems are the result of acute and chronic changes in the joint on a traumatic basis. The radiographic visualization of any important changes in traumatic temporomandibular joint arthritis that cannot be determined by careful clinical examination is doubtful.

Panographic radiography has become widely used as a screening procedure, as a full survey of the jaws, and as a method for expanding the visible anatomic area sur-

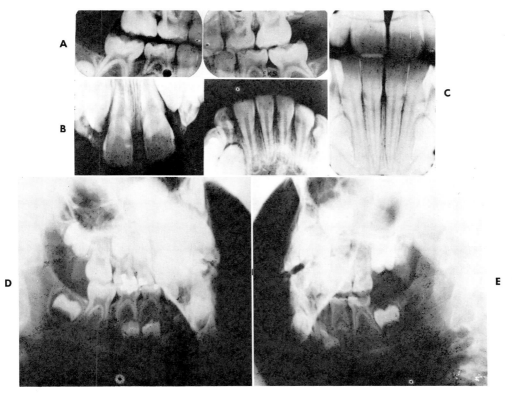

Fig. 12-41. *Radiographs for children.* **A,** Posterior bite-wing radiographs. **B,** Anterior occlusal films using No. 1 film. **C,** Anterior bite-wing radiographs. **D** and **E,** Lateral films of jaws.

rounding an area of radiographic change discovered on periapical films. Where precise detail is not required, it is an extremely valuable radiographic aid because of the inclusion of both maxilla and mandible in their entirety. Panographic radiography alone is not suitable for the detection of dental caries and periodontal disease in their early stages, nor will it provide the detail necessary to visualize early periapical changes. It should not be used as a substitute for routine periodic radiographic examination by means of periapical and bitewing films.

Special radiographic procedures

It is not within the scope of the general practice of dentistry to carry out specialized types of radiographic examinations.

Cephalometry requires special equipment and is primarily of interest to the orthodontist. Sialography requires special equipment and materials. Contrast medium is a valuable radiographic aid in certain pathologic situations; however, special skills must be developed for its use. None of these procedures should be carried out without the special training required to interpret them accurately.

RADIOGRAPHS FOR CHILDREN

The radiographic examination of children differs from that of an adult in that the basic requirement is the posterior bite-wing radiograph supplemented by lateral films of the jaw and anterior radiographs (Fig. 12-41).

The interpretation of radiographs of children is the same as the interpretation of radiographs of adults with the additional concern for presence or absence of permanent tooth buds and position of permanent tooth buds in relation to normal position in the jaw and in relation to eruption sequence (see Chapter 10).

RADIATION HAZARDS

Radiation hazards to the patient. It is well established that routine dental radiographs taken for diagnostic purposes do not endanger the patient. When a properly filtered x-ray machine, a diaphragm to limit the size of the x-ray beam, and fast x-ray film are used, the patient is exposed to an insignificant amount of x-rays. The Council on Dental Research of the American Dental Association has stated in effect that there is no justification for dental patients being concerned about being harmed by the use of x-ray examination and that curtailment of radiographic examinations would "impair proper diagnosis and treatment planning."

Radiation hazards to the dentist. A dentist who takes many radiographs is subject to exposure of varying quantities of radiation, depending on the care he takes to protect himself from direct and scatter radiation. Whenever possible, a lead-lined shield should be installed in the office behind which the dentist will be completely protected from x-rays. A dentist should never hold x-ray film routinely for patients, nor should it ever be necessary for him to hold x-ray film for a patient since there are many devices available that enable the patient to retain the film under any circumstance.

A study by Richards shows some interesting data on the amounts of radiation to which a dentist is exposed in various positions in relation to the patient being radiographed. Adequate protection from exposure is easily obtained by proper shielding and proper use of the x-ray machine and should be the concern of every dentist who uses x-rays. Radiation badges should be worn by dentists who do not use a shield. Such badges are a good means of evaluating how much radiation is being received by members of a dental office staff, especially those who operate the x-ray machine.

ILLUSTRATIVE CASE
Summary of history and clinical examination

A 27-year-old male presented with a chief complaint of vague pain on the left side of the face that had persisted for a period of 3 months. The patient had been examined by an internist and a neurologist without evidence of disease being found. The remainder of the medical history was noncontributory.

The dental history showed that the patient had received regular dental care; otherwise it was noncontributory.

Clinical examination revealed noticeable atrophy of the left temporal muscle. The oral mucosa was clear of lesions. The gingivae were uniformly pink and the gingival form was physiologic although there was evidence of recession of the free gingival margin and blunting of interdental papillae. The gingival sulcus depth was less than 3 mm. Teeth 15 and 16 were somewhat mobile and produced a dull percussion note. The existing restorations were functioning well and the carious lesions were minimal. The occlusal function was traumatic in the areas of the bridge abutments and in the right and left molar regions. The temporomandibular joints showed no significant findings. The clinical impression was as follows: (1) healthy mouth, minor caries, (2) dull percussion note on teeth 15 and 16 of questionable etiology, (3) occlusal trauma.

Radiographs of the complete mouth
(Fig. 12-42)

1. Continuity and thickness of lamina dura
   a. The lamina dura at the alveolar crest lacks continuity between teeth 3-4-5, 6-7, 15-16, 19-20-21, 27-28-29, 31-32.
   b. The lamina dura is not visualized around the roots of teeth 15 and 16.
   c. The lamina dura shows increased thickness on the mesial aspect of tooth 11 and on the distal aspect of teeth 22 and 27.
2. Widening of periodontal spaces
   a. Periodontal space widening is evident on the mesial aspect of tooth 6, the mesial aspect of tooth 9, the mesial aspect of tooth 11, the mesial and distal aspects of tooth 28, the distal aspect of tooth 22, the distal aspect of tooth 27. The periodontal space is widened in the interradicular area of teeth 19, 31, and 32. The periodontal space is thickened at the apex of tooth 22.

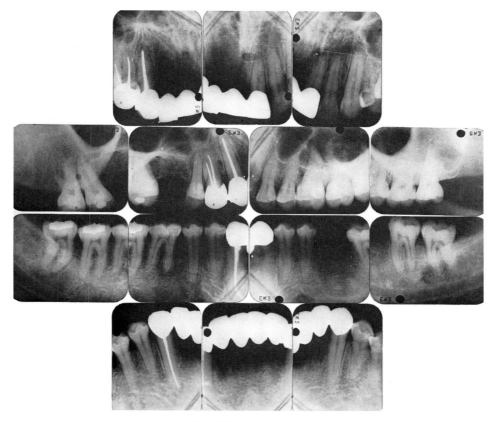

Fig. 12-42. See text.

b. The periodontal space is not evident around the roots of teeth 15 and 16.
3. Level of the alveolar crest in relation to the cementoenamel junction
   Level of the alveolar crest on individual teeth expressed in millimeters apical to the normal level of 1 to 1½ mm. apical to the cemento-enamel junction is as follows:
   Mesial aspect of tooth 5, 2 mm.
   Mesial aspect of tooth 6, 2 mm.
   Mesial and distal aspects of tooth 7, 2½ mm.
   Mesial and distal aspects of tooth 8, 1½ mm.
   Mesial and distal aspects of tooth 11, 1½ mm.
   Mesial aspect of tooth 19, 3 mm.
   Distal aspect of tooth 20, 3 mm.
   Mesial aspect of tooth 20, 1 mm.
   Mesial and distal aspects of tooth 21, 1 mm.
   Distal aspect of tooth 22, 1½ mm.
   Mesial aspect of tooth 22, 2 mm.
   Mesial aspect of tooth 27, 2 mm.
   Distal aspect of tooth 27, 1 mm.
4. Periapical radiolucency
   a. Tooth 22 shows a small radiolucent area to the apex.

b. Large area of relative radiolucency in the left maxillary tuberosity region with loss of trabecular detail and obliteration of the maxillary sinus outline.
5. Pathologic conditions of the teeth, none present; caries, none; calculus and overhangs, check tooth 8 clinically.
6. Pathologic conditions of the jaws
   a. Osseous radiolucencies—see area described in 4, B.
   b. Osseous radiopacities, none present.
7. Other dental findings—root canal filling on teeth 11, 12, and 22 show good adaptation to the walls of the root canals; root canals are completely filled to apex.

Posterior bite-wing radiographs (Fig. 12-43)

1. Continuity of lamina dura at alveolar crest
   Lamina dura lacks continuity between teeth 1, 2; 3, 4, 5; 15, 16; 19, 20, 21; 31, 32.
2. Alveolar crest level expressed in same manner as in complete mouth
   Mesial aspect of tooth 1, 1 mm.
   Distal aspect of tooth 2, 1 mm.

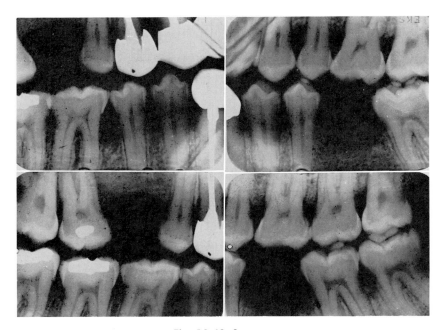

Fig. 12-43. See text.

Between teeth 3, 4, 5, 1 mm.
Between teeth 11, 12, not determined.
Mesial aspect of tooth 19, 3 mm.
Distal aspect of tooth 20, 3 mm.
Mesial aspect of tooth 20, 1½ mm.
3. Tooth crown form and formative defects of crown
   a. Bell-shaped crown form.
   b. No formative defects.
4. Pulp size
   a. Pulp horns prominent in vital bicuspids.
   b. Prominent mesial pulp horn on teeth 14, 19, 31.
   c. Pulpal calcification to a minor degree.
5. Existing restoration
   a. Heavy cervical margin on restoration of tooth 12.
   b. No recurrent caries.
6. Calculus
   None visualized.
7. Carious lesions
   Teeth 28^2, 29^1 (both incipient), 19^5, 31^5.

Summary of significant findings

1. Questionable radiolucent area is associated with teeth 15 and 16 and involving maxillary tuberosity.
2. Evidence of localized areas of resorption of alveolar crest; possible bifurcation involvement of teeth 31, 32.
3. Evidence of occlusal trauma.
4. Significant caries involvement on teeth 19, 31.

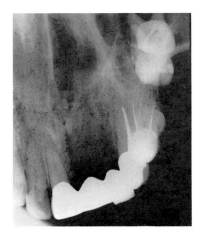

Fig. 12-44. See text.

Additional radiographs required (Fig. 12-44)

Maxillary posterior occlusal view of left side; supplemental radiographs shows area of distinct radiolucency involving maxillary tuberosity and possibly hard palate; lamina dura is absent from roots of tooth 16.

Further procedures indicated by radiographic examination

Referral to an oral surgeon for biopsy of area producing radiolucency.

Results reported from oral surgeon

Pseudoadenomatous basal cell carcinoma. Further medical investigation showed involvement of the left maxillary tuberosity, left pterygomaxillary fissure, left orbit, and base of skull by the neoplasm.

Comment

This case points out the significance of the procedures outlined in this chapter. The neoplasm might well have been overlooked if the loss of the lamina dura and the loss of anatomic characteristics of the tuberosity and maxillary sinus had not been noted. The sequence of examining radiographs and the notation of presence or absence of normal landmarks and details of bony architecture are extremely important in the recognition of many defects in radiographs of an apparently well-cared for patient.

REFERENCES

Barton, E. J.: Roentgenographic evidences of condylar neck fracture, Oral Surg. 8:58-63, 1955.

Baumann, L., and Rossmann, S. R.: Clinical, roentgenologic, histopathologic findings in teeth with periapical radiolucent areas, Oral Surg. 9:1330-1336, 1956.

Björk, A.: Cephalometric x-ray investigations in dentistry, Int. Dent. J. 4:718-744, 1954.

Editorial: Safety of dental roentgenography assured by modern technics and equipment, J.A.D.A. 56:113-114, 1958.

Ennis, L. M., Berry, H. M., and Phillips, J. E.: Dental roentgenology, ed. 6, Philadelphia, 1967, Lea & Febiger, p. 740.

Eselman, J. C.: Is the evidence on the radiograph reliable? J. Dent. Med. 11:216-219, 1956.

Goldman, H. M., Millsap, J. S., and Brenman, H. S.: Origin of registration of the architectural pattern, the lamina dura, and the alveolar crest in the dental radiograph, Oral Surg. 10:749-758, 1957.

Kronfeld, R.: Histopathology of the teeth and their surrounding structures, Philadelphia, 1949, Lea & Febiger.

Lilly, G. E., Steiner, M., Irby, W. B., and others: Oral health evaluation; analysis of radiographic findings, J.A.D.A. 71:635-639, 1965.

McCall, J. O., and Wald, S. S.: Clinical dental roentgenology, ed. 4, Philadelphia, 1957, W. B. Saunders Co.

Peterson, E. E.: Roentgenologic interpretation of anatomic lines of the maxillary sinus, J.A.D.A. 53:165-167, 1956.

Richards, A. G.: Roentgen-ray doses in dental roentgenography, J.A.D.A. 56:351-368, 1958.

Richards, A. G.: X-ray protection in the dental office, J.A.D.A. 56:514-519, 1958.

Robinson, H. B. G., Koch, W. E., Jr., and Kolas, S.: Radiographic interpretation of oral cysts, Radiog. Photog. 29:61-68, 1956.

Sherman, R. S.: Résumé of the roentgen diagnosis of tumors of the jawbones, Oral Surg. 4:1427-1443, 1951.

Sonesson, A.: Odontogenic cysts and cystic tumors of the jaws, Acta Radiol. (suppl. 81), 1-159, 1950.

Stafne, E. C.: Dental roentgenographic interpretation dealing with the pulp cavity and the maxillary sinus, J. Ohio Dent. Ass. 31:62-73, 1957.

Stafne, E. C.: Value of roentgenograms in diagnosis of tumors of the jaws, Oral Surg. 6:82-92, 1953.

Stafne, E. C.: Supernumerary teeth, Dent. Cosmos 74:653-659, 1932.

Thoma, K. H., and Goldman, H. M.: Oral pathology, ed. 5, St. Louis, 1960, The C. V. Mosby Co.

Turner, J.: Injury to the teeth of succession by abscess of the temporary teeth, Brit. Dent. J. 30:1233, 1909.

Updegrave, W. J.: The role of panoramic radiography in diagnosis, J. Oral Surg. 22:49-57, 1966.

Webber, R. L., Benton, P. A., and Ryge, G.: Diagnostic variations in radiographs, Oral Surg. 26:800-809, 1968.

West, R. K.: Differential diagnosis of abnormal dental radiopacities, J.A.D.A. 53:271-285, 1956.

Witkop, C. J.: Hereditary defects in enamel and dentin, Acta Genet. (Basel) 7:236-239, 1957.

13

Supplementary examination aids

The fact that many dentists do not use the services of a clinical laboratory for blood studies, urinalysis, and bacteriologic tests need not be interpreted as a failure of the dental profession to live up to the standards of the medical profession. For, although the literature is replete with laboratory tests for systemic disease, very few tests are practical for use in a dental office or dental clinic. In addition, although the general practitioner may have laboratory facilities available to him where competent technicians can carry out the tests desired, very few dentists feel the need for auxiliary examinations or believe that they are qualified to interpret the results. In many instances the latter feeling is justified because of the infrequent need for laboratory study interpretation.

Although the exclusion of an efficient and justified use of laboratory tests is not realistic, neither is the "shotgun" approach to laboratory diagnosis where the practitioner routinely uses multiple laboratory tests to supplement an obvious diagnosis of Vincent's infection, periodontitis, or herpetic gingivostomatitis. The expenses of extensive laboratory studies showing vague changes in serum calcium, serum phosphorus, serum cholesterol, sugar tolerance curves, and dynamic action of proteins appears to be unjustified in the diagnosis of "precocious advanced alveolar atrophy." Such findings do not enhance the obvious clinical diagnosis since no etiologic or differential diagnostic problem is usually present nor do such studies generally aid in treatment planning or the evaluation of the

progress of treatment of periodontal disease.

It is true that the practicing dentist should be informed of the clinical laboratory tests available for the conditions relevant to his field of endeavor. However, he should also be aware of his own limitations, the limitations of laboratory tests themselves, and the practicability and economic feasibility of performing the tests. The dentist's limitations should not be construed as an inability to interpret the laboratory findings, per se, but as an inherent drawback to the evaluation of such findings in view of the fact that the results of many tests are of little significance unless correlated with an examination of the whole body. Such an examination is in the province of the physician—not the general practitioners of dentistry. This in no way reduces the scope of dentistry or prevents the dentist from taking his place in a health service. It does mean that dental and medical cooperation must be encouraged by effective use of each profession's services. The limitations of the laboratory tests themselves must not be overlooked. There are tests, for example, sedimentation rate, that are so nonspecific that they only indicate the existence of some disorder. The limitations of this test are so extensive and the sedimentation rate is influenced by so many variable factors that its use appears to be of very dubious diagnostic and prognostic value (Yardumian), especially in dentistry.

The practicability of laboratory studies being carried out by the general practitioner of dentistry is an important consideration, even when there are obvious indications for their use. The infrequent indication for laboratory tests on blood and urine does not appear to justify the equipment and procedures necessary to carry out these tests in a dental office. The collection of specimens in a dental office presents difficulties that are not easily overcome. Even though the alternative of sending the patient to a clinical laboratory or physician seems obvious, this procedure also has drawbacks. For example, a history of polyuria, polydipsia, polyphagia, and loss of weight and the examination findings of multiple periodontal abscesses are sufficient to make a presumptive diagnosis of the classical case of diabetes mellitus without laboratory assistance. However, since the diagnosis has to be confirmed, the dentist has two alternatives: (1) refer the patient to a physician for further evaluation or (2) send the patient to a clinical laboratory for tests on the urine for "sugar" and on the blood for "sugar tolerance" or fasting blood sugar. In the first alernative the physician assumes all the responsibility for preparing the patient and evaluating the findings. In the second alternative the dentist assumes the responsibility for the interpretation and then the referral to a physician for confirmation and treatment of the diabetes. In many instances the physician will choose to do his own evaluating and testing. This is not only a "double" expense to the patient, it also discourages rapport between the dentist, the patient, and the physician. It must be pointed out that *occasional* interpretation of laboratory findings, especially of glucose tolerance curves, is not conducive to recognition of the many pitfalls that are inherent in such tests. The first alternative appears to be most rational.

The foregoing is not intended to discourage the use of laboratory tests; it is presented to point out the place of laboratory diagnostic aids in the practice of dentistry. There are many tests that are solely within the province of the dentist—not only for their interpretation, but also for their use in making a diagnosis and planning treatment. Such laboratory tests include those of value in the diagnosis of mouth diseases of local origin and of those diseases whose treatment is the primary concern of the dentist. Although this division of responsibility may appear to be rather vaguely defined at times, it will aid the general practitioner in determining what laboratory studies and their interpretations are in his field of endeavor.

The following situation is presented to point out the responsibility of the dentist in using laboratory diagnostic tests. A biopsy report indicates that a lesion is a giant cell tumor, and the pathologist has indicated that he has assumed that the patient has normal alkaline phosphatase and calcium levels of the blood. This reservation is made since the microscopic diagnosis of giant cell tumor does not rule out the possibility of osteitis fibrosa cystica generalisata. This report is an indication that the dentist should obtain the information needed to establish whether the lesion is of more than local significance. This is sufficient basis for determining the alkaline phosphatase and calcium levels of the blood. If the laboratory findings are abnormal, the dentist has a sound basis of referral to a physician for evaluation and treatment. Although this situation appears to be quite similar to the one concerning diabetes mellitus, two important differences exist. The preparation of the patient and the interpretation of the laboratory findings in a presumptive case of diabetes mellitus have many more inherent problems than an interpretation of the laboratory findings related to alkaline phosphatase and calcium levels. The other difference is quantitative—in most instances the alkaline phosphatase and calcium levels will be within the range of normal, for example, most giant cell tumors involving the jaws are of local origin and require only local treatment.

In other instances the indications for laboratory tests to be performed or interpreted by the dentist are even more apparent than the preceding situation. For example, a patient's history may strongly indicate a bleeding tendency; this is a positive indication for certain screening clinical laboratory tests to determine the presence or absence of a hemorrhagic disorder. The final evaluation and diagnosis should be left to the physician or hematologist.

It is not the purpose of this text to enumerate and describe all the tests that might be of diagnostic importance, especially those whose interpretation more rightly belongs to the physician or those that are impracticable to carry out or interpret in the office of the general practitioner of dentistry. The following list of clinical laboratory studies includes only those that are of practical value in oral diagnosis. The general dental practitioner should know when they are indicated and how to interpret the results. Although he may not carry out the tests in his office, he should know how to refer a patient to a clinical laboratory or a physician for the tests when they are indicated.

BACTERIOLOGIC STUDIES

Antibiotic sensitivity tests. Occasionally it may become necessary to know which antibiotic is most effective against a particular strain of bacteria causing a patient's illness. Laboratory methods for determining the effectiveness of antibiotics are only suggestive, since many variables that are present in vivo are not present in vitro. Since very few dental offices have the culture media and equipment necessary to culture a specimen, the specimen will have to be taken at the dental office and sent immediately to the clinical laboratory, or the patient will have to be referred to the laboratory or a physician for the collection of the specimen. If the specimen is sent to the laboratory, it must reach there in a condition suitable for cultivation. The following directions for collecting a specimen

are recommended: (1) use regulation tubes or bottles (sterile), (2) use regulation plugs to stopper tubes, (3) use only one applicator per tube, (4) collect specimen on a sterile cotton swab, (5) place swab in sterile test tube, (6) seat plug firmly in place, and (7) send specimen to laboratory without delay.

A sterile technic is absolutely necessary. Those practitioners unaccustomed to the procedure should use the facilities of the clinical laboratory. An antibiotic sensitivity test may be made by disk or tube dilution methods.

Methods. In the disk method one or more disks of filter paper containing antibiotics are placed in a Petri dish streaked with a culture of the specimen under consideration (Fig. 13-1). The width of the zone of inhibited growth around the disk indicates the degree of sensitivity of the organism to the antibiotic. The limitations of the test should be well understood. Antibiotic treatment is usually instituted without waiting for the results of the test and then changed if the test indicates the organism is not within the spectrum of the antibiotic used.

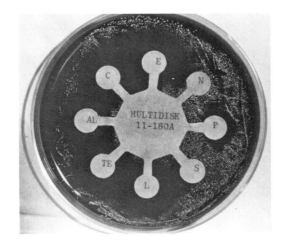

Fig. 13-1. Multidisk technique of testing for antibiotic sensitivity. On this blood agar plate inoculated with staphylococci, the different degrees of inhibition of growth is demonstrated by the clear zone around the effective disks.

Wound, abscess, lesion, and surgical incision cultures. When a wound, abscess, lesion, or incision site shows evidence of infection, it is sometimes advisable to identify the causative organism so that specific therapy can be instituted. One must remember that swelling after extractions and surgical procedures is not usually indicative of infection. Most wounds and surgical incisions are contaminated by bacteria; however, very few of them are infected. The significance of the culture will depend primarily on the clinical findings and the organisms present. Constitutional effects related to an infection must be evaluated; it may be necessary to establish the nature of the organism by laboratory examination of the blood. Since some types of bacteria do not survive changes in temperature or prolonged standing, it is impractical to send a specimen of venous blood to the laboratory to be cultured. A culture of venous blood should be inoculated directly into a culture medium.

To know what specific infecting agents to look for, the clinician needs to be acquainted with a very wide variety of diseases and their symptoms. In addition to this, it is necessary that he be familiar with the laboratory methods of isolating and identifying the infective agent. In general, blood cultures are rarely indicated in dental practice; more often, but not frequently by any means, cultures of incision and drainage sites and discharges from lesions are necessary to isolate or demonstrate infective organisms. (Smears rather than cultures may be used in some instances to identify an offending organism.) The specimen to be cultured is collected on a swab and placed in a dry sterile test tube. An aseptic technic should be followed, and the specimen should be sent immediately to the laboratory. A report may take 10 days; however, preliminary reports may be available in 24 to 36 hours.

Caries activity tests. Because of the association of lactobacilli to dental caries (Bunt-

ing and Parmerlee), an estimation of the number of lactobacilli in the saliva is thought to be useful in determining the degree of caries actively present in caries-susceptible individuals. However, all presently available tests have recently come under criticism (Socransky).

The lactobacillus count, the Snyder test, and the Fosdick test are the most frequently used methods for determining caries activity. A method outlined by Hadley is generally used for a quantitative estimation of lactobacilli present per milliliter of saliva. This test utilizes various dilutions of saliva in glucose acid broth spread over the surface of tomato agar plates (Fig. 13-2). The cultures are incubated at body temperature for 4 days and a quantitative estimate of the number of lactobacilli is made. Counts of between 1,000 and 10,000 lactobacilli per milliliter of saliva suggest a low caries activity. Counts of 50,000 lactobacilli per milliliter of saliva usually indicate a high caries activity. Rogosa and his co-workers have more recently devised a synthetic medium for the enumeration of oral lactobacilli that is used in many laboratories.

The Snyder test utilizes an acid medium containing bromcresol green, which, when inoculated with saliva, indicates the degree

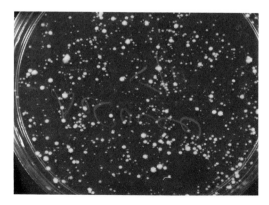

Fig. 13-2. Tomato agar plate with acidophilous colonies that are used to evaluate caries activity.

of acid production. A change in color of the medium within 24 hours is generally considered to be indicative of a high caries rate. Color changes delayed from 48 hours to 3 days indicate less caries activity, whereas no color change within 4 days is considered to be indicative of no caries activity.

Lactobacilli counts require equipment not usually found in the dental office. However, saliva need not be freshly obtained; specimens may be mailed in suitable containers to a dental school or state public health laboratory where this test is carried out. Because of its simplicity, the Snyder test can be carried out in the dental office. Saliva specimens need not be freshly obtained for this test either.

Caries activity tests are used to determine the degree of activity. This information is useful in determining the effect of preventive measures instituted by the dentist. By periodically checking caries activity, the effectiveness of caries control measures can be evaluated. Such tests are of particular use in the control of caries by restriction of carbohydrate intake. Lactobacilli counts, and hence dental caries activity, can be reduced by periodically restricting the amount of carbohydrate in the diet (Jay).

Root canal cultures. Cultures made from material obtained from root canals are valuable in determining the presence or absence of microorganisms. It is necessary that the dentist determine that a root canal is sterile before filling it. A culture is the best method for determining the presence of microorganisms in the root canal; radiographic findings of periapical involvement are not sufficient evidence to make a diagnosis of bacterial infection.

A culture consists of material taken aseptically from a root canal and inoculated directly into a suitable culture medium. Since a wide variety of organisms may be found in root canals, a culture medium must be used that is capable of growing the greatest variety. One of the best media for this and other requirements is glucose ascites medium. If penicillin is used in the treatment of the root canal, the bacteriostatic effect on the root canal sample can be overcome by the addition of penicillinase. Cysteine, semicarbazide, and sodium glycocholate can be used in culture media to overcome the bacteriostatic activity of streptomycin and dihydrostreptomycin. There are no practical methods for the inhibition of such antibiotics as chloramphenicol (Chloromycetin), polymyxin, bacitracin, and neomycin. Camphorated parachlorophenol is not inhibitory after 48 hours (Sommer, Ostrander, and Crowley). Glucose ascites culture medium tubes can be purchased ready for use.

Root canal cultures may be done in the general practitioner's office. The incubation of cultures present no serious difficulty since suitable incubators are quite inexpensive and occupy but little space. An aseptic technic for the collection and inoculation of the culture as described by Sommer and his colleagues is advocated. Paper points that have been inserted into the root canals are inoculated into the culture medium and incubated at 37.5° C. for 48 hours. Cultures should not be kept at room temperature for more than 8 hours. Any cloudiness in the tube is an indication of the growth of microorganisms.

True negative cultures should be obtained before filling canals. False negative cultures may occur because of inadequate samples. The sample to be inoculated should be taken from the apex of the canal. More than one negative culture should be obtained since the initial culture may not show evidence of microorganisms existing under dormant conditions. Three to four treatments of the canal may be necessary to obtain two successive negative cultures.

Fresh moist preparations, smears, and cultures. These tests are useful occasionally in confirming the presumptive diagnosis of oral candidiasis (moniliasis, thrush), tuberculosis, and actinomycosis. Their use in necrotizing gingivitis is of dubious value since fusospirochetal organisms are present in the mouths of most individuals. Their use in solitary lesions of Vincent's angina and cancrum oris (noma) is of occasional value.

The examination of the discharge from a lesion suspected of being actinomycotic can be accomplished by the use of a moist preparation. So-called sulfur granules, which are characteristic of actinomycosis, should be searched for in the pus or discharge. They can be seen best by washing the discharge with a saline solution in a Petri dish. The "sulfur granule" should be placed on a slide in a drop of saline solution and crushed with a cover glass. When examined under a miscroscope with the low-power objective, an entire fungus colony can be seen contained in a hard, sandlike granule. Macroscopically the granule may appear white, yellow, or black. Microscopically the crushed granule will show a mass of radiating filaments with "clubbed" ends. When stained with Gram stain, the central filaments will appear gram-positive, while the "clubs" will appear gram-negative.

If the clinical findings are positive for actinomycosis but the smear and/or biopsy is negative, an anaerobic culture technic using blood agar should be employed.

The material taken from suspected candidal (monilial, thrush) lesions can also be examined microscopically with a moist preparation. The heavy white growth (Fig.

13-3) can be removed from the mucous membranes with a scraper. The scrapings are placed on a glass slide with a 10 percent solution of KOH and heated gently and are examined under a low-power objective for round spores and short mycelia. This test has come into more clinical use with the widespread use of antibiotics. Cultures are the most specific method for the identification of a variety of microorganisms in the oral cavity (Fig. 13-4) and especially for the identification of *Candida (Monilia)* (Fig. 13-5).

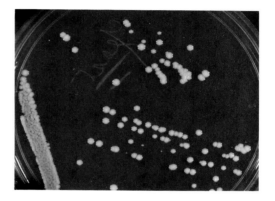

Fig. 13-4. Yeast colonies on Sabouraud's agar medium.

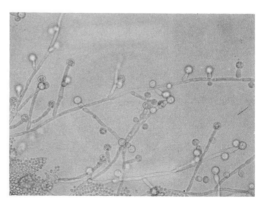

Fig. 13-5. Positive identification of *Candida (Monilia)* is made by growing organisms on corn meal agar.

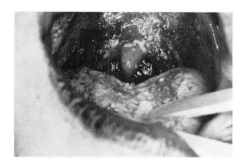

Fig. 13-3. *Thrush* involving soft palate and tongue.

It is not common for the general practitioner to have a microscope in his office. However, obtaining specimens presents no difficulty and they can be sent to a clinical laboratory for evaluation. From a practical standpoint, the actual staining of smears in a dental office appears to be outside the province of the general practitioner. Smears obtained from suspected tuberculous lesions should be fixed by gently warming the slide or by air drying and should be sent to the laboratory for an evaluation of the material for acid-fast organisms. Even though the smear is found to be negative, if the clinical findings are positive, guinea pig inoculations and biopsy procedures should be performed before ruling out tuberculosis. Smears are probably the least valuable in the diagnosis of a tuberculous lesion. Smears are also of little value in determining the presence of fusospirochetal organisms and necrotizing gingivitis. The clinical evidence is of much greater value than a stained bacteriologic smear. However, the smear may be of some value in a negative sense since necrotizing stomatitis does not occur in the absence of fusospirochetal organisms.

BLOOD STUDIES

Occasionally the general practitioner may find it necessary to evaluate certain clinical signs and symptoms of disease by examination of the blood. Of particular importance to the dentist are the principles of hematologic diagnosis associated with anemia and polycythemia, bleeding, infections, lymph node enlargement, and leukemias. It must be pointed out that the presence of the signs and symptoms of diseases responsible for changes in the blood, blood-forming tissues, and the lymph nodes are the main indications for blood studies. Therefore a presumptive diagnosis derived from the history and physical examination should indicate the need for a screening hematologic examination.

Pallor, anemia, bleeding, lymphadenopathy, and the cardinal manifestations of inflammation are only symptoms of disease, and their evaluation may require a thorough and complete examination of the body. The primary concern of the dentist should be the detection of the presence of such symptoms by the history and examination (to the degree his examination may extend). Inasmuch as most general practitioners will refer patients with these symptoms to a physician, the collection, examination, and evaluation of the blood should be left to the physician. This procedure may not be indicated in a few instances in which the presumptive diagnosis is not sufficiently clear to warrant a referral without a screening examination of the blood. In other instances a patient may be referred to a dentist by a physician for an evaluation of gingival bleeding. The dentist's findings may suggest the necessity for an examination of the blood. In this situation a hematologic screening examination for a hemorrhagic disorder should be instituted by the dentist. Frequently a patient gives a history of prolonged bleeding, and this information should be evaluated before dental treatment is instituted. Occasionally a history of extensive hemorrhage after extraction of a tooth is given. In most instances, such bleeding is caused by trauma of blood vessels; however, each case must be evaluated individually. Further questioning and a special search for signs of a hemorrhagic tendency should be carried out. A hematologic screening examination may be necessary to determine the presence or absence of a bleeding tendency. If the screening examination and the clinical findings correlate, the patient should be referred to his physician for a complete evaluation and diagnosis.

Hematologic diagnosis associated with anemia and polycythemia

The presence of an anemia is usually suspected by the dentist because of the subjective symptoms obtained in the interview of the patient and because of the presence of objective symptoms such as pallor, smooth tongue, Plummer-Vinson syndrome, and abnormal tongue sensations. Headache, vertigo, faintness, increased sensitivity to cold, tinnitus, weakness, and irritability are common subjective symptoms associated with anemia. Of particular importance to the dentist are anemias associated with excessive destruction of the blood, chronic diseases, plumbism, irradiation, and leukemias.

A simple anemia and polycythemia can be detected from the red cell count, the hemoglobin content, or the hematocrit determination. Since the objective and subjective findings referable to anemia may not be clear cut, these laboratory examinations of the blood may be necessary. However, these tests are only screening in nature; if the red cell count, hemoglobin content, or hematocrit findings are abnormal and substantiate the clinical findings, the patient should be referred to an internist so that the degree of polycythemia or anemia, the activity of the bone marrow, the morphology of the blood cells, changes in the white cells and platelets, and the cause of the anemia can be determined.

In a normal adult male the average red cell count is $5.4 \pm 0.8 \times 10^6$ per cubic millimeter; in the female the average count is $4.8 \pm 0.6 \times 10^6$ per cubic millimeter. The normal adult range of hemoglobin as determined by hemoglobinometry is 16 ± 2 Gm. per 100 ml. of blood in the male and 14 ± 2 Gm. per 100 ml. in the female. The normal hematocrit range for women is from 37 to 47 percent; for men, it is from 42 to 52 percent (Wintrobe). More extensive measurements of red blood cells take into consideration such characteristics as size, shape, and hemoglobin content; however, such measurements should be left to the hematologist. For screening purposes, the red cell count and hemoglobinometry or the hematocrit determination may be used.

Since many errors are possible in the determination of an anemia or polycythemia by red cell count and hemoglobinometry, the hematocrit determination should be used as a screening test. It is suggested that the reader review standard clinical laboratory diagnostic texts for a complete presentation of the characteristics of red cells and their hemoglobin content. Such a review will serve to point out the limitations of a screening examination and the complexity of evaluating extensive blood studies.

In a normal individual the clinical laboratory findings might be indicated as follows: hematocrit, 45 percent; red blood cell count, 5 million per cubic millimeter; hemoglobin, 15 Gm. per 100 ml. (red cells are normocytic as indicated by a normal mean corpuscular volume of 90 cubic microns). In a severe pernicious anemia there is macrocytosis indicated by an increased mean corpuscular volume; hematocrit, 14 percent; and a red cell count of 1 million per cubic millimeter. In a severe hypochromic anemia, the red cell is microcytic as indicated by a reduced or low mean corpuscular volume, hematocrit 14 percent, and a red cell count of 2 million per cubic millimeter. These latter findings warrant referral of a patient to a physician for complete evaluation, diagnosis, and treatment.

Hematologic diagnosis associated with bleeding

The indications for hemorrhagic study include consideration of a history of a bleeding tendency and the presence of petechiae, ecchymoses, and spontaneous bleeding from the mucous membranes. A history of prolonged bleeding can be quite well evaluated on the basis of previous episodes of unusual bleeding after extractions, cuts, and operations; ease of bruising; prolonged use of antibiotics and anticoagulants; and the presence of systemic disease such as nephritis, tuberculosis, or leukemia. A positive history of "easy bleeding" should indicate the need for a thorough examination of the lymph nodes for enlargement and of the mucous membranes for evidence of hemorrhage.

A screening examination of the blood of a patient with suspected hemorrhagic disease should include bleeding time, coagulation or clotting time, clot retraction time, tourniquet test, white cell count, differential white cell count, platelet count, and hematocrit determination. Although the performance and interpretation of these tests for screening purposes are within the dentist's responsibility, in most instances he will elect to refer the patient to a clinical laboratory or a physician for the tests and their interpretation. A screening examination may be useful to the general dental practitioner if it is needed to enhance a presumptive diagnosis of a hemorrhagic disorder so that a sound referral to a physician can be made. The routine use of blood screening studies is not indicated; such tests should be performed only when the findings of the clinical examination do not furnish sufficient evidence to warrant a referral without further evidence of disease. More complete examinations should be left to the physician, since their evaluation may require examination procedures outside the scope of the dentist's responsibility. For example, patients receiving bishydroxycoumarin (Dicumarol) and related anticlotting agents for the control of thromboembolic disease (coronary thrombosis) should not have teeth extracted until the prothrombin concentration is brought to an effective level. Since the anticlotting therapy is supervised by the physician, the determination of the prothrombin concentration is the physician's responsibility. Teeth should be extracted only when the dentist and the physician believe that the effective level of prothrombin concentration is such as to allow safe extraction of the teeth.

To further emphasize the limitations of a presumptive diagnosis of hemorrhagic disease based on clinical findings and a blood screening examination performed by the dentist, the answers to two basic questions should be considered in making the final diagnosis: (1) Is a primary disease present that is complicated by hemorrhagic manifestations? (2) Are the manifestations of the hemorrhagic disease primarily an abnormality of vascular response and clot formation? It is outside the scope of general dentistry to answer these questions completely. Thus, besides a history, an oral examination, and a blood screening examination, a minimal examination of a patient with a hemorrhagic disorder must include a complete physical examination, including examination of the stool and urine. Extensive clinical examinations and special tests relative to vascular disease and abnormalities of clot formation may be necessary to make a diagnosis.

With these considerations in mind it would be well at this time to determine what part the dentist should play in the evaluation of hemorrhagic diseases. First, the limitations of the oral examination must be considered; the dentist is not trained to make a complete physical examination of a patient. Second, the evaluation of urine and stool studies should be left to the physician making the complete physical examination; the infrequent need for such an evaluation does not justify the time required to "keep up" on all the ramifications of the results of such tests. Thus, the primary role of the dentist is to predict a tendency of a patient to bleed during or after a dental operation and to cooperate with the hematologist or physician in evaluating the operative risk of patients who have a history and the signs of a primary or secondary hemorrhagic disorder. For example, a patient with the signs and symptoms of a hemorrhagic disorder may present to the dentist for treatment of spontaneous hemorrhage in the mouth, extraction of teeth, or treatment of gingival disease. If the presumptive diagnosis is borderline and if the clinical findings of the dentist hardly warrant a referral to a physician for evaluation but do warrant further evaluation, the dentist can carry out screening tests related to vascular response and clot formation. If the results of these tests are positive, the dentist has a sound basis for referral to a physician for a complete work-up of the patient. Dentists interested in collecting blood specimens and carrying out the laboratory procedures should consult detailed accounts of the procedures. One should bear in mind that the history and examination are more important in the prevention of hemorrhagic problems than are laboratory tests. The limitations and interpretation of basic screening laboratory tests for abnormal vascular response and clot formation should be understood by the dentist if such tests are to be used by him.

Bleeding time is the time required for hemostasis to occur in a standard wound of the capillary bed. With the Duke method the normal range of time is 1 to 6 minutes. The Ivy method is somewhat more standardized than the Duke method since it is done on the volar surface of the forearm below a blood pressure cuff held at 40 mm. Hg. Many difficulties are encountered in producing a standard wound. Poor tissue tone resulting from senile changes, altered vascular response, and abnormal clot formation can prolong the bleeding time. Bleeding time is prolonged in thrombocytopenic purpuras but variable in nonthrombocytopenic purpuras. It is normal in hemorrhagic states such as scurvy and allergic nonthrombocytopenic purpura since the only abnormality is a decrease in capillary resistance. Other tests of bleeding time are also in use (Frankel and Reitman).

Coagulation time or clotting time is a screening test to determine plasma coagulation defects and anticoagulation activity. The normal time depends on the test method used. The normal range of the clotting time as determined by the Lee-White method is 4 to 12 minutes. Coagulation time measured by the capillary tube method

is unreliable and should not be used. A prolonged clotting time does not indicate a specific abnormality and should be used only in relation to plasma coagulation defects. An increased clotting time does not in itself indicate specifically an absence of fibrinogen, a deficiency of prothrombin accelerator, or the presence of hemophilia, since many factors must be evaluated in the interpretation of a prolonged coagulation time.

Partial thromboplastin time is a screening test for hemophiliac states; it is somewhat more sensitive than the coagulation time. The normal partial thromboplastin time is 45 seconds or less.

One should keep in mind that the coagulation time test will only detect patients who are less than 2 percent of normal. The partial thromboplastin time test will detect patients who are less than 20 percent of normal. Therefore the tests should not be regarded as "sensitive" to patients with less than severe hemorrhagic problems.

Clot retraction time is a test of the ability of the clot to retract adequately in a given interval of time. Coagulation time takes into account the time required for the clot to form, whereas clot retraction time takes into account its ability to retract and capability of closing a wound. Clot retraction occurs normally in 1 hour. Good clot retraction is usually associated with normal platelet counts. Clot retraction may be affected by platelets, decreased fibrinogen, anemia, polycythemia, and hyperglobulinemia.

The tourniquet test is a measure of capillary fragility. This test is considered to be a test of the vascular factors in hemostasis. It is performed by applying positive pressure methods with a tourniquet or blood pressure cuff that produces an increased venous pressure for 5 minutes halfway between systolic and diastolic pressure. The cuff is placed above the elbow. If no petechiae appear after 5 minutes, the pressure is raised to 100 mm. and continued for another 5 minutes. The test should be discontinued if numerous petechial spots begin to appear. In normal subjects only a few scattered petechiae may appear. This test does not indicate a specific diagnosis. It may be positive in scurvy, severe primary or secondary thrombocytopenia, and other systemic vascular abnormalities.

In addition to these tests, a white cell count and a white cell differential count should be a part of the screening examination. A leukopenia in severe cases of hemorrhage is highly suggestive of an abnormality of the marrow.

These screening examinations will serve to point out a hemorrhagic diathesis. Additional special tests are necessary to determine the precise defects causing the hemorrhagic conditions, namely, a deficiency of platelets, a deficiency of one or more of the factors of plasma necessary for coagulation, and circulatory anticoagulants. The latter has practical significance to the dentist who is contemplating the extraction of teeth or other procedure likely to produce hemorrhage. The measurement of prothrombin activity is of diagnostic and prognostic significance not only in diseases of the liver and hemorrhagic diathesis, but also in the control of the prothrombin level when Dicumarol is being used in the treatment of thromboembolic disease. Although the hematologist or physician may be responsible for testing the prothrombin activity and instituting treatment, the dentist should be informed on the limitations and interpretation of the tests to have a better understanding of the problems involved. The prothrombin test is valuable in detecting the absence of prothrombin as a cause of hemorrhagic diathesis and in the study of response to vitamin K therapy. The prothrombin level should be determined whenever disease of the liver or biliary system is present and surgical procedures are contemplated.

Two methods of determining prothrombin activity in terms of its concentration in percent of normal are used: the one-stage procedure of Quick and the more complete but less practical two-stage procedure. The interpretation of prothrombin time requires a knowledge of the factors other than prothrombin deficiency that may cause prolongation and a knowledge of the sources of error in the test. By the Quick method the prothrombin time is prolonged in afibrinogenemia and in deficiencies of "prothrombin accelerators." The prothrombin concentration is usually normal in other hemorrhagic diseases. To prevent thrombotic accidents, the prothrombin time is usually maintained at approximately 30 to 40 seconds or the prothrombin concentration between 4 and 8 percent of normal (Ham). Since individuals may vary widely in their response to Dicumarol therapy, periodic estimations of prothrombin activity are necessary.

No attempt has been made to mention all the hemorrhagic diseases. The patient's history and the clinical findings are usually sufficient to alert the examiner to the possibility of the presence of such disease. Thus, the stress should be upon the detection of the signs and symptoms rather than on blood studies necessary to make a diagnosis since the latter is rightly in the field of the hematologist. Also, unexpected hemorrhage occurring during surgical procedures is more often caused by leukemia, aplastic anemia, or systemic disease that has been overlooked than by a primary hemorrhagic disease such as hemophilia (Miller).

An uncommon hemorrhagic diathesis of interest to the dentist is scurvy. The clinical manifestations of hemorhage occurring from the mucous membranes of the mouth, especially the gingivae in the presence of local traumatic factors, are not particularly specific. Therefore, if scurvy is suspected, the diagnosis can frequently be made on the basis of the history of an inadequate diet. Bleeding time and all other special tests are normal except capillary fragility. Thus the history and the cessation of bleeding after ingestion of orange juice and vitamin C are of primary consideration in the diagnosis of scurvy. Quantitative determinations of the ascorbic acid content of the blood and urine appear to be unnecessary except in rare instances.

Hematologic diagnosis associated with infections

Blood studies are occasionally indicated in the presence of fever. An elevation of temperature in patients seen by the dentist can usually be related to tissue injury. In most instances the cause of the fever will be clinically evident—necrotizing gingivitis, herpetic gingivostomatitis, abscesses, and dry socket. Only rarely will the dentist see patients with fever from a drug sensitivity reaction, neoplasia, generalized infections, or immunity reactions. A white cell count and white cell differential count should be made when a fever is present in the absence of distinctive clinical signs of disease, and when the systemic reaction exceeds that expected for the degree of tissue injury present.

In the adult, the normal range of circulating leukocytes is between 5,000 and 10,000 cells per cubic millimeter. The leukocyte count is affected by many factors other than tissue injury. Leukocytosis associated with exercise, paroxysmal tachycardia, pain, and other factors such as physical and mental rest can usually be differentiated from that associated with tissue injury by the increase in young cells that accompany the latter.

The leukocytosis most commonly seen in oral disease is that of neutrophilic leukocytosis. Pyogenic infections caused by coccal organisms are likely to produce neutrophilia. The extensive destruction of tissue and liberation of protein as well as the presence of organisms may produce leukocytosis in acute necrotizing gingivitis (Vincent's infection). Leukopenia is much less likely to be observed in relation to diseases seen in the practice of dentistry. Changes

in the eosinophilic leukocyte count may be manifest in allergic disorders, angioedema, skin diseases (with oral manifestations), or parasitic infections. An increase in the number of lymphocytes occasionally occurs in diseases with associated oral manifestations. An increase in the number of monocytes occurs in bacterial infection such as tuberculosis and in such disorders as Hodgkin's disease.

Hematologic diagnosis associated with lymph node enlargement

Blood studies may occasionally be indicated in lymph node enlargement of the neck and submaxillary region. Most instances of enlargement seen by the dentist can be related to regional tissue injury.

Blood studies are indicated if lymphadenopathy is thought to be related to primary lymph node disease or lymphoma, leukemia, or syphilis. An examination of the peripheral blood will generaly distinguish the lymph node enlargement of the lymphomas from the leukemias because of the characteristics of the blood cells of the latter. A serologic test for syphilis is indicated when lymphadenopathy (bubo) is present and accompanied by the characteristic lesions of syphilis—chancre and mucous patches. In the chronic forms of lymph node enlargement, especially in the differentiation of lymphomas, a biopsy of the node may be necessary. If lymphadenopathy is not related to infection in the mouth such as syphilis, herpetic stomatitis, and necrotizing gingivitis, and the peripheral blood is not characteristic of leukemias, lymph node enlargement should be considered as the result of metastatic neoplasm or lymphoma until proved otherwise.

Hematologic diagnosis associated with leukemias

The most common symptoms of leukemia seen by the dentist are referable to gingival changes (enlargement and hemorrhage) and enlargement of lymph nodes. Acute and chronic forms of leukemia differ considerably in their clinical manifestations; however, very little clinical difference in the various forms of acute leukemias or the chronic leukemias may be seen.

The onset of acute leukemia is usually abrupt, and not infrequently the first obvious sign of the disease is gingival bleeding or prolonged bleeding after the extraction of a tooth. The initial symptoms may arise from leukocyte infiltration of the gingivae and lymph nodes. Lymph node enlargement is usually not so obvious as that seen in chronic leukemia. Gingival enlargement resulting from infiltration of immature leukocytes occurs in response to local irritation. Ulceration and superimposed Vincent's infection may be present. Differentiation of the various types of acute leukemia cannot be made on the basis of clinical symptoms alone and is frequently difficult even with a blood examination. The blood examination will generally reveal a severe anemia, decreased platelet count, prolonged bleeding time, poor clot retraction, and a positive tourniquet test. The leukocyte count may reach 100,000 cells per cubic millimeter but may be less than 10,000 cells per cubic millimeter.

The onset of chronic myelocytic leukemia is insidious; the most common symptoms are related to anemia, loss of weight, weakness, slight fever, and, later, a tendency to bleed. Lymph node and gingival enlargement from leukocyte infiltration is seldom apparent. The blood picture early in the disease is primarily one of leukocytosis of the myeloid series with a "shift to the left." As the disease progresses, myelocytes predominate. The leukocyte count may range from 100,000 to 500,000 cells per cubic millimeter. Anemia may be absent in the earlier stages but becomes profound as the disease progresses. The platelet count is usually normal except in the terminal stages when hemorrhagic manifestations and the signs of thrombocytopenic purpura are found.

The clinical findings in chronic lymphocytic leukemia are enlargement of the lymph nodes and manifestations of anemia. The blood picture is that of an overwhelming increase in lymphocytes. Sometimes the level may reach 250,000 cells per cubic millimeter. As with myelocytic leukemia, the platelet count decreases as the disease progresses; hemorrhagic disorders may develop (see Chapter 2).

Hematologic diagnosis associated with chemotherapy

Many patients with neoplastic disease are being treated with a variety of chemotherapeutic agents. This form of therapy is being most intensively used in the treatment of leukemia, but other types of neoplastic disease are being treated by this method. Agents such as nitrogen mustard, urethan, cyclophosphamide, and many others are being used for this purpose.

All of these drugs have a depressant effect upon bone marrow; so the patients develop an agranulocytosis that has early manifestations in the oral cavity. The mucosa becomes smooth and shiny with some intensification of color. The changes progress rapidly to superficial ulcerations of the type typical of neutropenia (Fig. 13-6). Superficial ulcers are present in the vestibular mucosa, and there are also gingival ulcerations associated with the palatal aspects of the upper central incisors (Fig. 13-6, *A*). A copy of the patient's chart shows the white blood cell count in the left column; the administration of the nitrogen mustard is recorded on the right side with the dates indicated (Fig. 13-6, *B*). The correlation of drug administration and the fall in the white blood cell count is apparent.

Serologic tests

The clinical diagnosis of syphilis, except in the most typical cases, is unreliable. Even when a syphilitic chancre is suspected by its clinical characteristics and from the

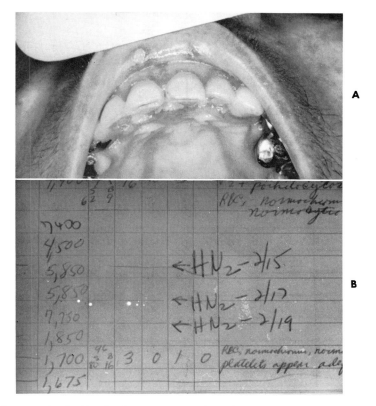

Fig. 13-6. *Neutropenia.* **A,** Mouth of a patient on chemotherapy. **B,** Chart indicating drug administration.

history, clinical laboratory procedures are the most reliable and valuable methods for a positive diagnosis. These procedures include smears from the lesion, cultures, biopsy, and serologic tests.

In the presence of a lesion with the characteristics of a primary chancre (Fig. 2-15, *A*), the examiner should take precautions against infection by wearing rubber gloves. The test to be used depends upon the stage or localization of the disease. The presence of syphilis can be detected by finding the *Treponema pallidum* in the discharge from the lesion (dark-field examination), recognizing rather characteristic tissue changes, identifying the causative organisms by biopsy, and recognizing immunologic responses by serologic methods.

Early syphilitic lesions of the skin and the demonstration of the spirochetal organism by dark-field examination or dry smear may be the only proof of a primary syphilitic infection. Mucous patches (Fig. 7-53, *B*) may show organisms regardless of the stage of the disease. In the secondary stage of the infection, complement fixation or precipitation tests are the most valuable. Primary chancres of short duration, up to 1 week, will rarely give a positive serologic test. In tertiary syphilis, serologic tests are almost always positive. False negatives are possible in any stage. Biologic false positive serologic tests may be present in yaws, leprosy, certain febrile diseases, malaria, and collagen diseases.

Complement fixation and flocculation tests. A correct serologic diagnosis of syphilis is usually based on two approved tests.

Specimens to be evaluated are sent to public health laboratories. If the dentist is accustomed to collecting blood specimens, he may send them directly to the nearest public health laboratory. In other instances a referral to a clinical laboratory or physician for the test may be made. Whether the tests used are based on complement fixation (Wassermann) or flocculation (Kahn) is less important than their execution and interpretation. Although serologic tests were originally reported as negative or positive (1+, 2+, 3+, or 4+), this scheme of reporting led to erroneous interpretation. Recent qualitative reporting of reactions is signified by negative, doubtful, or positive. Quantitative reporting is based on the greatest dilution at which the tested serum produced a positive reaction. For example, a serum that gives a positive reaction in the undiluted state is reported as 1:1; if the highest dilution of the serum with saline is 1:32, the reaction is reported as 1:32. Contraction of the term "dilution" to "dil" is sometimes used and the 1 dropped; for example, a 1:32 dilution would become 32 dils.

Alkaline phosphatase, calcium, phosphorus, and serum protein determinations. The dentist is sometimes called upon to interpret the values for serum calcium, phosphorus, and phosphatase in relation to diseases of the jawbones. It is assumed that the reader is familiar with basic concepts of the metabolism of calcium and phosphorus in bone.

Alkaline phosphatase is elevated whenever bone matrix is being formed in excess and when diseases of the liver and biliary system prevent the excretion of bile. Thus the presence of liver disease must be considered and evaluated in the presence of changes in the serum concentration of alkaline phosphatase, calcium, and inorganic phosphorus. The dentist is primarily interested in the changes of the concentration of these factors in relation to diseases of the bone, more especially the jawbone.

The serum alkaline phosphatase activity of normal adults is 1.5 to 4 Bodansky units. A Bodansky unit is equivalent roughly to 2.5 King-Armstrong units and 0.8 Gomori unit. The level in children from 2 years of age to late childhood ranges from 5 to 14 Bodansky units. The activity of serum alkaline phosphatase should be considered in conjunction with the serum levels of phosphorus and calcium.

Inorganic phosphorus is found mainly in bone in combination with calcium. The level of serum inorganic phosphorus is influenced by the functional state of the kidney, by the parathyroid and growth hormones, and by vitamin D. Renal disease may produce phosphate retention; parathormone increases the excretion of phosphorus and mobilizes calcium and phosphorus from the bone; vitamin D aids in the absorption of calcium from the gastrointestinal tract and the excretion of phosphorus by the kidneys. The normal adult level of serum inorganic phosphorus is 3 to 4.5 mg. per 100 ml. Children tend to have a slightly higher concentration.

Calcium is found principally in bone. It exists mainly in two states in the blood serum—ionized calcium and protein-bound calcium. The concentration of serum calcium in normal individuals varies from 9 to 11.5 mg. per 100 ml. Approximately 5 mg. per 100 ml. are ionized and most of the remainder is present as protein-bound calcium (a small amount 0.25 to 0.5 mg. per milliliter, is also present in the form of an un-ionized but diffusible citrate). A change in the concentration of serium calcium may be caused by a rise in protein-bound or ionized calcium.

The serum concentration of calcium, total serum protein, inorganic phosphorus, and alkaline phosphatase activity should be determined in individuals who show radiographic evidence of bone disease and clinical evidence of systemic disease. The radiographic findings alone may suggest the diagnosis and the need for blood studies.

Occasionally the dentist is the first to see bone lesions. The radiographic findings correlated with the history may be the basis of a presumptive diagnosis of a bone disorder. Occasionally bone lesions will be biopsied when the history and radiographic findings do not obviously suggest a systemic disorder of bone metabolism. Such a situation occurs in giant cell tumors of the jaws. The histopathologic features of the lesion as determined by biopsy may be the first indication that the lesion is other than of local origin. Therefore a diagosis of giant cell tumor of the jaw requires that the blood studies mentioned be carried out to determine whether the lesion is local or systemic in origin, for example, giant cell tumors associated with hyperparathyroidism.

Metabolic disorders of bone such as Paget's disease and diseases characterized by increased serum proteins such as multiple myeloma and sarcoidosis generally show clinical evidence of systemic disease and diffuse radiographic pictures suggestive of a systemic disorder (Fig. 13-7). These findings should suggest the need for clinical laboratory examination of the blood. Blood

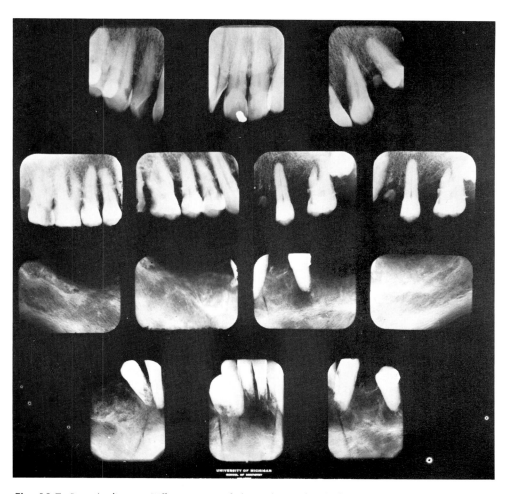

Fig. 13-7. *Paget's disease.* Diffuse nature of the radiographic findings suggests systemic disease.

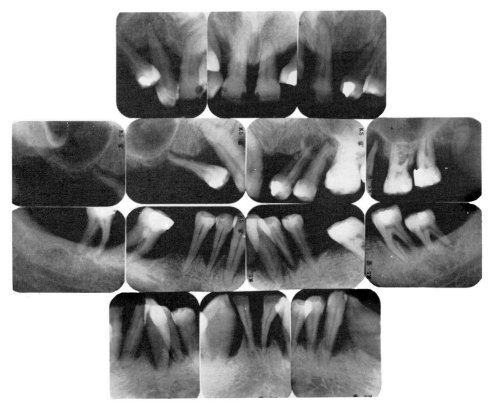

Fig. 13-8. *Advanced periodontal disease.* Blood and urine studies are not indicated on basis of radiographic findings of periodontitis alone.

and urine studies are not indicated in periodontitis (Fig. 13-8).

• • •

The dentist's responsibility regarding the patient has been discussed previously. The dentist should be familiar with the interpretation and implication of the results of the blood studies. The reader is referred to texts on clinical medicine, oral medicine, and clinical laboratory diagnosis for the complete details of decreases and increases in alkaline phosphatase, inorganic phosphorus, and serum calcium in diseases of the bone. The final diagnosis of systemic bone disease should be left to a competent physician, since a complete physical ex-

amination, radiographic examination, blood study, and urinalysis may be necessary.

URINE STUDIES

Urinalysis should not be considered a routine part of the examination of a patient. The dentist only rarely will have occasion to require urinalysis and then only as a screening procedure.

Probably the most frequent use of urinalysis by the dentist relates to a suspicion of diabetes mellitus. However, the dentist who believes that a negative or positive test for "sugar" in the urine is an appreciable evidence that his patient does or does not have diabetes mellitus might better obtain the knowledge for proper interpretation before he uses the test. Not infrequently the clinical examination and history may warrant the presumptive diagnosis of diabetes mellitus. Occasionally a dentist may feel that he should obtain a clinical laboratory report on the patient's urine for "sugar" to substantiate the diagnosis. Unfortunately the presence or absence of melituria alone cannot be depended upon as an indicator of diabetes mellitus. Although persistent melituria will most often be found to be glycosuria and a manifestiation of diabetes mellitus, it also occurs in the presence of a lowered renal threshold associated with otherwise normal subjects, in pregnancy, and in patients with chronic renal disease. Transient glycosuria occurs frequently in persons without diabetes under conditions of stress or after ingestion of a high-carbohydrate meal. Even glycosuria associated with ketonuria is not always pathognomonic of diabetes mellitus.

If it is observed that a urine contains substances capable of reducing copper or ferricyanide solutions, glycosuria is suggested. It must be determined that the reducing substances are sugar, and diabetes mellitus must be considered. The diagnosis can be made only after a high fasting blood sugar of 150 mg. percent or more or an impaired glucose tolerance has been demonstrated. It must be pointed out again that many patients with diabetes mellitus exhibit only minor symptoms and do not excrete sugar in the urine. Thus a urine screening test for sugar may overlook a significant number of persons with this disease. However, if a screening procedure for blood sugar is used, more adequate coverage can be expected. An effective screening test consists of determining the blood glucose level on a single sample of blood taken 3 hours after ingestion of a breakfast containing 100 Gm. of carbohydrate. If the value is within normal limits (70 to 110 mg. per 100 ml. of blood), diabetes mellitus is excluded (Thorn and Forsham). This is merely a screening test. If positive, the

patient must be referred to a physician for additional tests and evaluation. The question of referring the patient to the physician in the first place instead of after tests are performed has been discussed previously.

BIOCHEMICAL PROFILES

A new concept in diagnostic medicine is related to the use of the SMA® 12/60 analyzer to produce "biochemical profiles." Twelve-test biochemical panels can lead to early diagnosis of diseases having vague or absent symptoms and provide a record of chemical values for the normal patient. From the biochemical tests certain profiles are sufficiently characteristic to suggest a specific diagnosis or groups of differential diagnoses. A graphic display of the biochemical data permits pattern recognition (Fig. 13-9, *A*). The shaded areas represent the normal range for each of the test values. Not all variations from the normal ranges shaded on the graph represent abnormalities (Fig. 13-9, *B*). The medication a patient may be using can cause an interference in the analytical measurement or influence the test values because of an altered physiologic response.

CONTACT SENSITIVITY TESTS

Patch tests for agents producing contact stomatitis are of little practical value. The simplest method for determining the presence of an agent causing a contact mucositis of the mouth is to refrain from using the suspected agent. If the stomatitis disappears after withdrawal and reappears when the agent is used again, it is reasonably established as the offending agent. Only rarely is it necessary to actually patch test the oral mucosa to determine what components of an agent may be responsible for stomatitis. It is fairly well known that some part of a denture, or certain ingredients of toothpaste, mouthwash, or almost any substance, for that matter, may be responsible for an untoward reaction. A history of their use, the clinical appearance of the reaction of the tissues to the agents, and remission after withdrawal of the agent make the identification possible.

Patch testing of the skin is not reliable as a substitute for testing the oral mucosa, since the oral mucosa and the skin very often differ widely in their response to

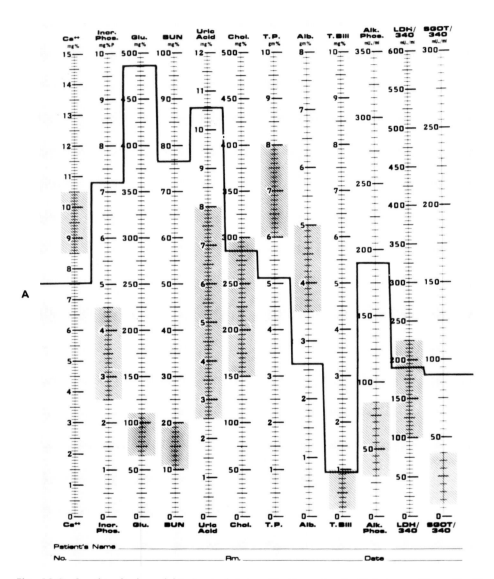

Fig. 13-9. Graphic display of biochemical tests with diagnosis. **A,** Diabetes mellitus with Kimmelstiel-Wilson disease and secondary hyperparathyroidism. The elevated glucose is a reflection of the primary disease. The elevated BUN, uric acid, and inorganic phosphorus and the low protein reflect the chronic renal involvement. The low calcium level is caused by both hypoproteinemia and hyperphosphatemia. The elevation of alkaline phosphatase is related to secondary hyperparathyroidism. The enzyme is heat labile, and therefore it is of osseous origin. **B,** Normal pattern of old age with hypoproteinemia and hypocalcemia.

sensitizing agents. One must keep in mind that such a simple procedure as skin testing may result in untoward systemic effects in susceptible subjects. Scratch tests of the skin have no general practical or important value in the general practice of dentistry. They are unreliable in many instances, and

severe systemic reactions can occur. Unless the dentist is prepared to meet these emergencies in his office, he should refer the patient to a competent allergist.

Patch testing is of no value in determining the causative agent in stomatitis medicamentosa. Cessation of the stomatitis when

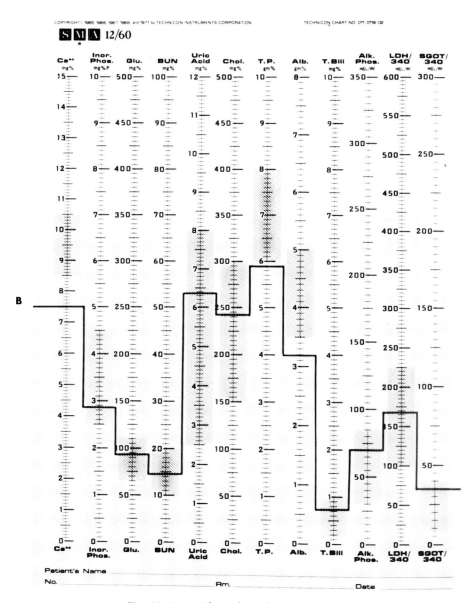

Fig. 13-9, cont'd. For legend see opposite page.

the suspected agent is withdrawn is fairly good evidence of the nature of the agent. Readministration of a drug to observe the possibility of a recrudescence may produce severe systemic reactions. This method of testing should be used with caution.

BIOPSY

Of the various supplementary diagnostic aids, biopsy is one of the most valuable. Because histologic changes provide the basis for a high degree of accuracy in determining the nature of a lesion, biopsy is frequently used to confirm a presumptive diagnosis made on clinical and radiographic findings.

Some clinicians have the impression that biopsy is used only as a means of recognizing neoplastic disease and therefore use it only to a limited degree. However, it may be used to verify the presence of specific inflammatory or granulomatous processes, blood dyscrasias, certain metabolic disorders, developmental disturbances, reactive lesions, and so on. It is also of value in determining the type of treatment to be instituted in certain diseases and in evaluating the progress of treatment. Further, it is a valuable self-teaching diagnostic aid. The repeated microscopic vertification or correction of clinical impressions improve diagnostic acumen.

Biopsy should always be used to verify the presence and nature of neoplastic disease. Since the type of extent of treatment of a neoplasm are dictated by the microscopic findings, biopsy is therefore imperative before treatment is instituted.

Taking a biopsy is relatively simple, inexpensive, and painless. The removal of tissue to be examined microscopically can be accomplished in a dental office with a limited armamentarium by anyone who has basic surgical training and an understanding of the anatomy of the area from which the specimen is to be removed.

The armamentarium needed for biopsy consists of the following:

1. Antiseptic to apply at the injection and biopsy sites
2. Local anesthetics and syringe
3. Scalpel
4. Small pointed scissors
5. Tissue forceps
6. Surgical hemostats
7. Sponges
8. Sutures
9. Needle holder
10. Wide-mouthed bottle containing 10 percent formalin 15 times the volume of the specimen
11. Periosteal elevator ⎤
12. Bone bur   ⎪
13. Bone chisel   ⎬ for intraosseous lesions
14. Mallet   ⎪
15. Curettes   ⎦
16. Syringe for aspiration (10 to 20 ml. capacity and large-bore needle)
17. Biopsy punch—rarely used in dental practice

Specific indications for biopsy. Specific indications for biopsy are as follows:

1. Any ulcer that has not shown evidence of healing in a period of 3 weeks.
2. Any tumescence suspected of being a neoplasm.
3. Any persistent hyperkeratotic lesion.
4. Any tissue surgically excised.
5. Any tissue spontaneously expelled from a body orifice.
6. Material from a persistent draining sinus, the source of which cannot be readily identified, together with some of the lining of the sinus.
7. Any intraosseous lesion that cannot be positively identified radiographically.

Precautions and contraindications for biopsy. Permission to take a biopsy should always be obtained from the patient. This is usually not difficult if the value of the biopsy procedure is explained. The following precautions and contraindications should be observed:

1. Pigmented lesions that suggest the presence of melanin should never be removed by the incisional method. They should be excised, with a wide margin of the normal tissue surrounding the lesion.
2. Lesions that are purplish in color and appear to be filled with blood are probably vascular in origin, and incision would result in extensive hemorrhage. Consequently, such lesions should not be biopsied as an office procedure. When possible, the entire lesion should be removed in the initial procedure.
3. The specimen should be removed with a minimum of manipulation of the area.

4. Local anesthetics should never be injected into the lesion.
5. The lapse of time between taking the specimen and reporting the diagnosis should be as short as is possible and practical. If the lesion is suspected of being a neoplasm, provision for treatment immediately after receipt of a positive report is imperative.

Some observers have suggested that the removal of tissue from a neoplasm may cause dissemination of the cells, resulting in early metastasis; others have shown that this is not true. However, unnecessary rough manipulation and palpation of a lesion is much more dangerous than performing a biopsy. Certainly the minimal dangers incident to removal of a biopsy specimen far outweigh the dangers of attempting any type of treatment without definite diagnosis. Under no circumstances should the treatment of a neoplasm be attempted without a positive diagnosis by microscopic means whether the lesion is far advanced or in early stages of its development.

Selection of the biopsy specimen. The tissue specimen should be removed from a site and in such a manner as to provide the pathologist with a representative piece of tissue in a state suitable for microscopic examination. The following rules should be observed in obtaining a biopsy specimen:

1. From the standpoint of the pathologist, the whole lesion provides the most desirable specimen. This should pertain in all cases where the lesion is small and where removal of an adequate specimen would take practically the entire lesion.
2. In large lesions the specimen should be removed from the most easily accessible area and from an area that represents the characteristic portion of the lesion.
3. Thin deep sections taken from the substance of the lesion across the border into the normal tissue are more desirable than large shallow specimens taken from the surface. Surface specimens often provide only necrotic tissue or crust and do not represent the deeper, more typical character of a lesion.
4. If several lesions are present, the specimen should be taken from the most representative.
5. If the lesion is intraosseous, the cortical plate of bone should be removed and, along with the material curetted from the interior of the lesion, submitted for examination.

Removal of tissue. The tissue specimen may be obtained by any one of the following methods:

Complete excision

When a lesion is small, it can be excised in its entirety with some of the surrounding tissue; thus the entire lesion serves as the biopsy specimen.

Incision

When a lesion is extensive and complete removal would entail a complicated surgical procedure, an adequate specimen for observation of the pathologic character of the entire lesion can be obtained by the removal of a small portion of the lesion and some of the surrounding tissue by incision.

Aspiration

This method is used for large masses that are relatively inaccessible and for lesions whose clinical character suggests that they are soft or semifluid in consistency. Aspiration is done by inserting a large-gauge needle into the softer parts of the mass. Strong negative pressure is created which draws fluid and cells into the needle. More than one sample may be necessary to demonstrate positively the character of a disease process.

Paracentesis

This is withdrawal of fluid from a body cavity through a large needle by negative pressure.

Punch

A tissue punch is inserted into the center of a lesion and a small plug of tissue removed. This method is sometimes used for lesions that are surgically inaccessible.

Curettage

This is the removal of small bits of tissue with a sharp instrument. Curettement is used to remove tissue from a bony cavity, a sinus tract, or a body space such as the maxillary antrum.

Tissue smears

Smears from tissue surfaces are sometimes used when a lesion is ulcerated and surgically inaccessible. They can be taken on Gelfoam or similar material that can be fixed and sectioned without disturbing the material obtained.

The method chosen for obtaining the tissue specimen is dependent on the size, location, and character of the lesion. A small lesion elecated above the surface in a region in which the tissue is flexible, such as in the buccal mucosa, can be removed by complete excision as shown in Fig. 13-10.

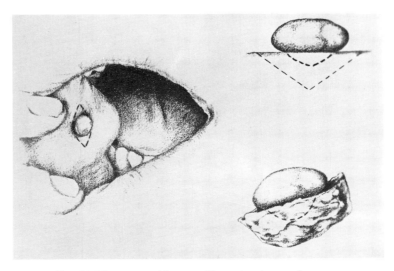

Fig. 13-10. *Excisional biopsy* of lesion involving soft tissue.

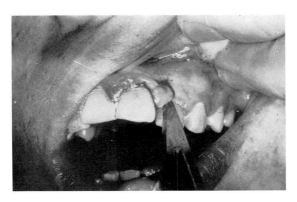

Fig. 13-11. *Gingival biopsy.* Elliptical incision for removal of interdental papilla, free gingival margin, and base of crevice.

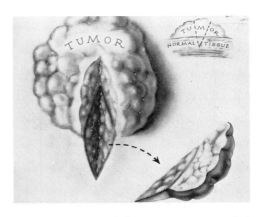

Fig. 13-12. *Incisional biopsy.* Specimen includes normal and pathologic tissue.

This leaves a small oval-shaped defect that can be closed easily with a couple of sutures.

In a small, elevated lesion in an area in which the tissue is not flexible, such as the gingiva or palate, two elliptical-shaped incisions (which surround the lesion) should be made at such an angle that they meet beneath the base of the lesion and the specimen removed with tissue forceps. The resulting wound can be closed smoothly with a few sutures. The removal of gingival tissue for biopsy of gingival enlargement is best accomplished by elliptical incisions. The specimen should includes the interdental papilla, free gingival margin, and base of crevice (Fig. 13-11). The wound may be dressed with Ward's surgical dressing.

It is desirable that the specimen removed from a large lesion be thin, deep, and ellipsoidal in shape. The incisions should converge deep in the lesion and extend to its full depth if possible. The specimen should be removed with tissue forceps, and it

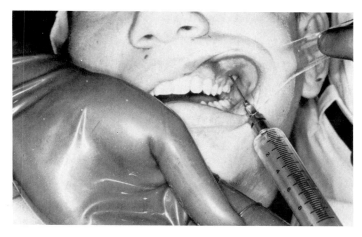

Fig. 13-13. *Aspiration of cyst.* Slightly compressible bulging of buccal plate over first molar, indicating a possible cyst. Aspiration with exfoliative cytology may be helpful in establishing true character of intraosseous lesion.

should be grasped lightly in only one location to prevent crushing. The resulting wound should be closed with sutures (Fig. 13-12).

In a large friable fungating lesion in which the site of tissue removal would be difficult to close with a suture, the specimen can be removed with an electric scalpel. However, the specimen must be larger than that obtained with a steel scalpel to compensate for coagulation that takes place at the margin of the specimen.

In an intraosseous lesion, an incision should be made through the periosteum, the periosteum stripped away to expose the cortex, and the cortex of bone over the lesion removed by the use of bone burs, chisels, or a combination bur and chisel, with care taken to prevent disturbing the underlying tissue. A portion of the lesion then is removed through the cortical opening with sharp curettes. The soft tissue should be sutured over the defect.

In aspiration biopsies a large needle is inserted into the center or softer part of a lesion and strong suction created to bring material into the needle or syringe (Fig. 13-13). The small amount of material obtained can be expressed from the needle

onto a piece of Gelfoam for each in handling. If the quantity of fluid is large, it can be expressed into a test tube containing a fixative. If cultures are also desirable, some of the material should be placed in a sterile plugged test tube or in a Petri dish.

Handling of the tissue specimen. In the laboratory the material is usually sectioned by the paraffin embedding method, which can be completed in 24 hours. Calcified material will require decalcification and will take a longer period to prepare. If immediate diagnosis is necessary, the material can be prepared by the frozen section technic in 10 minutes. This method produces extensive distortion and is much less accurate than the paraffin method and is rarely required for oral specimens. The following instructions should be followed:

1. The tissue should be removed with a sharp instrument and with a minimum of manipulation. If tissue forceps are used, they should not grasp that portion of the lesion selected to show the character of the process. The specimen should not be grasped more than once since crushing the forceps distorts the cells and makes the tissue unsatisfactory for microscopic examination.
2. The specimen should be placed immediately into a fixative. It should not be left in the air to dry.

3. The container for the fixative should have a wide mouth to permit the specimen to be dropped into the fixative. A specimen should never be placed in a dry container and the fixative poured over it, since it may adhere to the side of the container and prevent the fixative from penetrating the adhered surface.
4. Ten percent formalin (4 percent formaldehyde) is a good universal fixative. Bouin's solution, mercuric chloride, or other special fixatives may be used.
5. The specimen container should have a leak-proof cap and should be clearly labeled with the patient's name.
6. If more than one specimen is removed from a patient, they should be placed in separate, clearly identified containers.
7. A history bearing the patient's name, age, and sex, name of operator, and pertinent information about the lesion should be attached to the outside of the specimen container.
8. The specimen should be sent or mailed to the pathology laboratory immediately.

• • •

Any abnormal tissue removed from the oral cavity should be biopsied to verify clinical impressions. In many instances what appears to be a lesion of little significance is found to be one of a more grave nature when the histologic features are studied. When the more exact nature of the lesion is known, proper therapy that benefits the patient and protects the operator can be instituted. For patients who have a cancer phobia, the histologic examination provides a means of eliminating the phobia. Legally the treatment of a lesion without the aid of biopsy can be construed as malpractice.

EXFOLIATIVE CYTOLOGY

Numerous writings extrol the use of exfoliative cytology as a simple and reasonably accurate method for the detection of

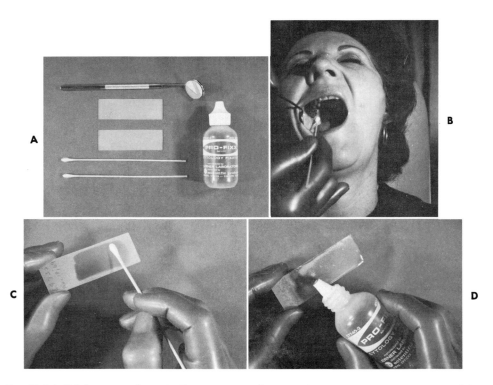

Fig. 13-14. *Exfoliative cytology.* **A,** Equipment. **B,** Obtaining the specimen. **C,** Smearing the slide. **D,** Fixing the specimen.

oral disease (Fig. 13-14). The exfoliative cytology technic has been used effectively as a means of detecting disease in remote areas of the body not accessible to biopsy as well as a screening technic for cancer of the cervix. It also has been suggested as a method for the diagnosis of oral disease. The use of exfoliative cytology as a diagnostic technic has advantages and disadvantages. The advantages includes the following:

1. A limited amount of equipment is needed.
2. The procedure is simple and can be accomplished without anesthetic or surgical instruments.
3. The time involved is much shorter than that in any other method.
4. It does not induce the same degree of anxiety or arouse intense fear of cancer in the patient.
5. It is a simple and inexpensive laboratory procedure.

The disadvantages of exfoliative cytology are the following:

1. It detects only surface lesions.
2. If the surface of the lesion is heavily keratinized, the typical character of the lesion will not be demonstrated by the limited material.
3. Treatment cannot be predicated on a positive smear—a biopsy is still necessary to verify the positive lesion.
4. There are many disease processes other than cancer that produce "white lesions" that are not precancerous, nor can they be diagnosed from exfoliated cells.
5. In other areas of the body, exfoliated cells are retained in body secretions, but in the oral region they are continually washed away.
6. The technic, although simple, frequently is not adequately accomplished so that material is not representative.
7. A negative report on such material provides a false security of having adequately surveyed the area or lesion.
8. A positive smear indicates the need for a biopsy; the negative smear means very little.
9. Exfoliative cytology is inadequate as a screening procedure.

Materials. The materials needed in the office include the following:

1. Ethyl alcohol, 95 percent
2. Glass slides (preferably full-surface frosted slides)
3. Paper clips
4. Plain lead pencil
5. Metal or wooden spatula or cotton-tipped applicator
6. Mailing container

Although 95 percent ethyl alcohol is the ideal fixative, 70 percent alcohol may be substituted if the need arises. Wooden spatulas or cotton-tipped applicators should be moistened before use, preferably in physiologic saline solution. Any type of cardboard or plastic mailing container is satisfactory if it is adequate to protect the slides en route to the cytology laboratory. Several types of containers are available commercially.

Method. If exfoliative cytology is to be used as a diagnostic procedure, the following method of obtaining and handling the material is recommended.

1. The patient's full name should be written on one end of each of two slides, and a paper clip should be placed on that end of the slide.
2. If cellular debris and exudate are excessive, the lesion should be wiped moderately clean with a piece of gauze.
3. The lesion should be scraped with the instrument of choice (a metal spatula and a cotton-tipped applicator moistened in a saline solution) and the material should be spread immediately on the slide.
4. If the spatula is used, the material should be placed on one slide and another drawn across it. If the cotton-tipped applicator is used, the material should be smeared on both slides with the applicator.
5. As soon as the material is placed on a slide, it shold be immersed immediately in fixative, since the slightest air drying will cause

distortion of the cells and will make interpretation difficult or impossible. The slides should be fixed for at least 30 minutes and then air dried.

6. Next, the slides are prepared for shipment together with the clinical information available. This information should include, at least, the name and address of the sender and of the patient, the age, sex, and race of the patient, the duration and location of the lesion, and its description.

Aspiration. Aspiration is a means of obtaining material from a body cavity, a cystic space, or a lesion containing fluid. The fluid obtained through a large-bore needle by negative pressure will provide varying numbers of individual cells or aggregates of a few cells. The material so obtained may be handled in a variety of ways to permit the study of cellular detail for diagnostic purposes.

The obtained material may be smeared on a slide and treated in the same manner as the smears prepared for exfoliative cytology. The material, if abundant, may be fixed and then centrifuged. The compressed sediment may then be processed as solid tissue and sectioned for study. When the material is of limited quantity, it may be placed on a piece of cellulose sponge or some other similar porous material that will be unaffected by tissue-processing procedures. The material can be processed and cut by the same method as tissue with the cells entrapped in the mesh of the sponge. This procedure in reality is a type of exfoliative study and provides the same aid to diagnosis.

PULP VITALITY TESTS

The excitability of the dental pulp is related to the physiologic state of this tissue—the principle upon which the determination of abnormalities of the pulp has been based. Clinical procedures utilizing mechanical, chemical, thermal, and electrical stimuli have been used. Each method has certain basic limitations. Mechanical stimulation with an explorer or bur is difficult to evaluate and is considered to be unreliable.

Chemical stimulation has even greater drawbacks and has never been widely used. Both thermal and electrical excitation have been used with considerably more success in determining the biologic state of the dental pulp. These two methods can be regulated fairly well and are of considerable value when their limitations are well understood.

Several types of electric current have been used: faradic, galvanic, alternating, and condensor discharge current. Serious attempts have been made by diagnosticians to assess the physiologic condition of the pulp accurately by the establishment of a positive and direct correlation between the quantitative exciting factors (voltage, current, frequency, wave form, and so on) and the irritability of the pulp tissue. However, the clinical use of a pure quantitative factor and the determination of the excitability of the dental pulp have not progressed to the point of consistent results. It is not surprising that many instruments have been designed in an attempt to relate voltage or current accurately with the irritability of the pulp tissue.

The physiologic basis for the use of electrical stimulation is based upon the fact that pain is a specific sensory experience mediated through nerve structures that are separate from those that mediate other sensations such as touch, pressure, heat, and cold. No sensation other than pain can be elicited from the dental pulp. Electrical pulp testing is an algesimetric method based upon the fact that pain can be elicited from the pulp by electrical stimuli. Procedures for determining pain threshold of the teeth are difficult to evaluate because the methods used do not closely associate the stimulus with the tissue changes causing the pain.

The minimal stimulus necessary to cause excitation of the free nerve endings and to register pain is called a *threshold stimulus*. The response or reaction of a patient to an excessive stimulus is a subjective sensation;

it is a complex physiopsychologic process involving the cognitive functions of an individual and represents an emotional and physiologic expression resulting from the perception of pain. The dual aspect of pain—threshold stimulus and reaction to pain—is of experimental value only; it is of no clinical value because of the intricate relationship between the two factors. Hence, under clinical conditions it is better to consider only the factors that can be easily measured—*pain perception threshold*. This factor is defined as the lowest perceptible intensity of pain caused by a pain threshold stimulus; this is the amount of stimulus necessary to induce threshold pain (Bonica).

Under normal circumstances the threshold for the perception of pain is approximately the same in the same subject at varying times of the day. One must remember that although this threshold does not vary appreciably, the threshold for reaction to pain varies widely. The patient's mentation and attitude may cause the reaction threshold to vary considerably. Age, sex, emotional security, fatigue, drugs, and race may also alter it.

The following conditions are necessary for a reaction to a stimulus to occur: (1) there must be an adequate stimulus that transcends the excitment threshold of the free nerve endings, (2) the stimulus must be conducted by the nerve tracts to the brain, and (3) the tissue must be capable of being excited. Obviously the blocking of the nerve transmission caused by anesthetics, nerve resections, nerve injuries, or nerve lesions will prevent the stimulus from producing a painful sensation. Changes in the excitability state of the nerve tissue may result from injury to the pulp. Probably other factors may be related indirectly to the excitability of the teeth. The teeth of young persons, especially maxillary central incisors with apices that are open, may fail to show response to what might ordinarily be considered painful stimuli. The reaction

of the patient to pain varies greatly and may be only slightly correlated with the intensity of the stimulus. It is apparent that the electrical stimulus of choice should be the one that is the most indicative of stimulus intensity.

The problems of electrical pulp testing are numerous. They include high resistance and variations of resistance in the teeth, periodontal membrane reaction, difficulty in determining the difference in pain perception and reaction to pain, limitations of the testing apparatus and its clinical application, and inability to establish a direct relationship between the threshold value and the pathologic process viewed microscopically.

Attempts have been made to separate the response of the periodontal membrane from the response of the pulp by utilizing the difference in the frequency necessary to stimulate the two contiguous tissues and the difference in the excitation thresholds of the teeth and periodontal membrane. Under normal conditions the threshold of excitation of the periodontal membrane is about 200 to 400 microamperes (Björn), and the excitation threshold of pulp is about 15 to 20 microamperes. Ziskin and Wald considered that frequencies between 1,000 and 5,000 cycles per second separated the pulpal and periodontal responses in some instances. The use of ultrahigh frequency alternating current for the stimulus is of no value. An increase in the frequency of excitation current produces a rise in the pain threshold to the point that no excitation occurs (Björn).

For an electric pulp tester to be completely effective in correlating pathologic pulp changes and changes in the excitability of the pulp, it is necessary that the tester indicate induced pain without tissue damage by a stimulus whose intensity can be accurately measured and that can be used in a predictable manner accomplished by means of a relatively simple neuroreceptive conductive and perceptive mechanism.

As previously mentioned, several problems make this goal difficult, if not impossible, to obtain at the present time. Serious attempts, directed toward both instrument design and instrument use, have been made to eliminate most of the problems.

One of the principal problems in instrument design is related to the construction of an instrument that will be simple, easy to use clinically, and safe. Many types of apparatus have been developed to apply and measure an electrical stimulus to the tooth for the purpose of determining the excitability state of the dental pulp tissue. The two most practical accepted methods are measurement of the current or measurement of the voltage necessary to produce the lowest perceptible intensity of pain. Accordingly, the pain threshold is considered to be raised when more stimulus energy is required to induce threshold pain; conversely, when less energy is required, the pain threshold is said to be lowered. Thus the rationale for using an electrical pulp tester as a diagnostic aid in determining the state of the pulp depends on two important factors: (1) in order for the determination of the threshold stimulus to be of value, the stimulus (current or voltage) must be exactly defined, and (2) there must exist predetermined physiologic and/or pathologic states to correlate with alterations in the threshold stimulus; this implies that the stimulus be standardized and that normal thresholds of other teeth be known or be determined.

The excitation of the teeth by electrical stimulation is dependent upon the current passing through tissue that is capable of responding to a stimulus. Hence excitation depends on current density; this varies with the total current, the placement and size of the electrodes, and the conductivity of the tissues. It becomes obvious that the absolute threshold of excitation of the pulp is obscure at best. The duration of the stimulus is also related to the excitation. In general, the shorter the duration of the exciting

stimulus, the greater the intensity required to produce a response. The time of the application of the stimulus must be a certain minimum for a given current; otherwise there is a possibility of producing tissue damage. Electrical stimuli of reasonable intensity do not produce tissue changes, and repeated applications of the stimulus are possible without loss of uniformity of response—all other factors remaining equal (Goetzel, Burrill, and Ivy). However, prolonged stimulation at high current intensity results in irreversible damage to the tooth (Hardy, Wolff, and Goodell). The current in a pulp tester should be utilized according to its form, strength, and duration. For uniform results the form should be easy to define and constant and the current duration should not be so short that the strength is unnecessarily high nor so long that excessive amounts of energy are applied to the tissues.

The physiologic effect of an electrical stimulus depends upon current strength. This factor is related to the voltage and the electrical resistance in the current circuit. There is considerable variation in the resistance of teeth and in the resistance between the pulp-tester electrode and the tooth. Measurement of voltage would then tend to measure the resistance of these two factors rather than simply the threshold stimulus. Pulp testers utilizing voltage measurements are of clinical value when the operator is familiar with the necessity for keeping conditions under which the tests are made as nearly uniform as possible. Though there appears to be little agreement among investigators as to which aspect of an electrical stimulus should be measured to indicate stimulus intensity, Björn and Ziskin and Wald consider current strength to be the important decisive factor.

To eliminate the variations in the resistance of the dental tissues and the resistance between the electrode and tooth and also to protect the tooth against accidental excessive current, pulp testers generally are constructed so as to have a high internal resistance. In these instruments it is the voltage applied that determines the current strength and not changes in the external circuit. This is possible because resistance changes in the external circuit are minor when compared to the high resistance of the internal circuit of the pulp tester.

In general, whenever an electrode of a pulp tester is applied to the lip, finger, gingiva, or cheek, a stimulus is usually felt at a very low threshold. The threshold for excitation of the finger or lip is more than 50 times that of many teeth; however, the electrical resistance of the skin is very low compared with that in the teeth and the stimulus is usually felt at a very low intensity. Inasmuch as the dental pulp has only specific stimuli receptors for pain and the cheek and lip and periodontal structures have other receptors present for cold, heat, and pressure sensations, it is to be expected that certain current strengths may produce two sensations. Therefore, it is possible that a current may produce only a tickling sensation in soft tissues of the lip and cheeks whereas the same application may produce pain in the dental pulp. As was previously pointed out, current voltage, wave form, frequency, and other factors play a considerable part in what the reaction and threshold of stimulus will be for any given instrument. The proper use of an electrical pulp tester dictates that the patient respond only to those stimuli that produce pain—not to those that produce tickling sensations or other types of responses.

Pulp testers in use. The Burton Vitalometer is an electrical pulp tester that employs an interrupted high frequency wave produced by a mechanical generator. This tester provides for an internal circuit resistance of over 3 million ohms, which limits the actual current in the external circuit to about 4 microamperes. An applied interrupted voltage that is used to stimulate the

pulp may be increased or decreased by sliding an indicator along an arbitrary scale; this sliding indicator operates the secondary coil of an inductorium. A mechanical magnetic breaker system in the primary coil of the inductorium alters the output of the tester from 60 cycles to 400± cycles per second. The Burton Vitalometer is connected in the manner indicated in Fig. 13-15. The patient holds the capacitor and the operator manipulates the inductorium (sliding scale) while holding the electrode on the tooth. The vibrator mechanism is actuated when the contact button is pressed. The contact button is moved from the lowest point on the scale to that point which first elicits a response from the patient. The arbitrary scale is numbered from 1 to 16. The value of each figure must be calibrated for each tooth being tested by comparing it with that of adjacent teeth or with similar teeth on the opposite side of the arch. Low readings on the scale are

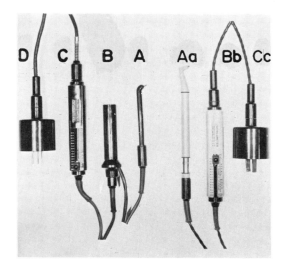

Fig. 13-15. *Types of Burton Vitalometers.* The Vitalometer on the right is a new model (No. 205MB) that eliminates the patient-held electrode, **B**, by incorporating the capacity tube, **B**, into the tooth electrode, **Aa. A**, Tooth electrode. **Aa**, Tooth electrode with included capacity tube. **B**, Patient's hand electrode. **C, Bb**, Inductorium. **D, Cc**, Power generators. (Courtesy Burton Manufacturing Co., Santa Monica, Calif.)

usually indicative of a hyperexcitable pulp; high readings usually indicate a hypoexcitable or "dead" pulp. The significance of each reading cannot be fully evaluated without the correlation of clinical findings.

The Pelton and Crane Company manufactures the Vitapulp pulp tester, which uses a 7-volt mercury battery as its power source for a transistorized circuit. The circuit uses three transistors—two employed as a multivibrator oscillator and the third as a buffer. The voltage is increased by a small iron-core transformer. The stimulus produced delivers a maximum of 350 peak volts at about 400 cycles per second. Actual loading of the instrument in use reduces the peak voltage to about 250 volts. The Vitapulp uses a voltage-divider rheostat to vary the intensity of the stimulus. A separate switch button assures that the circuit is not activated unintentionally or left on when not in use.

The Ritter pulp tester (Fig. 13-16) delivers a current of about 400 cycles per second of short duration to a tooth electrode. The intensity of the current can be regulated by a circular dial attached to the handle of the instrument. An arbitrary scale of 0 to 10 is afforded to indicate the degree of current tolerated by the patient. A neon light is present in the circuit to indicate whether current is being delivered to the tooth. The operator holds the handle of the pulp tester in one hand and completes the circuit by contacting the patient with the other hand. The manufacturer recommends that a drop of toothpaste rather than water be applied to the tooth electrode tip to ensure adequate electrical contact. The electrode is maintained in constant contact with the tooth, and the regulating dial located on the top of the instrument handle is moved slowly from 0 upward until the patient indicates a tingle or a sense of warmth. Readings in the region of 10 without eliciting a response indicate a hypoexcitable or devital pulp.

The Parkell Dentotest Vitalometer is a fully transistorized, battery-operated instrument. The source of power is a 4-volt mercury battery with an operating life of about 90 hours. A rheostat varies the current applied to the tooth from 20 microamperes to 220 microamperes. The Dentotest operates on a frequency of 9,000 cycles per minute (Fig. 13-17).

Test considerations. The following considerations should be taken into account when testing with an electric pulp tester.

1. The patient should be informed of the nature of the test.
2. The teeth to be tested should be dried.
3. Adequate electrical contact between the tooth and the electrode must be made.
4. An excessively applied stimulus is likely to

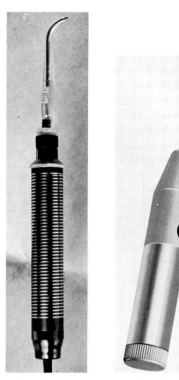

Fig. 13-16   **Fig. 13-17**

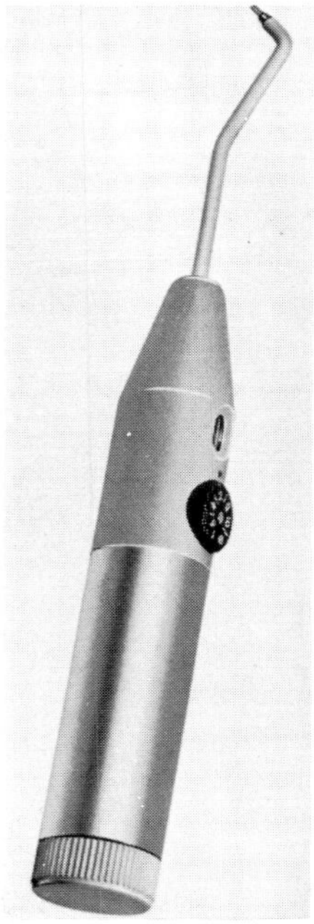

Fig. 13-16. *Ritter pulp tester.* (Courtesy Ritter Co., Inc., Rochester, N. Y.)

Fig. 13-17. *Parkell Dentotest Vitalometer.* (Courtesy Parkell Products, Inc., Long Island City, N. Y.)

result in a false positive test because of leakage.

5. The electrode should be placed on sound tooth structure.
6. The electrode should not touch or be in proximity to the gingiva.
7. Molar teeth may require tests at more than one point.
8. Electrical conduction through proximal inlays and continuous bridgework should be avoided.
9. Teeth with full gold, porcelain, or acrylic coverage cannot be tested with an electrical stimulus.
10. Pulp tests should substantiate the findings from the history and clinical examination.

The patient should be fully informed of the nature of the test. Since many patients are apprehensive of electrical apparatus, they are likely to respond to the test prematurely. Excessive pain is to be avoided. The tooth should be thoroughly dried to prevent leakage of the current to the soft tissues. When leakage occurs, the patient experiences an unnecessary pain and false positive readings can occur. The electrical contact between the electrode and the tooth may be enhanced by wetting the electrode with a saline solution. Unless an adequate electrical contact is made, an excessive current may have to be applied and a false hypoexcitable or devital pulp may be suggested by the test.

The electrode should be placed on sound tooth structure—never on restorations (Fig.

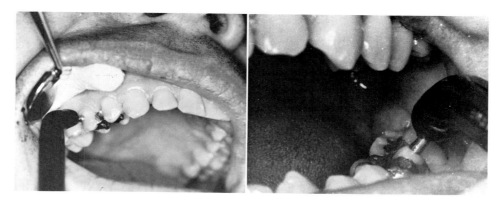

Fig. 13-18. *Pulp testing.* Application of Vitalometer tip on tooth with restoration.

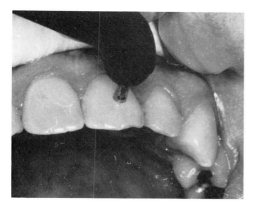

Fig. 13-19. *Pulp testing.* Vitalometer tip is placed well away from gingiva to prevent gingival response.

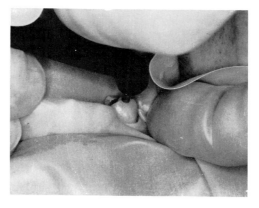

Fig. 13-20. *Pulp testing.* Rubber dam for isolation of tooth to be tested.

13-18). Placing the electrode on undermined enamel should be avoided. Occasionally large restorations may extend beneath the outer surface of the tooth being examined—the electrode should not be placed over these areas but over areas where sound tooth structure exists between the pulp and the surface of the tooth.

The electrode should be placed so as to avoid leakage to the gingiva (Fig. 13-19). Placement close to the gingiva may result in leakage via the small amount of moisture left on the surface of the tooth, especially if the electrical resistance path to the pulp is greater than that to the gingiva. Leakage is quite likely to occur when the electrical stimulus is intense.

Multirooted teeth may have to be tested at more than one point since the pulp may be vital in one portion of the tooth and devital in another. One should remember that larger teeth, namely, molar teeth, generally require more stimulus to elicit a painful response than do smaller teeth. Comparisons of vitality readings should be made between the same kind of teeth.

Occasionally the electrical resistance between adjacent teeth will be less than that of the tooth being tested because of approximating restorations. This occurs frequently when large restorations are present. This situation can be avoided by use of a rubber dam to isolate the tooth being tested (Fig. 13-20). Although this shortcoming cannot be overcome with fixed bridgework, it can be minimized by proper placement of the electrode, for example, on exposed surfaces where abutment teeth are three-fourths crowns.

All tests should be correlated with the clinical findings. If a tooth appears to be involved apically as indicated by the radiographic examination but the electrical test is positive, the examiner should review his technic to assure himself that leakage or other shortcomings have not occurred. The shortcomings of electrical vitality tests should be well known to the examiner. In most instances, false positive or false negative tests are the fault of the person making the test, not the testing device.

Thermal tests. Thermal tests are frequently of value in testing changes in the pulp. Since the patient may experience pain in the pulp upon drinking hot coffee or cold water, thermal tests may be more effective than electrical tests in duplicating the natural cause of the pain. They are especially useful for teeth with full gold, porcelain, or acrylic coverage.

The correlation between pain caused by thermal stimulation and the state of the pulp is not specific or constant. Teeth that are sensitive to heat may not be sensitive to cold; those sensitive to cold may not be sensitive to heat; teeth may be sensitive to both heat and cold. To correlate these changes with histopathologic changes of the pulp is often misleading. Irrespective of the type of stimulus used, the clinical findings must be correlated with the pulp test findings.

Heat thermal tests may be accomplished by heating a small ball of gutta-percha on the end of a plastic instrument and touching it to the tooth being tested (Fig. 13-21). The tooth should be wet to prevent the gutta-percha from sticking. The material should be applied lightly to the surface until the degree of tolerance by the patient can be determined. Since conduction of

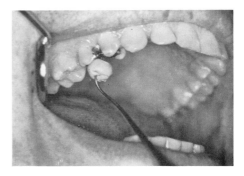

Fig. 13-21. *Pulp testing.* Thermal test using hot base plate gutta-percha.

heat is slow but accumulative, it is possible for excessive heat to be applied unless the examiner is careful, especially in the presence of large restorations.

Cold thermal tests may be performed with cold air, ice, or cotton soaked in ethyl chloride (Fig. 13-22). Ethyl chloride should never be sprayed directly on the teeth. Since the transfer of heat away from the pulp is delayed, the application of the cold should be accomplished slowly to avoid excessive cold and a severe painful stimulus. Probably the most specific relationship that exists between the state of the pulp and the reaction to thermal change is that associated with an acute suppurative pulpi-

tis or acute alveolar abscess. In these conditions the patient will experience severe pain when heat is applied and gain relief when cold is applied. In most instances he has discovered this for himself and is treating the pulp symptomatically by keeping ice on the offending tooth and avoiding heat.

Interpretation of pulp tests. The principles of interpreting pulp tests are the same for both electrical and thermal stimulation. Because of the individual variations that exist in the response of a diseased pulp to any kind of painful stimulus, no specific histologic picture can be anticipated clinically or microscopically even if the tooth

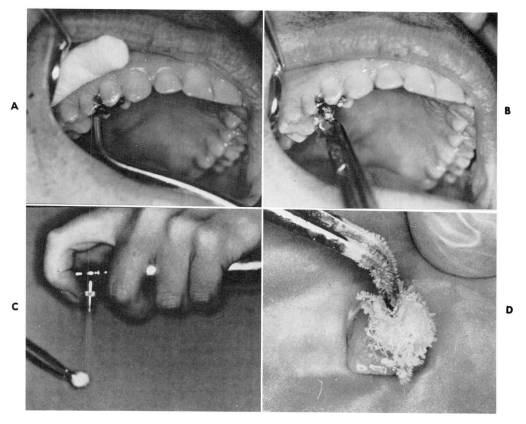

Fig. 13-22. *Pulp testing.* **A,** Thermal pulp test with cold air. **B,** Thermal pulp test with ice. **C** and **D,** Thermal pulp test with ethyl chloride applied to cotton pledget; ethyl chloride should not be sprayed directly on the tooth.

is extracted for study. Thus, it must be emphasized that it is impossible to make a differential diagnosis of the histopathologic features of pulp disease on the basis of pulp tests and clinical radiographic examinations alone. The clinical diagnosis is made on the basis of history, physical examination, radiographic examination, and the findings from the electrical or thermal tests. If all of these are used correctly, an accurate diagnosis of devital or vital pulp usually can be made. The diagnosis of hyperplastic pulpitis (pulp polyp) is obvious clinically. Aside from the common clinical findings relative to acute suppurative pulpitis and acute alveolar abscess already mentioned, no other unequivocal clinical diagnosis of pulp disease can be made without exposure of the pulp.

The acuteness of pulp disease for practical purposes must be based on the severity of the pain and the suddenness of onset. This does not imply any particular degree of pulp damage, for the symptoms of partial pulpitis may be the same as those of total pulpitis. From a practical standpoint, acute clinical symptoms of pulp disease in adult teeth with closed foramens generally indicate the death of the pulp. As far as pulp testing results are concerned, it is well known that pulp destruction from severe inflammatory or circulatory disturbances will produce a rise in the threshold of excitation. It is also well known that the threshold of excitation may be lowered in the early stages of inflammation. However, one should remember that the threshold value may be affected by factors having nothing to do with the excitability of the tooth per se (Björn).

The diagnosis of chronic pulp disease can only be made clinically on the basis of a history of chronicity or recurrence and the absence of acute symptoms. A history of an acute episode of pulpitis followed by less severe episodes may also occur. In some instances a state of mild, chronic, recurrent, or latent pulpitis may be detected

on the basis of history alone. On occasion a tooth will suddenly give signs of pulp disease after it is restored or used as an abutment tooth. Not infrequently the exacerbation of such latent disease will be caused by the occlusal trauma. In many of these situations acute exacerbations result in failure of extensive reconstructions. This can be avoided many times by a complete history, physical examination, radiographic examination, and vitality test of the teeth prior to reconstruction. Unfortunately not all cases of latent pulpitis can be determined in advance.

Summary. These salient features of pulp testing should be kept in mind:

1. A maximum stimulus without reaction is always indicative of a partial or totally necrotic pulp, and root canal therapy is indicated (assuming the pulp test is correlated with the clinical findings and the tests are accurately done).
2. A "normal" reaction to pulp testing either by electrical or thermal stimulation may not necessarily indicate a healthy pulp, since retrogressive changes may not affect the threshold of excitation.
3. A raised threshold of excitation does not necessarily indicate a diseased pulp.

Some of the confusion arising from the diagnosis of pulp changes and excitation threshold can be eliminated by taking an adequate history and making a careful physical and radiographic examination. Thus, no one method of examination should be done to the exclusion of all others.

STUDY CASTS

Study models can be an important aid in diagnosis and treatment planning when the patient is away from the dental office. Articulation of study casts will materially aid the examiner in evaluating occlusal function and allow trial adjustments to be made and the effect noted before actually carrying out the procedure in the mouth. Articulation of models and the preparation of a grinding chart may be quite valuable in the occlusal adjustment of a difficult case. The mounting of casts in an articulator is also helpful in studying the preparation of the mouth for prosthetic appliances. The examination of unmounted casts by visual inspection and by a surveying instrument may reveal factors that will interfere with the seating of fixed appliances or with the insertion and removal of removable appliances. This information will help the examiner decide what appliance is most appropriate and what changes should be made during the preparation of the mouth to more effectively utilize a particular appliance. Study casts can be surveyed by the use of a paralleling surveyor to determine the most advantageous path of insertion and removal of an appliance; the amount and location of retention can be determined by the use of a surveyor. Further, study casts serve as excellent visual aids in informing a patient of his dental problems.

Articulation of casts

The articulation of study casts on an adjustable articulator is an important procedure in the functional analysis of occlusal relations. Although errors of reproducing the complicated movements of the human jaws are inherent in any method of mounting, the simple procedure presented here will be of considerable value in diagnosis and treatment planning in spite of its limitations. A clinical functional analysis of occlusal relationships should be carried out prior to mounting study casts. This analysis has already been described (see Chapter 10).

The mounting procedure should be as follows:

1. Determination of the conventional hinge axis
2. Preparation of the bite fork with wax
3. Positioning of the bite fork in the mouth
4. Positioning and locking of the face-bow
5. Transfer of the face-bow to the articulator and mounting of the maxillary cast
6. Preparation of wax recording of centric relation
7. Transfer of the recording to the articulator and mounting of the mandibular cast
8. Preparation of protrusive wax recording
9. Transfer of the recording to articulator and adjustment of condylar guidance

Conventional hinge axis. The true hinge axis cannot be determined without the use of a kinematic face-bow. If used properly, the Hanau face-bow is sufficiently accurate to record a hinge axis that is reasonably close to that of the true terminal hinge axis. Such a hinge axis is called a conventional hinge axis. The error between a true hinge axis and a conventional hinge axis may be kept to a minimum if the opening between the teeth is limited to ½ to 1 mm. If pronounced premature occlusal interferences prevent this, a preliminary adjustment of these areas should be made. Since the determination is also dependent upon the ability of the patient to relax his muscles during hinge axis closure, muscle spasms, pain in the teeth, and temporomandibular joint pain will have to be relieved before the registration can be accomplished. Symptomatic treatment with muscle relaxants may be of value.

The conventional hinge axis is determined by measurement (Fig. 13-23, *A*). A millimeter rule is placed on the face so that it forms a line from the middle of the tragus of the ear to the corner of the eye, and the axis is marked 13 mm. in front of the anterior border of the tragus. After marking the point, the dentist should evaluate it for accuracy by palpation of the condyle while the patient makes small up-and-down movements of the mandible.

Use of bite fork. The Hanau bite fork is made for use with occlusion rims that may hinder its use with natural dentition; therefore it should be related to the study casts to determine whether it will cause an interference. Modification of the center prong and shape of the fork may be necessary to avoid impingement on the teeth.

The bite fork is wrapped with two or three layers of medium hard base plate wax that has been softened. The thickness and form of the wax should be related to the

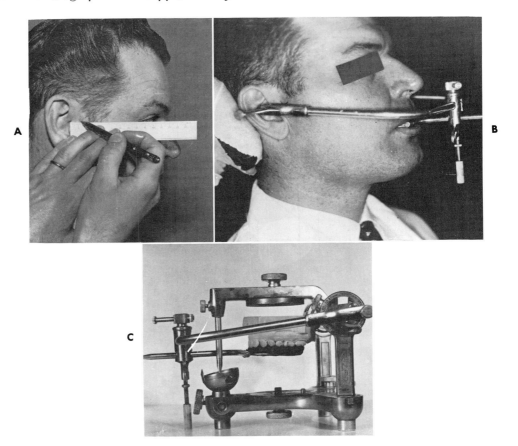

Fig. 13-23. *Articulation of casts.* **A,** Location of hinge axis. **B,** Placement of face-bow. **C,** Mounting maxillary cast on articulator.

study cast to determine if sufficient wax is present to prevent the teeth from going through to the metal fork. Pronounced overbite and convex occlusal planes require more wax than do straight occlusal planes to prevent impingement on the metal fork. The wax should be uniformly soft throughout; this can be accomplished by placing the waxed fork in warm water. The fork is positioned in the mouth so that its handle is sufficiently displaced laterally to avoid contact with the incisal pin of the articulator when the cast is mounted. The patient is instructed to bite until sufficient occlusal imprints have been made to provide stability. The waxed fork is then chilled

thoroughly and removed, and all excess wax and soft tissue impressions are removed with a sharp knife. The waxed fork is placed on the casts to determine stability. Rocking of the models on it indicates an improper relationship and the bite should be taken again. The wax should be trimmed along the incisal and buccal surfaces of the teeth. The waxed fork is chilled and placed back in the patient's mouth in its original position, and the patient is instructed to hold it while the face-bow is centered (Fig. 13-23, *B*). The ends of the condyle pins of the face-bow should be centered on the ink markings that have been previously made on the face to mark

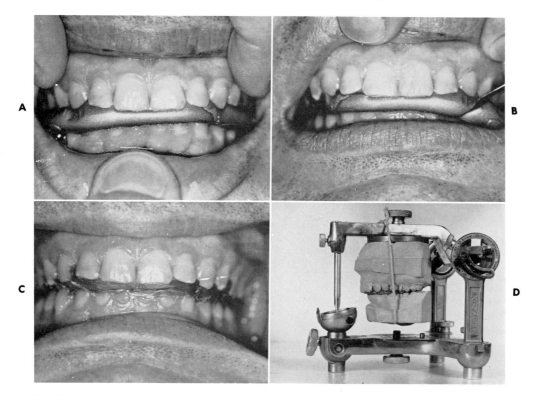

Fig. 13-24. *Articulation of models.* **A,** Wax in position to record centric relation. **B,** Trimming excess wax. **C,** Completion of wax bite. **D,** Positioning mandibular cast on articulator with wax bite.

the conventional hinge axis. They should just touch the surface of the skin and no pressure should be exerted on the tissues. Their position should be checked after the face-bow has been fixed in position, since movement may occur during the tightening procedure. The face-bow is then transferred to the articulator and the maxillary cast is mounted (Fig. 13-23, *C*). Since the ordinary face-bow does not have an infraorbital pin for orientation to the Frankfort horizontal plane, the occlusal plane is set arbitrarily. The bite fork is leveled with the notch on the incisal pin.

Registration of centric relation. Centric relation may be registered with plaster or wax. Wax is more commonly used because of its ease of manipulation and because of

the margin of error that can be tolerated between the cast and wax bite. Plaster is quite accurate but it cannot clear undercuts. It flows into the embrasures and requires considerable trimming before the impression can be seated on the casts. One distinct advantage of plaster warrants mention. When it is used there is less tendency for the patient to displace the jaw than when wax is used because plaster offers no resistance to closure of the jaws. Though displacement of the jaw can be minimized when wax is used if the wax is uniformly soft, the difficulty with the plaster flowing into undercuts and requiring considerable trimming cannot be minimized easily. Whether wax or plaster is used is primarily up to the clinician. The use of wax is discussed here merely because of its more common usage.

In addition to the disadvantages of wax mentioned are its tendency to harden before the registration can be completed and the difficulty in chilling it completely before removal. The latter can be partly overcome by the use of wax containing aluminum. This type of wax tends to heat more evenly, retain heat longer, and chill more quickly. The experienced operator may find that ordinary plate wax with a medium hard base serves his requirements as well.

To register centric relation, the patient's muscles must be relaxed as completely as possible. Trial movements of the mandible in hinge axis closure should precede the actual registration so that the patient may be trained to assist in the procedure. When this has been accomplished, the wax registration can be made.

The wax to be used is prepared by making a narrow roll (½ inch) of two or three thicknesses of base plate wax. The form of the wax can be determined by softening the roll and adjusting it to the curvature and length of the maxillary cast. The roll is immersed in warm water until it is uniformly warm throughout; it is then positioned in the patient's mouth.

The mandible is guided and controlled by light pressure on the patient's chin in the direction of the joint so that there is no displacement from hinge axis movement during the final 1 to ½ inch of closure (Fig. 13-24). Centric relation registration should be recorded with 1 to 0.5 mm. of wax or space between the teeth just prior to initial occlusal contact. As soon as the operator is satisfied that this position has been reached in the wax bite, he should trim the excess wax from the teeth so that the labial and buccal incisal edges of the maxillary teeth are visible (Fig. 13-24). The wax should then be chilled and removed from the mouth, and any wax that has touched soft tissue should be removed. At least three recordings should be taken for a comparison

of results. The amount of wax used and the interocclusal space present just prior to initial occlusal contact should be relatively the same.

A method for visualization and comparison of wax bites is demonstrated in Fig. 13-25. The casts are marked with vertical lines on their anterior and posterior parts. The casts should be in maximum occlusal contact—centric occlusion. The operator should compare the position of the midline in the mouth in centric relation and in centric occlusion. If deviation of the midline occurs on opening 1 to 0.5 mm., the amount should be indicated on the mandibular cast. If two wax registrations are identical, the most posterior displacement of the lines on the mandibular teeth will be the same for the two wax bites. The amount of displacement is not important since the thickness of the wax may alter the actual linear displacement. The important consideration is that the displacement posterior to the mandibular lines be proportioned on the same sides for two wax registrations. In general, if the closure is within 1 to 0.5 mm., the variation in the width of the wax bite will be of no significance. Therefore, if true centric relation is registered in two different registrations, the most posterior displacement of the mandibular lines on like sides of the cast will be the same. Any change from this will indicate a displacement of the mandible from true centric relation during closure.

No wax pattern should be used that shows perforation of the wax, since this indicates that the initial occlusal contact has been recorded and some displacement of the mandible probably has occurred. There is no simple and completely accurate way in which to determine whether a wax bite has recorded true centric relation. A comparison of wax bites is of some assistance, but even then an experienced operator may have difficulty in obtaining a proper registration. Even the experienced operator may on occasion have to remount his cases several times before being satisfied that he has the proper centric relation recorded. For the beginner the mounting of a case for study may present a problem, but some of the sources of error may be eliminated by careful attention to details. The stone models must be as nearly perfect as possible, and all extraneous plaster and imperfections should be removed. The patient should be thoroughly relaxed and trained in the method of centric relation closure, and the wax should be uniformly soft throughout.

Protrusive registration. The wax roll is prepared in the same manner as for centric relation registration. The thickness of the wax roll may have to be increased in the molar region to compensate for a large interocclusal space caused by a pronounced overbite of the maxillary incisors.

The patient should be trained to bite straight forward about 4 to 5 mm. Lateral displacement or Bennett movement should be avoided. After the patient is trained to bite in the desired position, the uniformly soft wax roll is inserted in the mouth. The closure should be stopped 1 to 0.5 mm. short of initial tooth contact. The wax is chilled and trimmed the same as in centric relation registration.

Mounting of the mandibular casts. The accepted centric wax registration is used to

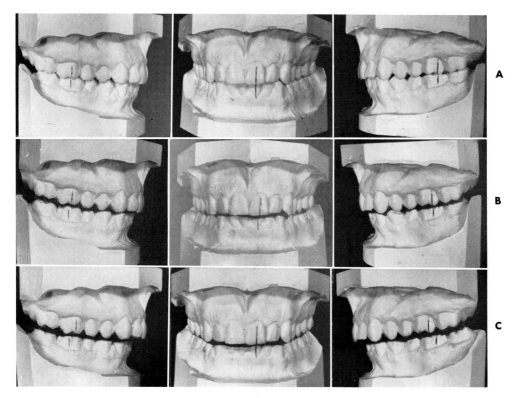

Fig. 13-25. *Determination of correct wax bite.* **A,** Series of casts in acquired centric occlusion. **B,** Series of casts showing incorrect wax bite; note discrepancy in comparison lines; these points of reference must be compared with the mouth. **C,** Series of casts showing correct wax bite. Posterior displacement on both sides of the mouth should be the same for two consecutive bites. Center line deviation, if any, should be the same for two consecutive wax bites.

position the mandibular cast to the maxillary cast. It may be held in position by wax or string (Fig. 13-24, *D*). Before the mandibular cast is fixed to the mounting ring, the incisal pin of the articulator is adjusted sufficiently (2 to 3 mm.) to compensate for the thickness of the wax registration. The centric lock is closed and locked to prevent displacement of the articulator arm. The mandibular cast is then fixed to the mounting ring (Fig. 13-26). After the plaster has set, the next step is to transfer the protrusive bite recording to the articulator.

Adjustment of condylar guidance. The

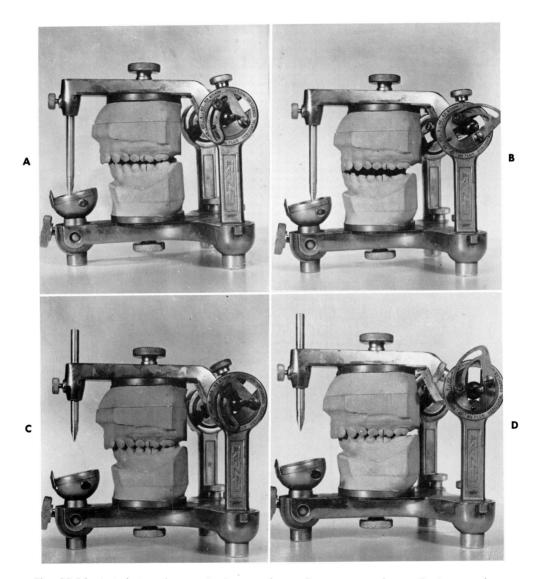

Fig. 13-26. *Articulation of casts.* **A,** Centric relation. **B,** Protrusive relation. **C,** Centric relation without wax bite in place; note the posterior displacement of reference line on the mandibular cast; condyle axis is locked, and teeth are occluding on premature contacts only. **D,** Acquired centric occlusion. Difference in position of casts in **C** and **D** represents "slide in centric."

centric lock is opened, the condylar guidance screws are loosened, and the incisal pin is raised or removed. The protrusive registration is then positioned and fittted firmly to the maxillary and mandibular casts. The condylar guidance adjustments are moved forward and backward while the maxillary and mandibular casts are held firmly in position in the wax. The movement of the condylar guidance will cause the maxillary cast to rock in the wax. The condylar guidance should be locked in a position half-way between its forward and backward position where no rocking of the cast takes place. Each side is checked individually and then rechecked after the first position on each side is determined. The variation in the condylar guidance angulation should not vary more than 2 to 4 degrees from one side to the other if the temporomandibular joints are normal. Negative readings are generally the result of an inadequate registration. The lateral guidance is computed with the formula on the undersurface of the base of the Hanau articulator.

If the centric lock is tightened, the incisal pin is raised, and the casts are brought into contact, one will find that the casts are in centric relation, and the initial occlusal contact should be the same as that seen in the mouth (Fig. 13-26). With the centric locks free, the casts should articulate in the acquired centric occlusion (Fig. 13-26, *D*). If the articulation is closed in centric relation, incomplete occlusal contact is made until sliding of the maxillary cast on the articulator occurs; this represents a slide in centric.

When the mounting has been completed, the operator should determine whether he has a reasonably accurate centric relation registration. The most frequent sign of an improper registration is the presence of space between the molar teeth without the presence of any initial contact even in the position of centric occlusion. One method for demonstrating an inaccurate mounting is to loosen the screw on the maxillary arm about two turns so that the maxillary cast can be placed manually into centric occlusion, that is, maximum interdigitation of the teeth. Once in this position (with the condylar guidance locks loosened), the maxillary and mandibular casts are held tightly together with one hand. With the other hand, the maxillary mounting ring nut is tightened; any shift of the maxillary cast should be noted. With an incorrect mounting the maxillary cast will shift laterally or upward so that there is an opening between the molar teeth. When this occurs it is apparent that no centric stops in centric occlusion would be present—an unusual situation if true in the patient's occlusion. Lateral movements should be made with a comparison of the excursions of the teeth with facets worn on the teeth. When the teeth do not occlude in any position or with these facets, it is apparent that the mounting is incorrect. The comparison of these excursions on the facets can be best seen in working relationships.

• • •

A functional occlusal analysis can be made by an experienced clinician without the aid of an articulator; however, many of the details can be analyzed more conveniently when the patient is not in the dental chair. Occasionally the occlusal interferences may be so complex as to require a more detailed study than can be accomplished when the patient is in the dental chair. The articulation of casts may make it possible to determine if satisfactory treatment can be achieved by grinding alone or if other forms of treatment will be necessary. In some instances the clinician may wish to make the occlusal adjustment on the models before the treatment is carried out on the patient so that the extent and limitation of the grinding may be determined. When occlusal rehabilitation is being considered, articulation of casts is very advantageous in planning the proposed reconstruction. It may be helpful in the preparation of abutments, in the trial use of pontics and facings, and in the determination of the type of restoration that can be used. Occasionally when orthodontic treatment is indicated, articulation of the casts is helpful in determining what the alignment of the teeth will be after orthodontic treatment and what the functional possibilities are. Thus, the articulation of stone casts can be used (1) as a diagnostic instrument, (2) as a planning instrument, and (3) as an instrument for carrying out technical work in connection with prosthetic occlusal reconstruction or full dentures.

USE OF SURVEYOR

No attempt will be made to present all the details of the use of a surveyor. A few of the principles of its use as they relate to diagnosis will be given. Consult suitable references at the end of this chapter for the application of the surveyor to specific cases.

The surveyor is primarily used to determine what preparation of the mouth will be necessary to reduce to a reasonable limit the amount of interference to the insertion of an appliance (Fig. 13-27). Thus the cast may be used in a preliminary survey to determine the degree of nonparallelism of surfaces to be used. Surveying of the cast may indicate the necessity for reduction of tooth contours by disking, the placement of parallel restorations, the extraction of excessively malposed teeth, and the surgical correction of connective tissue and bone that present severe undercuts (Applegate, 1940).

In addition, the surveyor is important in determining the path of insertion and removal of appliances. The position and type of clasp that may be used should be designed with the aid of a surveyor to determine the proper amount of retention to avoid excessive lateral movement of the retaining teeth during insertion and re-

moval of an appliance. The surveyor is also used to determine the position and placement of adequate guiding planes. Guiding planes on opposing parallel tooth surfaces are necessary to assure that the appliance

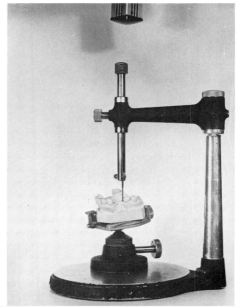

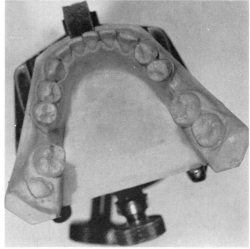

Fig. 13-27. *Cast survey.* Surveying casts to determine parallelism prior to preparation of the mouth for prostheses; this procedure aids in formulating the treatment plan.

will be given a positive direction for removal and insertion.

The principles of the use of a surveyor for diagnostic purposes are centered around the advisability of using a particular appliance with the conditions that affect retention present, path of insertion and removal, and the alignment of the teeth and surfaces relative to parallel guiding planes. This information is necessary before treatment planning can be undertaken. Since the preparation of the mouth for a prosthetic appliance should be planned in advance, a survey of the casts will greatly facilitate this part of treatment. The survey as it relates to the preparation of the mouth should be an integral part of treatment planning.

STOMATOMICROSCOPE

A diagnostic aid in limited use currently is the stomatomicroscope. This diagnostic aid is an adaptation of the colposcope, which has been used in gynecologic examinations and surgery for several years.

The stomatomicroscope is limited in flexibility, reducing its usefulness for examining posterior areas of the mouth. Because of the limitations imposed by the optical system, only 8 to 16 magnifications are practical for clinical use. As the magnification is increased, the depth of focus is reduced, as is the working distance between the objective and the tissue. In addition, the field of visualization is reduced. All these restrictions interfere with retaining orientation of the area being examined (Fig. 13-28).

DISCLOSING SOLUTION

Disclosing solution is a valauble aid in detecting the location of plaques on the teeth, in demonstrating the presence of plaques to patients, in determining the efficiency of home-care procedures, and in detecting irregular and rough surfaces that habitually take up stains. Various types are available. Most contain iodine in some form. Refer to *Accepted Dental Therapeutics* for complete details of their constituents. The following disclosing solution contains no iodine, and no known sensitivity reactions to it have occurred.

Bismark, brown	3 Gm.
Alcohol, ethyl 95%	10 ml.
Glycerin, USP	120 ml.
Anise	1 drop

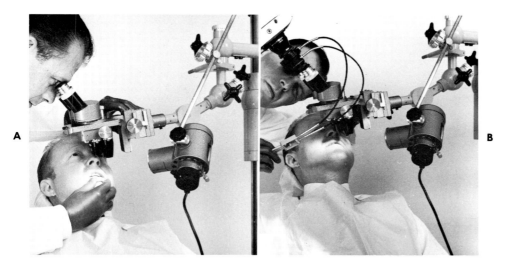

Fig. 13-28. *Stomatomicroscope.* **A,** Examination with stomatomicroscope. **B,** Camera attachment.

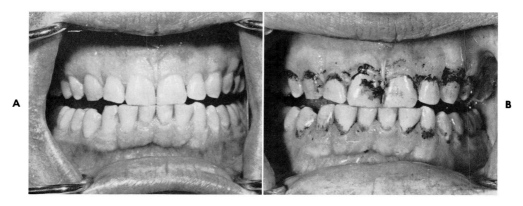

Fig. 13-29. *Disclosing solution.* **A,** Before application. **B,** After application; showing areas of plaques.

The disclosing solution is placed on the teeth with a cotton applicator. The patient is instructed to rinse his mouth with water to remove the excess solution. The solution will stain readily all the tooth surfaces on which soft mucinous plaques are present (Fig. 13-29). Margins and porous cracks, imperfect margins, and rough porous acrylic and silicate restorations are often temporarily stained.

REFERENCES

Aduddell, A. C., and Reynolds, R. L.: Pulp testers. (In press, 1972.)

American Dental Association: Accepted dental therapeutics, ed. 35, Chicago, 1973-1974, The Association.

Applegate, O. C.: Essentials of removable partial denture prosthesis, Philadelphia, 1954, W. B. Saunders Co.

Applegate, O. C.: Use of a paralleling surveyor, J.A.D.A. **27:**1397-1407, 1940.

Björn, Hilding: Electrical excitation of teeth and its application to dentistry, Sven. Tandlak. Tidskr. (suppl.) vol. 39, 1946.

Bonica, J. J.: The management of pain, Philadelphia, 1953, Lea & Febiger.

Broshear, A. D.: Innervation of the teeth, J.A.D.A. **23:**662, 1936.

Bunting, R. W., and Parmerlee, F.: The role of Bacillus acidophilus in dental caries, J.A.D.A. **12:**381, 1925.

Fosdick, L. S., Hansen, H. L., and Epple, C.: Enamel decalcification by mouth organisms and dental caries. A suggested test for caries susceptibility, J.A.D.A. **24:**1275, 1937.

Frankel, S., Reitman, S., and Sonnenwirth, A. C. (editors): Gradwohl's Clinical laboratory methods and diagnosis, ed. 7, St. Louis, 1970, The C. V. Mosby Co.

Goetzl, F. R., Burrill, D. Y., and Ivy, A. C.: A critical analysis of algesimetric methods with suggestions for a useful procedure, Quart. Bull., Northwestern Univ. Med. School **17:**280-291, 1943.

Goss, A. N.: Infra-red thermography in oral diagnosis, Mich. Dent. Ass. J. **51:**180-184, 1969.

Hadley, F. P.: A quantitative method for estimating Bacillus acidophilus in saliva, J. Dent. Res. **13:**415, 1933.

Ham, T. H. (editor): A syllabus of laboratory examinations in clinical diagnosis, Cambridge, 1950, Harvard University Press.

Hardy, J. D., Wolff, H. G., and Goodell, H.: Pain sensations and reactions, Baltimore, 1952, The Williams & Wilkins Co.

Jay, P.: The reduction of oral Lactobacillus acidophilus counts by the periodic restriction of carbohydrate. Amer. J. Orthod. (Oral Surg. Sec.) **33:**162, 1947.

Kaletsky, T., and Furedi, A.: Further studies on the reliability of various types of electric pulp testers, Dent. Cosmos **78:**732-742, 1936.

Koss, L. G.: Diagnostic cytology and its histopathologic bases, Philadelphia, 1961, J. B. Lippincott Co.

Martin, H., Ferris, C., and Mazzella, W.: An evaluation of media used in electrical pulp testing, Opt. Acta (London) **27:**374-378, March, 1969.

McDaniel, K. F., Rowe, N. H., and Charbeneau, G. T.: Tissue response to an electrical pulp tester, J. Prosth. Dent. **29:**84, Jan. 1973.

Miller, S. E., (editor): A textbook of clinical pathology, ed. 4, Baltimore, 1952, The Williams & Wilkins Co.

Mumford, J. M., and Björn, H.: Problems in electrical pulp testing and dental algesimetry, Int. Dent. J. **12:**161-179, July, 1962.

Pfaffman, C.: Afferent impulses from the teeth

due to pressure and noxious stimulation, J. Physiol. **97**:207, 1939.

Preston, J. A., and Troxel, D. B.: Biochemical profiling in diagnostic medicine, Tarrytown, N. Y., 1971, Technicon Instruments Corp.

Reiss, H. L., and Furedi, A.: Significance of the pulp test as revealed in a microscopic study of the pulps of 130 teeth, Dent. Cosmos **75**:272-281, 1933.

Rogosa, M., Mitchell, J. A., and Wiseman, R. F.: A selected medium for the isolation and examination of oral lactobacilli, J. Dent. Res. **30**:682-689, 1951.

Rovin, S.: The role of biopsy and cytology in oral diagnosis, Dent. Clin. N. Amer. 429-434, July, 1965.

Sandler, H. C., and Stahl, S. S.: Exfoliative cytology as a diagnostic aid in detection of oral neoplasms, J. Oral Surg. **16**:414, 1958.

Selbach, G. J., and von Haam, E.: The clinical value of oral cytology, Acta Cytol. **7**:337-345, 1963.

Snyder, M. L.: A simple colorimetric method for the estimation of relative numbers of lactobacilli in the saliva, J. Dent. Res. **19**:349, 1940.

Socransky, S. S.: Caries-susceptibility tests, Ann. N. Y. Acad. Sci. **153**:137-146, 1968.

Sommer, R. F., Ostrander, F. D., and Crowley, M. C.: Clinical endodontics, Philadelphia, 1956, W. B. Saunders Co.

Thompon, E. O.: Constructing and using diagnostic models, Dent. Clin. N. Amer. 67-84, March, 1963.

Thorn, G. W., and Forsham, P. H.: Diabetes mellitus. In Harrison, T. R. (editor): Principles of internal medicine, Philadelphia, 1950, McGraw-Hill Book Co., chap. 59.

Tiecke, R. W., and others: Oral cytology, J.A.D.A. **75**:855-861, 1961.

Todd, J. C., Sanford, A. H., and Stilwell, G. G.: Clinical diagnosis by laboratory methods, ed. 12, Philadelphia, 1962, W. B. Saunders Co.

Veterans Administration Cooperative Study, 1962: Oral exfoliative cytology, Washington, D. C., 1963, U. S. Government Printing Office.

Wintrobe, M. M.: Clinical hematology, ed. 6, Philadelphia, 1967, Lea & Febiger, pp. 1287, xxv.

Wolff, H. G., and Wolf, S.: Pain, Springfield, Ill., 1948, Charles C Thomas, Publisher.

Yardumian, K.: Physiochemical factors influencing the red cell sedimentation rate, Amer. J. Clin. Path. **7**:105-119, 1937.

Ziskin, D. E., and Wald, A.: Observations on electrical pulp testing, J. Dent. Res. **17**:79, 1938.

14

Synopsis of diagnostic procedures

The synopsis of diagnostic precedures presented here is not only a review of the minimal elements of the case history and clinical examination, but also may be used as a basis for the screening and the incomplete or emergency examinations. The principles for an incomplete type of examination given in Chapter 1 should be reviewed.

The health questionnaire is often used in the complete type of examination as an adjunct to the case history, but is the primary screening instrument in the other types of examinations. The examiner still must evaluate the chief complaint and details of the present illness. The health questionnaire is usually given to the patient prior to considering the chief complaint and details of the present illness. After obtaining the chief complaint and present illness, the examiner should go directly to that portion of the clinical examination pertinent to the chief complaint; however, at some time during the clinical examination the screening elements of the general and oral clinical examinations should be undertaken. Thus the health questionnaire acts as a screening instrument for the case history, and the modified clinical examination acts as a screening procedure for disturbances potentially related to the chief complaint.

A health questionnaire should cover an optional field of information; that is, it should be designed to be taken in a reasonable length of time but provide consistent clinical data to alert the examiner to meaningful avenues of inquiry. Some questions must be broad in scope, whereas others must be specific. A proper combination of questions that have been tested clinically for the most appropriate yield of informative data has been one of the important advances of oral diagnosis in clinical dentistry.

In addition to being an adjunct to the complete history, especially the initial examination of a patient, the health questionnaire may be used as an interim history. A patient may use the original questionnaire to determine whether changes in systemic or oral health have occurred.

The health questionnaire is not a substitute for a complete history even when combined with a printed form for recording data from a clinical examination. However, such forms give some assurance that certain essential data is always obtained and recorded.

The general health of a patient is of significance to the hygienist and to the dentist under whose supervision she is working. Many times ill health may directly affect the tissues of the mouth or the ability and inclination of a patient to carry out home-care instructions. It is assumed that the hygienist will make use of any history that the dentist has previously taken and will inform him of any interim changes that may be present either as the result of answers to the screening questions or because of changes that she has observed.

Most often the questionnaire is given to the patient prior to the beginning of the interview so that the clinician may review the answers at the time the chief complaint and present illness are being evaluated. The significance of the questions in the health questionnaire is found beginning on p. 351.

The following outline can be used to review the sequence of procedures used in obtaining the case history and carrying out the general and oral clinical examinations:

1. Completion of the health questionnaire by patient
2. Case history
   a. Chief complaint
   b. Present illness
3. Evaluation of the health questionnaire by clinician
4. Clinical examination
   a. General
   b. Oral
      (1) Soft tissues
      (2) Periodontium
      (3) Teeth
      (4) Occlusion
      (5) Temporomandibular joints

HEALTH QUESTIONNAIRE

Name _____ Sex _____ Age _____

Address _____

Telephone _____ Height _____ Weight _____

Date _____ Occupation _____ Marital status _____

Name of physician _____

Directions

If your answer is YES to the question asked, put a circle around "Yes."

If your answer is NO to the question asked, put a circle around "No."

Answer all questions. You may comment on answers that require explanation by writing in the space between questions.

Answers to the following questions are for our records only and will be considered confidential.

1. Do you think that your teeth are affecting your general health in any way?	Yes	No
2. Are you dissatisfied with the appearance of your teeth?	Yes	No
3. Are you worried about receiving dental treatment?	Yes	No
4. Do you have difficulty in chewing your food?	Yes	No
5. Are you being treated for any condition by a physician now?	Yes	No
6. Are you taking any medicines now?	Yes	No
7. Have you been examined by your physician within the last year?	Yes	No
8. Has there been any change in your general health in the last year?	Yes	No
9. Have you lost weight without dieting in recent months	Yes	No
10. Have you ever been seriously ill?	Yes	No
11. Have you ever been hospitalized?	Yes	No
12. Have you ever had a major operation?	Yes	No
13. Have you ever had a blood transfusion?	Yes	No

14. Have you had any of the following diseases:

Rheumatic fever	Yes	No	Tuberculosis	Yes	No
Inflammatory rheumatism	Yes	No	Venereal disease	Yes	No
Jaundice (yellow skin and eyes)	Yes	No	Heart attack	Yes	No
Diabetes (sugar disease)	Yes	No	Stroke	Yes	No
High blood pressure	Yes	No			

15. Have you ever been told by a physician that you have a heart murmur?	Yes	No
16. Do you ever have asthma or hay fever? (Underline which one.)	Yes	No
17. Do you ever have hives or skin rash?	Yes	No

Continued.

18. Have you ever experienced an unusual reaction to any of the following drugs:

Aspirin	Yes	No	Sulfonamides (sulfa)	Yes	No
Penicillin	Yes	No	Barbiturates (sleeping pills)	Yes	No
Iodine	Yes	No	Other medicines	Yes	No

19. Have you ever experienced an unusual reaction to a dental anesthetic? Yes No
20. Do you bleed for a long time when you cut yourself? Yes No
21. Have you ever had any injury to your face or jaws? Yes No
22. Have you ever had surgery or x-ray treatment for a tumor, growth, or other condition in your mouth or on your lips? Yes No
23. Do you have frequent, severe headaches? Yes No
24. Do you have any complaints regarding your eyes? Yes No
25. Do you have any ear trouble? Yes No
26. Do you have frequent colds? Yes No
27. Do you have sinus trouble? Yes No
28. Do you have nosebleeds? Yes No
29. Do you have frequent sore throats? Yes No
30. Are you a mouth breather? Yes No
31. Do you have any sensitive teeth? Yes No
32. Have you had a toothache recently? Yes No
33. Do you have bleeding gums? Yes No
34. Do you have frequent canker sores or cold sores? Yes No
35. Have you ever had a severe sore mouth? Yes No
36. Is it difficult for you to open your mouth as wide as you would like? Yes No
37. Does your jaw click when you chew? Yes No
38. Do you have any chest pain on exertion? Yes No
39. Are you ever short of breath on mild exertion? Yes No
40. Do your ankles swell Yes No
41. Do you have a persistent cough? Yes No
42. Do you ever cough blood? Yes No
43. Has your appetite changed recently? Yes No
44. Are there any foods you cannot eat? Yes No
45. Do you have any difficulty swallowing? Yes No
46. Do you have frequent indigestion? Yes No
47. Do you vomit frequently? Yes No
48. Do you have kidney trouble? Yes No
49. Do you urinate more than six times a day? Yes No
50. Are you thirsty much of the time? Yes No
51. Have you ever had painful and swollen joints? Yes No
52. Do you have any numb or prickling areas on your skin? Yes No
53. Do you ever have fits or convulsions? Yes No
54. Do you have a tendency to faint? Yes No
55. Do you bruise easily? Yes No
56. Do you have any blood disorder such as anemia (thin blood)? Yes No
57. Does hot weather bother you more than it does other people you know? Yes No
58. Are you excessively nervous? Yes No
59. Do you get tired easily? Yes No
60. (Women) Are you pregnant at the present time? Yes No

Patient's signature _____

SIGNIFICANCE OF QUESTIONS IN HEALTH QUESTIONNAIRE

Below are the same questions that are found in the sample questionnaire with the significance of each question stated briefly. More detailed information relating to each of the subjects will be found in Chapter 3.

1. **Do you think that your teeth are affecting your general health in any way?** This question establishes the relationship between general and oral health. Also, it tends to bring to light any notions that the patient may have that the condition of his mouth is influencing another health problem of a more generalized nature, such as rheumatism or indigestion.

2. **Are you dissatisfied with the appearance of your teeth?** Often esthetic considerations are paramount in the patient's mind. This question gives him an opportunity to express his concern about the appearance of his teeth.

3. **Are you worried about receiving dental treatment?** This question provides the patient with an opportunity to admit that he is apprehensive about receiving dental treatment. It also gives the dentist an opportunity to identify individuals who require sedation prior to a dental appointment.

4. **Do you have difficulty in chewing your food?** The patient's appraisal of the functional status of his mouth may be evaluated here. Quite frequently the patient is able to point to a specific situation that has reduced his functional effectiveness.

5. **Are you being treated for any condition by a physician now?** The influence of medical treatment on the practice of dentistry is significant from the standpoint of the diagnosis of the condition for which the patient is under treatment and because of the reactions and side effects produced by the many new drugs that are continually being introduced into the practice of medicine. It is imperative that the dentist have a fundamental knowledge of systemic illnesses and of some of the methods of treatment that are employed currently in medical practice, particularly those that involve treatment with drugs. The influence of certain dental procedures on patients who have systemic illnesses is well established, and the hazards that are encountered in connection with some of the drugs being employed in medical treatment are well known. If the patient is unaware of his systemic condition but is aware that he is receiving a form of medical treatment, a written statement from his physician is appropriate prior to instituting dental treatment.

6. **Are you taking any medicines now?** This question is closely related to the previous question and is intended to determine specifically what drugs a patient is taking. If the patient does not know the name of the drug, it is possible to identify the drug either by calling the physician or the pharmacist or by referring to the proper publication that illustrates most of the drugs according to the manufacturer's identification.

7. **Have you been examined by your physician within the last year?** Individuals who have been examined within the past year should be questioned about the reason for seeking medical examination. If the patient is in the habit of receiving annual examinations, it provides an opportunity to establish on the dental record that the patient is in good general health, or it provides an opportunity to bring to light important findings from the medical examination.

8. **Has there been any change in your general health in the last year?** An affirmative answer to this question may indicate an improvement in general health or the onset of a significant illness. In either event, it is of interest, if not always of importance, to the dentist to be aware of the general condition of his patient. Many times a patient will give a subjective appraisal of his general health in answering this question affirmatively and will not base the affirmative answer on a professional diagnosis. In

such cases, it is advisable to recommend a physical examination by a physician rather than to give advice to a patient relative to his general health.

9. **Have you lost weight without dieting in recent months?** There are numerous illnesses that are accompanied by weight loss, particularly in their more advanced stages. Characteristically, diabetes is accompanied by weight loss if the disease goes undetected. In the case of diabetes, the affirmative answers to Questions 9 and 50 would be of significance. Other illnesses that are accompanied by a weight loss are tuberculosis, cancer, and the blood dyscrasis. Unexplained rapid weight loss of 10 pounds or more should always be investigated.

10. **Have you ever been seriously ill?** It is difficult to define the term "seriously ill" used in this question, but it may be explained as referring to an illness that has required hospitalization for more than 1 week or that has been life threatening. In any event, the purpose of this question is to point to illnesses in the individual's past history that are indicative of permanent impairment of health. Impairment of health may require that special precautions be taken during dental treatment. In some instances, the illnesses described by a patient as serious may be recurrent or chronic in nature.

11. **Have you ever been hospitalized?** The reasons for an affirmative answer to this question are commonly the result of tonsillectomy, adenoidectomy, and childbirth. The question is asked to determine the possible history of an illness that may be defined as serious, resulting in hospitalization of the patient. When the question is answered affirmatively, it is necessary to inquire further as to the cause and length of time of hospitalization and whether or not there was any important event, such as serious reaction to a drug, that took place during the hospitalization.

12. **Have you ever had a major operation?** The purpose of this question is not to have the patient enumerate his scars and their history. If answered affirmatively this question should be followed by questions on what procedure was carried out, whether local or general anesthesia was used, how well the procedure was tolerated, whether or not healing was uneventful and, if not, what complications occurred, and if any drug allergies or idiosyncrasies were encountered. It may be significant to know that an individual has had a major operation for a malignant neoplasm prior to planning treatment.

13. **Have you ever had a blood transfusion?** Most blood transfusions are given as part of supportive care during major surgery; however, an affirmative answer to this question may uncover repeated blood transfusions that are being received in the treatment of a blood dyscrasia.

14. **Have you had any of the following diseases?**

Rheumatic fever: The importance of a history of rheumatic fever or rheumatic heart disease is well known. The special precautions that must be taken are clearly indicated whenever dental procedures that produce bleeding are to be carried out. This is especially true of the extraction of teeth and scaling of teeth. The dental profession may not have a true appreciation of the hazard of subacute bacterial endocarditis, because in most instances the disease does not develop for 2 or more weeks after the production of a bacteremia. The connection between subacute bacterial endocarditis and a dental procedure may be quite remote and yet quite significant.

Inflammatory rheumatism: Inflammatory rheumatism is a term that was used for a number of years to indicate rheumatic fever. Today it may be interpreted by patients as indicating rheumatoid arthritis or even what the layman refers to as rheumatism.

Jaundice (yellow skin and eyes): The significance of a history of jaundice is twofold, particularly when the disease causing jaundice is recent. If jaundice is precipitated by hepatocellular disease or cirrhosis, it is particularly significant to the dentist because of the possibility of reduced prothrombin production, with a resultant hemorrhagic tendency.

When a history of viral hepatitis is given, the dentist should protect himself from encountering the blood of his patient directly, since the disease may be transmitted through infected blood. Special precaution must be taken against transmission of the disease by improperly sterilized syringes or other instruments.

Diabetes (sugar disease): Diabetes is classified as adult and juvenile. The blood sugar level tends to be better controlled in patients in the adult diabetic group than in juvenile diabetic patients, in whom the level shows tendencies for fluctuation to the point that insulin shock is not an infrequent occurrence. In general, diabetic patients are more susceptible to infection than nondiabetic patients. In addition, infection has a great influence on the insulin requirements of the diabetic individual. It is entirely possible for a diabetic patient to slip into diabetic coma while receiving daily doses of insulin if he has an infection. Another consideration in diabetes is the timing of the dental appointment. It is advisable to take diabetic patients soon after a meal, unless, of course, use of a general anesthetic is anticipated. The timing of dental appointments shortly after meals tends to avoid the possibility of insulin shock. It is advisable to have a source of sugar on hand, since most diabetic patients can feel the onset of insulin shock and may have time to receive sugar by mouth to elevate the blood sugar level and prevent insulin shock.

High blood pressure: High blood pressure is an important consideration in dentistry, particularly in the use of vasoconstrictors. In general, it is believed that vasoconstrictors in the quantity contained in dental anesthetics are of no great significance in individuals with hypertension. On the other hand, the apprehension to which the individual is subjected prior to a dental appointment and during dental procedures may be of great significance. It has been shown that proper sedation for individuals with hypertension prior to stressful dental procedures reduces greatly the degree of increase in blood pressure related to apprehension.

Tuberculosis: If a patient gives a history of tuberculosis, he should also give a history of receiving a checkup every 6 months. If this is not the case, the dentist is justified in deferring treatment of the patient until it has been verified by x-ray films and by other means that his disease is inactive.

Venereal disease: A history of venereal disease is probably more easily obtained on a questionnaire than by interview and may be of significance in some instances in which clinical findings suggest a possibility either of gonococcal temporomandibular joint arthritis or lesions of secondary or tertiary syphilis in the oral cavity. Whenever a history of venereal disease is obtained, the possibility of reinfection should be considered even though medical treatment has been received for the disease at one time or another.

Heart attack: Heart attacks today are commonly treated by the use of anticoagulant drugs. The drugs that are taken by mouth reduce the production of prothrombin. The prothrombin level is usually controlled by monthly determinations of prothrombin time. It is important to know whether this test is done by means of the Quick method or other methods, since the values may differ significantly and may therefore influence the interpretation of the laboratory test. Many individuals today are being maintained on anticoagulants for an indefinite period. Such individuals may not consider themselves as taking a medication or being treated by their physician, since the therapy that they are receiving has become longstanding and routine.

Stroke: The history of stroke can be important in the same respect as the history of heart attack, since anticoagulant drugs also are used in the treatment of cerebrovascular accident. The paralysis associated with stroke frequently is also important with particular reference to insertion and removal of dental appliances and the maintenance of adequate oral hygiene.

15. **Have you ever been told by a physician that you have a heart murmur?** The concern of the dentist is in determining whether a heart murmur is functional or organic in nature. So-called functional heart murmurs may be disregarded as far as premedication for the prevention of bacterial endocarditis is concerned. Since organic heart mumurs are based on a defect in the endocardium that renders the affected individuals susceptible to subacute bacterial endocarditis, premedication is indicated prior to extractions, scaling of teeth, and other procedures that interrupt tissue continuity.

16. **Do you ever have asthma or hay fever?** (**Underline which one.**) This question is intended to reveal a history of allergy to pollens, dusts, and animal danders. It is important to note that the individuals who give a history of asthma are more likely to experience a severe asthmatic reaction to aspirin than are nonasthmatic patients.

17. **Do you ever have hives or skin rash?** In general, hives or skin rash is associated with food and drug allergies. The reactions are nonspecific, and in many cases a thorough search of ingested foods or chemical agents is necessary to determine the allergen.

18. **Have you ever experienced an unusual reaction to any of the following drugs?** This question should identify persons who have had serious reactions to one or more drugs. In all probability if any drug is given to enough individuals, an allergic manifestation or idiosyncrasy will develop in one of them.

Aspirin: Aspirin is a widely used drug that produces a great many allergic reactions, including a severe asthmatic reaction. This reaction is usually nonreversible and may be precipitated by as little as 5 grains of aspirin. Aspirin also may produce generalized urticaria as well as angioedema.

Penicillin: Penicillin, another widely used drug, is a notorious allergen. The reactions to penicillin range from mild skin rash to a fatal anaphylactoid type of reaction. Any suggestion in the history of a previous allergic reaction to penicillin contraindicates the future use of the drug, no matter how mild the reaction might have been, since successive allergic reactions to drugs tend to increase in severity.

Iodine: Iodine is not a potent sensitizer, but in some individuals it is capable of producing a skin rash. The topical use of iodine in dentistry precipitates few allergic reactions.

Sulfonamides (sulfa): The sulfonamide drugs are a group of drugs that in the past have been known to produce a wide variety of untoward reactions, both allergic and toxic. The allergic reactions attributed to sulfonamide drugs vary as widely as do allergic reactions to penicillin. A number of sulfa drugs are still prescribed for the treatment of urinary tract infections. Sulfonamides are available in combination with antibiotics for treatment of other infections.

Barbiturates (sleeping pills): Barbiturates can precipiate dermatitis medicamentosa. They have been known to produce stomatitis medicamentosa also. It is interesting to note that cross-sensitiveness among the various barbiturates do not exist with any frequency, so that it is possible to prescribe an alternate barbiturate if the patient develops a sensitivity to the one initially prescribed.

Other medicines: The entry "other medicines" is included in Question 18 so that the patient may include drugs to which he has had an unusual reaction that are not listed on the questionnaire.

19. **Have you ever experienced an unusual reaction to a dental anesthetic?** Most unusual reactions to the local anesthetics that are used in dentistry are mild syncope and occur on a psychogenic basis rather than on an allergic basis. However, true allergies and idiosyncrasies to dental anesthetics do exist. Procaine seems to be a more potent sensitizer than lidocaine. Cross-reactions occur in the drugs related to procaine, rendering a person sensitized to procaine also sensitized to butacaine and butethamine hydrochloride (Monocaine). Frequently the psychogenic reactions to dental anesthetics can be avoided by proper sedation of the patient prior to dental appointments and by use of a reassuring approach. It is extremely important to recognize a history of true allergic reaction or idiosyncrasy to a dental anesthetic in order to avoid an uncomfortable or even serious experience.

20. **Do you bleed for a long time when you cut yourself?** Questions 55 and 56 are related to Question 20. These questions are an attempt to disclose a history of a hemorrhagic disease. If there is a possibility that a patient may bleed excessively, a further detailed history should be obtained, along with the appropriate laboratory studies to reveal whether a hemorrhagic diathesis exists.

21. **Have you ever had any injury to your face or jaws?** Injuries to the face or to the jaws in the history may be related to delayed manifestations involving the temporomandibular joint or previously injured teeth. Acute traumatic temporomandibular joint arthritis often can be related to injuries to the jaws in which the temporomandibular joints were involved through severe stresses placed on the joint region. It is not unusual for teeth to become devitalized and remain asymptomatic after injuries to the face or jaws. Injuries to the teeth may result from automobile accidents are other traumatic incidents that the patient may not relate to the oral or facial region be-

cause of more serious injury to other parts of the body.

22. **Have you ever had surgery or x-ray treatment for a tumor, growth, or other condition in your mouth or on your lips?** A history of surgery for a tumor in the oral region, particularly a malignant one, may modify the approach to the clinical examination in that it requires particular attention to the possibility of metastases to the regional lymph nodes and also the possibility of recurrence at the primary site. Irradiation therapy for tumors in the oral region presents certain hazards in dental treatment, particularly where surgical procedures are indicated. It is well known that irradiation therapy involving bone reduces the vitality of bone through reduction in vascularity. Osteoradionecrosis may result from trauma to previously irradiated bone. Dental extractions from irradiated bone are strictly contraindicated.

• • •

From this point on in the questionnaire, the questions are intended to elicit symptoms that may indicate disease processes in the various systems of the body. These questions comprise a part of the history referred to as the systems review.

• • •

23. **Do you have frequent, severe headaches?** Most of the headaches about which individuals complain are the result of tension. True histamine and migraine headaches occur less frequently. Hypertension may be the basis of recurrent, severe headaches. Most headaches caused by tension are frontal in location. Histamine and migraine headaches are extremely severe and blinding, whereas hypertensive headaches tend to be occipital in location. It is possible that a unilateral headache, particularly in the temporal region, may be related to temporomandibular joint disease or to muscular spasm in the muscles of mastication.

24. **Do you have any complaints regarding your eyes?** The most common complaint registered is the necessity for wearing glasses. Of significance to the dentist is the patient with glaucoma, since the use of antisialagogues is contraindicated in such patients. Antisialagogues tend to further increase intraocular pressure, which is already elevated in glaucoma. Occasionally an ophthalmologist will refer a patient to the dentist for examination to rule out foci of infection associated with the teeth as a possible source of an inflammatory process in the eye. It is unusual to find any relationship between dental foci of infection and inflammatory processes of the eye, but the ophthalmologist wishes to rule out all possibilities in his search for a causative factor.

25. **Do you have any ear trouble?** Because of the proximity of the temporomandibular joint to the ear, complaints originating in the temporomandibular joint may be attributed to a disease process in the ear. An otologist may ask for dental consultation to rule out the possibility of dental or temporomandibular joint disease in a patient who complains of pain in the ear without evidence of an inflammatory process involving the middle or outer ear.

26. **Do you have frequent colds?** Frequent colds can be described as more than three or four during one winter. A continuous cold during the winter is suggestive of allergy to house dust or of vasomotor rhinitis.

27. **Do you have sinus trouble?** A history of acute sinusitis is rather significant in some individuals because it is possible for a toothache to develop in the teeth that approximate the maxillary sinus. Teeth with roots close to an infected sinus may become sensitive to biting pressure. In general, chronic sinus problems do not affect the adjacent teeth in any way, nor do the teeth contribute to chronic disease processes in the maxillary sinuses.

28. **Do you have nosebleeds?** Nosebleeds may result from frequent trauma to the nasal mucosa. Another local cause of nosebleeds is a nasopharyngeal tumor that has invaded a blood vessel. More generalized causes of nosebleed are hypertension and blood dyscrasias. Nosebleeds in an adult patient, if they are more than a simple show of blood occurring when the individual blows his nose, should be investigated thoroughly to determine the cause of bleeding.

29. **Do you have frequent sore throats?** Frequent sore throats are often the result of habitual mouth breathing. Frequent sore throats may be seen in individuals with enlarged tonsils and adenoids. Tongue thrusting habits have been attributed to frequent sore throats in children, since the child can swallow more comfortably if the tongue is thrust forward during the act of swallowing.

30. **Are you a mouth breather?** Mouth breathers many times complain of a dry mouth. They are also susceptible to periodontal disease in the anterior part of the mouth resulting from the irritation of continual drying of the gingival tissues. It is entirely possible that a mouth breathing habit may be the result of nasal congestion, which may be corrected by medication. On the other hand, the correction of a mouth breathing habit may necessitate surgical intervention to clear nasal obstructions.

31. **Do you have any sensitive teeth?** A positive response to this question should be followed by additional questions such as "To what are your teeth sensitive? Heat, cold, or biting pressure?" The placement of a new, large metal restoration may elicit one or all three of these types of sensitivity; however, in the absence of the placement of a new restoration, sensitivity to cold suggests hyperemia of the dental pulp and the possibility that the situation is reversible. Sensitivity to heat suggests an irreversible process in the dental pulp, whereas sensitivity to biting pressure suggests an involvement of the periodontal membrane either as the result of trauma to the tooth

in question or as the result of periapical inflammation secondary to a devital pulp. The complaint of sensitive teeth should be pursued until the cause of the complaint is determined.

32. **Have you had a toothache recently?** This question is related to the previous question and is included in the questionnaire to identify painful areas in the patient's mouth that have occurred in the recent past and that might not be recalled unless the patient is reminded.

33. **Do you have bleeding gums?** If the patients answers this question affirmatively, he should be asked whether the bleeding is spontaneous at any time or whether it is necessary for him to stimulate bleeding, for example, through use of a toothbrush. If spontaneous hemorrhage is experienced by the patient, it is necessary to determine whether or not the gingival tissues are painful. On clinical examination, it is necessary to look for evidence of necrotizing ulcerative gingivitis, and in the absence of these findings, blood dyscrasias should be suspected. Many laymen feel that it is normal for the gingiva to bleed to some extent when the teeth are brushed, and it is the tendency for many dentists to ignore gingival bleeding on toothbrushing as evidence of periodontal disease. Nevertheless, under normal conditions the gingival tissues should not bleed when the teeth are brushed or during any other procedure related to the maintenance of oral hygiene.

34. **Do you have frequent canker sores or cold sores?** Canker sores or cold sores may be defined as frequent if they occur more than four to six times a year. Frequently recurring lesions that can be identified as those produced by the herpes simplex virus may be a source of constant oral discomfort for the patient. The determination of whether to treat lesions resulting from the herpes simplex virus must be based on the severity of the discomfort and the degree of incapacitation they produce. Infrequently recurring herpetic lesions can

be treated on a local basis. The injection of immune serum globulin has proved to be a satisfactory method of delaying recurrence of frequently recurring herpetic lesions.

35. **Have you ever had a severe sore mouth?** An affirmative answer to this question leads to more specific questions to determine the number of times that a sore mouth has been experienced, to a detailed description of what is meant by a severe sore mouth, and to a consideration of the possible diagnosis or causative agent. A variety of disease processes may result in a severe sore mouth, such as primary herpetic gingivostomatitis, Vincent's infection, erythema multiforme, stomatitis medicamentosa, and others.

36. **Is it difficult for you to open your mouth as wide as you would like?** This question is an attempt to discover any functional limitations in the movement of the mandible. An affirmative answer to this question should be followed by a question about the progressive or static character of the limitation of opening of the mouth. It is also important to note whether the limitation of mandibular movement is of recent onset or is long standing and whether movement is restricted because of pain or mechanical obstruction.

37. **Does you jaw click when you chew?** An affirmative answer to this question suggests altered relationship in the components of the temporomandibular joint during functional movements of the mandible. The examiner should determine during what excursion or in what position of the mandible the noise occurs in the temporomandibular joint region. He should further determine whether or not pain is experienced in relation to clicking in the temporomandibular joint.

38. **Do you have any chest pain on exertion?** Chest pain (angina pectoris) on exertion suggests insufficiency of blood supply to the myocardium. If an affirmative answer to the question is obtained and the patient has not sought medical advice for

the complaint, he should be urged to see his physician at an early date. Nitroglycerin is given routinely for control of anginal pain. The administration of nitroglycerin sublingually just prior to a stressful dental procedure may prevent the patient from experiencing angina pectoris during the procedure.

39. **Are you ever short of breath on mild exertion?** The patient who complains of shortness of breath may do so for a number of reasons, one of the most important of which is cardiac failure. An overweight individual with a normally functioning heart often becomes short of breath on mild exertion. Cardiac insufficiency or heart failure is further indicated if the patient is unable to sleep all night in a recumbent position or if he must prop himself up with several pillows to breathe more easily.

40. **Do your ankles swell?** Dependent edema frequently occurs in patients with heart failure and in those with chronic nephritis. The relationship of this question to Question 39 is apparent, and a combination of affirmative answers to these two questions should stimulate the dentist to consider a medical consultation for his patient to rule out heart failure.

41. **Do you have a persistent cough?** A persistent cough may be the result of chronic irritation from smoking, carcinoma of the lung, tuberculosis, or bronchiectasis. A chronic cough that is productive of sputum suggests that presence of an inflammatory process with the production of an exudate. A chronic nonproductive cough is suggestive of bronchogenic neoplasm.

42. **Do you ever cough blood?** Hemoptysis may be the result of tuberculosis, bronchiectasis, or lung cancer. The most common cause of hemoptysis in the United States is bronchiectasis, whereas the most common cause of hemoptysis in the world is tuberculosis.

43. **Has your appetite changed recently?** A sharp increase in appetite may be suggestive of hyperthyroidism or diabetes. A significant decrease in appetite may be suggestive of hepatitis, gastrointestinal cancer, and several other generalized disease processes.

44. **Are there any foods you cannot eat?** Individuals will most commonly avoid certain foods because of peptic ulcer, gallbladder disease, or allergy to certain foods.

45. **Do you have any difficulty swallowing?** Difficulty in swallowing may be related to anxiety, globus hystericus, pharyngeal carcinoma, or cardiospasm.

46. **Do you have frequent indigestion?** The most common causes of indigestion are peptic ulcer and gallbladder disease.

47. **Do you vomit frequently?** Frequent vomiting may be the result of functional disease, hiatus hernia, or esophageal diverticulum. It is important to determine whether actual stomach contents are regurgitated into the mouth. Persons who vomit frequently may show evidence of the decalcifying effect of hydrochloric acid on the enamel of the teeth.

48. **Do you have kidney trouble?** Chronic renal disease often results in anemia at some point in the course of the disease. In patients with advanced chronic renal disease, compensatory hyperparathyroidism may occur with mobilization of calcium from bone, including the bones of the jaws.

49. **Do you urinate more than six times a day?** Increased frequency of urination may be the result of functional disease, renal disease, prostatic hypertrophy, or diabetes. The increased frequency of urination related to diabetes is also accompanied by an increase in thirst.

50. **Are you thirsty much of the time?** An affirmative answer to this question accompanied by an affirmative answer to Question 49 is strongly suggestive of diabetes. The suspicion of diabetes is even stronger if there has been a recent loss of weight and an increase in appetite.

51. **Have you ever had painful and swollen joints?** If this question is answered

affirmatively, the examiner should determine whether the patient is referring to single or multiple painful and swollen joints. Most often the involvement of a single joint with pain and swelling is the result of trauma. Pain and swelling in multiple joints may be the result of rheumatic fever, rheumatoid arthritis, or osteoarthritis. The involvement of the temporomandibular joint in the generalized arthritides must always be considered.

52. **Do you have any numb or prickling areas on your skin?** Anesthesias and paresthesias of unexplained origin may be the result of injury to the nerve trunk or possibly a tumor located more centrally that interferes with the transmission of nerve impulses along a nerve trunk. When areas of anesthesia and paresthesia are localized to the facial region, it is important to outline the area of involvement in an effort to determine the distribution of the nerve that is being affected. If explanations are not possible on a local basis, it may be necessary to refer patients with the complaint of paresthesia or anesthesia to a neurologist for more extensive investigation of the defect in transmission of nerve impulses. It is not unusual for anesthesia and paresthesia to result from the extraction of mandibular molar teeth when the roots are closely related to the mandibular canal. In most instances, the anesthesia or paresthesia disappears in a matter of a few days or weeks after the extraction site is healed.

53. **Do you ever have fits or convulsions?** The purpose of this question is to identify the individual with epilepsy so that special care may be taken in his management during dental appointments. It is entirely possible for an epileptic patient to experience a seizure in spite of the fact that he has received his daily medication when he is placed under the additional stress of a visit to the dental office. Consultation with the patient's physician is helpful in determining if increased dosages of the anticonvulsive drugs are advisable during

the period in which the individual is receiving dental care.

54. **Do you have a tendency to faint?** The main purpose in this question is to identify the individual who has a tendency to experience syncope reaction after the administration of local anesthetics in the oral region. It is entirely possible that individuals who experience petit mal seizures may describe them as a tendency to faint without any relationship to stressful procedures or time of day.

55. **Do you bruise easily?** This question has already been related to Question 20. The purpose in listing a history of bruising easily is to determine whether unusual capillary fragility exists. In many instances, mature women will answer this question affirmatively without actually having an exceptional degree of capillary fragility.

56. **Do you have any blood disorder such as anemia (thin blood)?** It is well known that persons with anemia experience more difficulty during stressful procedures and may be more susceptible to shock than do normal patients when additional loss of blood occurs during a surgical procedure. This question is also directed at revealing any other blood dyscrasias that might exist.

57. **Does hot weather bother you more than it does other people you know?** Individuals with hyperthyroidism complain about the heat and prefer a lower room temperature than that thought comfortable by other members of their family. It is important to recognize the patient with hyperthyroidism to avoid surgical procedures and to encourage them to seek prompt treatment. Surgical procedures may precipitate thyroid storm in the hyperthyroid individual.

58. **Are you excessively nervous?** Excess of "nervousness" may be simply the result of the current "age of anxiety." Increase in thyroid activity produces increased "nervousness." In the former cause, "nervousness" may be controlled by seda-

tion; in the latter, medical consultation is imperative.

59. **Do you get tired easily?** Ease of tiring may be the result of advancing age, insufficient rest, or decrease in thyroid function, as well as a host of other generalized diseases. The onset of leukemia or infectious mononucleosis may be accompanied by ease of tiring.

60. (**Women**) **Are you pregnant at the present time?** Awareness of early pregnancy is important in the recognition of gingival changes associated with pregnancy and commonly referred to as pregnancy gingivitis. It is also important to avoid ex-posing the patient to x-rays and stressful procedures during the first trimester of pregnancy if it is at all possible. The quantity of x-rays used for exposing dental films is not harmful to the pregnant patient or the developing embryo. Most dental procedures are not stressful enough to cause difficulty during early pregnancy; nevertheless, the first trimester of pregnancy is the period during which abortion is most likely to occur. An attempt may be made months later by a patient who has received exposure to dental x-rays to relate the exposure to a congenital anomaly in the infant.

Figs. 14-1 to 14-13 follow.

Illustrated synopsis of the clinical examination

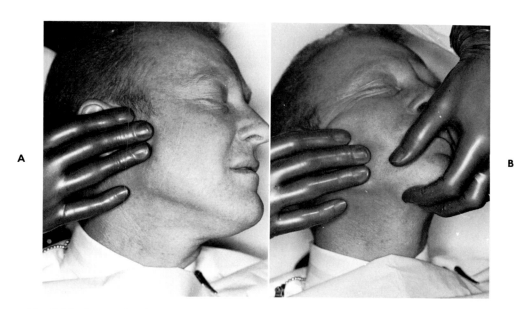

Fig. 14-1. *Extraoral palpation.* **A,** Preauricular nodes and parotid gland. **B,** Prevascular nodes.

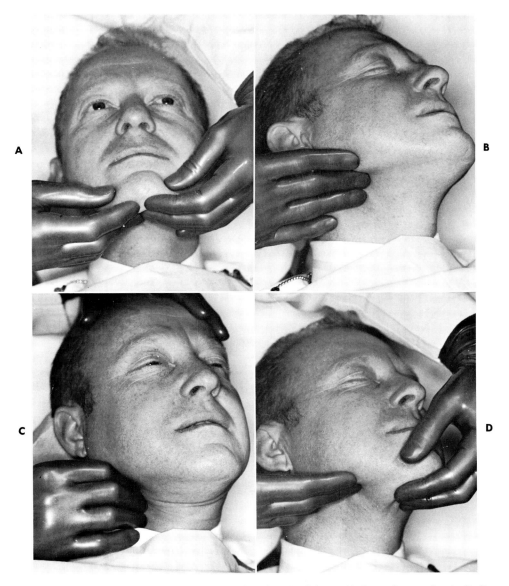

Fig. 14-2. Extraoral palpation. **A,** Submental nodes. **B,** Submandibular salivary gland. **C,** Superior cervical nodes. **D,** Jugular nodes.

A B C

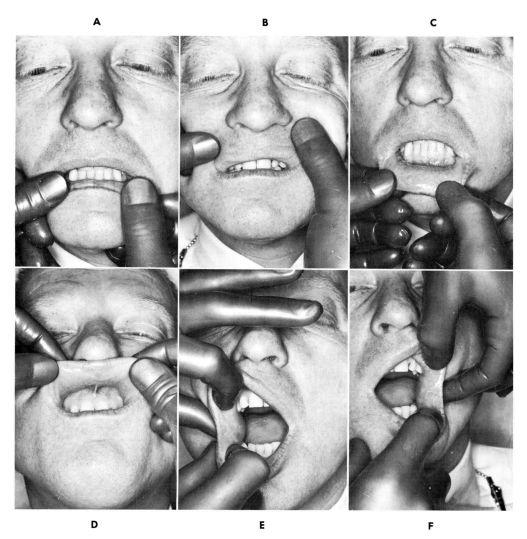

D E F

Fig. 14-3. *Inspection.* **A,** Lower vermilion of lip. **B,** Upper vermilion of lip. **C,** Lower labial mucosa. **D,** Upper labial mucosa. **E** and **F,** Lateral vestibular mucosa.

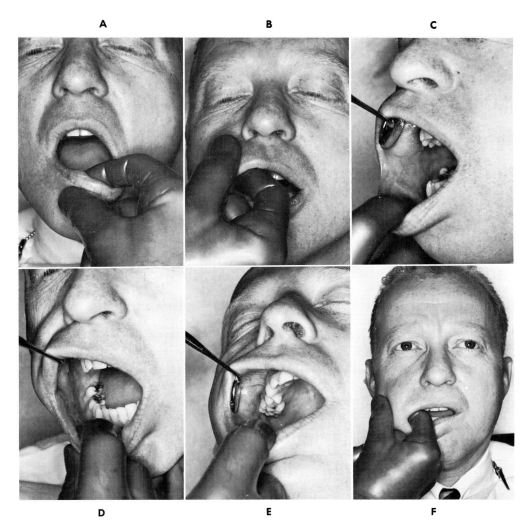

Fig. 14-4. *Inspection and palpation.* **A,** Lower lip. **B,** Upper lip. **C,** Buccal mucosa. **D,** Lower mucobuccal fold. **E,** Upper mucobuccal fold. **F,** Palpation of buccinator area.

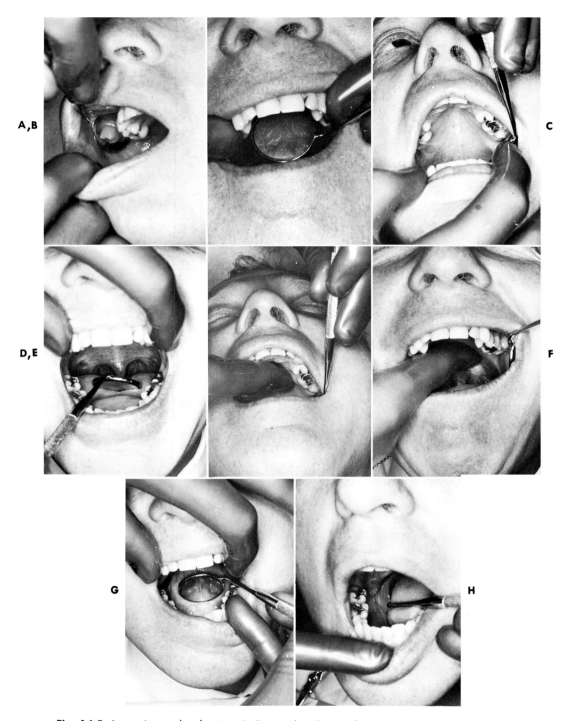

Fig. 14-5. *Inspection and palpation.* **A,** Retromolar. **B,** Rugal area. **C,** Hard palate. **D,** Soft palate, uvula. **E,** Palpation, hard palate. **F,** Palpation, soft palate. **G,** Floor of mouth. **H,** Lateral lingual space.

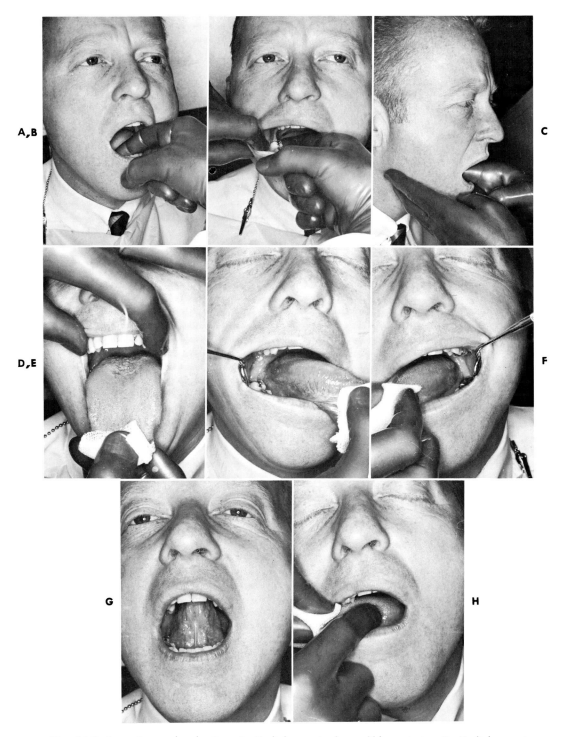

Fig. 14-6. *Inspection and palpation.* **A,** Medial aspect of mandible, anterior. **B,** Medial aspect of mandible, posterior. **C,** Bimanual palpation, floor of mouth. **D,** Inspection, dorsum of tongue. **E,** Inspection, right lateral aspect of tongue. **F,** Inspection, left lateral aspect of tongue. **G,** Inspection, ventral aspect of tonque. **H,** Palpation of tongue.

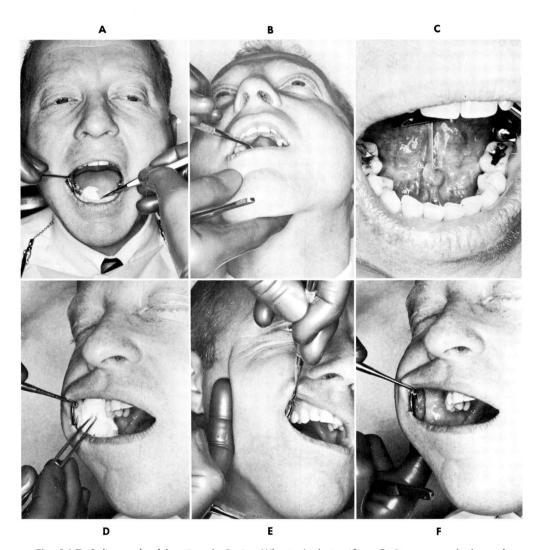

Fig. 14-7. *Salivary gland function.* **A**, Drying Wharton's duct orifices. **B**, Pressure applied to submental area. **C**, Clear saliva appearing at caruncle. **D**, Drying Stenson's duct orifice. **E**, Pressure applied to duct externally. **F**, Appearance of saliva at duct orifice.

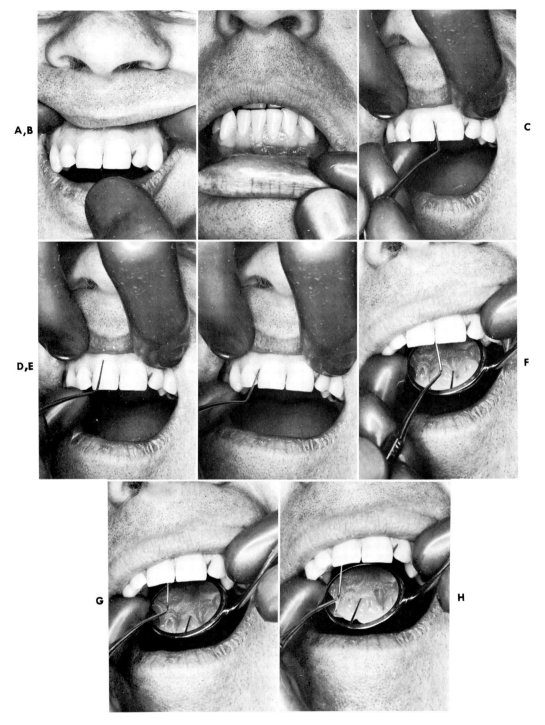

Fig. 14-8. *Gingival examination.* **A** and **B**, Inspection for color and form. **C** to **H**, Probing gingival sulcus.

A   B   C

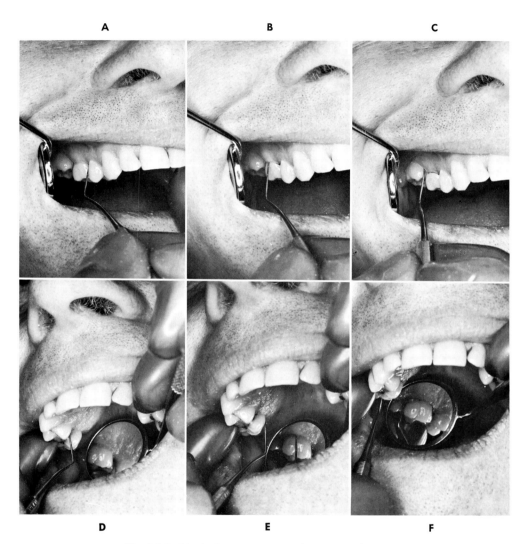

D   E   F

Fig. 14-9. *Gingival examination.* Probing gingival sulcus.

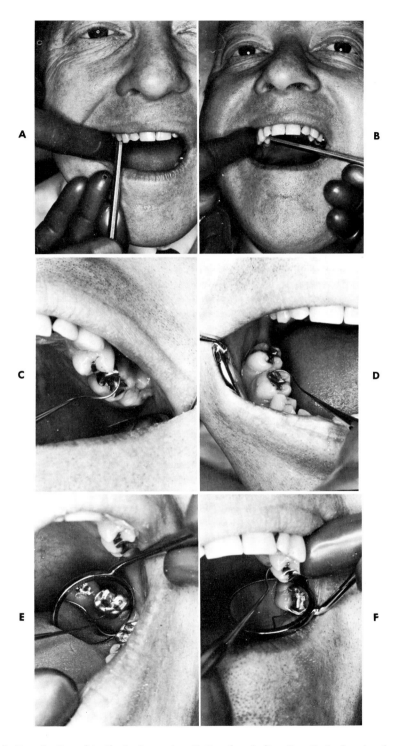

Fig. 14-10. *Examination of teeth.* **A,** Percussion. **B,** Test for vitality. **C** to **F,** Exploration for caries.

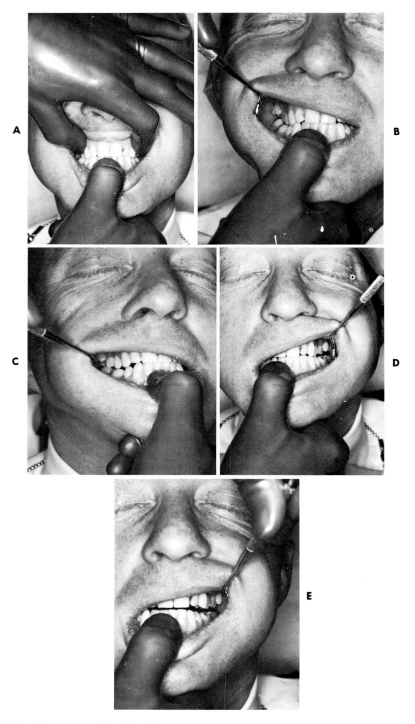

Fig. 14-11. *Examination of occlusal function.* **A,** Centric. **B,** Right working position. **C,** Right balancing position. **D,** Left working position. **E,** Left balancing position.

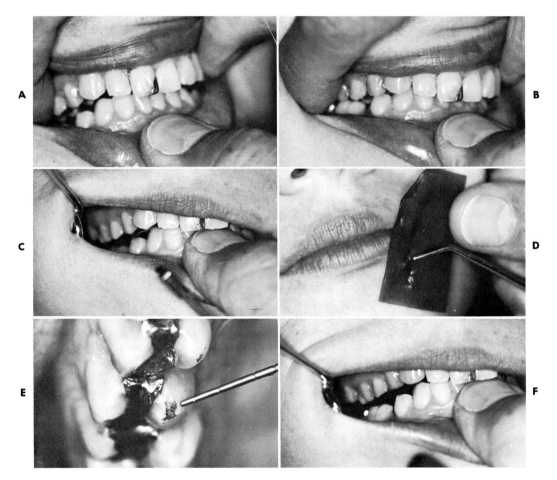

Fig. 14-12. *Location of centric prematurity.* **A,** Centric relation. **B,** Centric occlusion. **C,** 28-gauge green wax in place. **D,** Perforation of wax by premature contact. **E,** Articulating paper in place. **F,** Premature contact on second bicuspid.

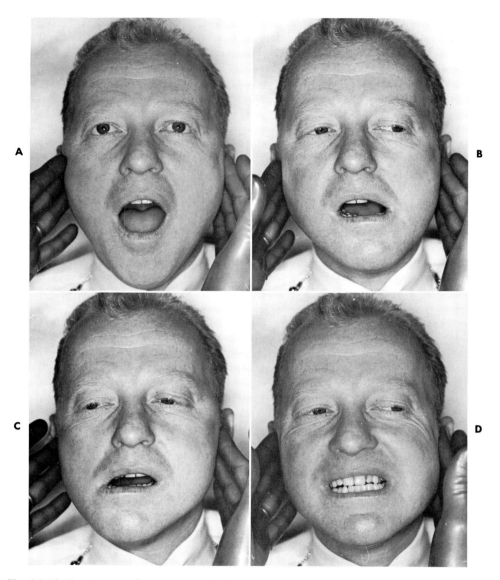

Fig. 14-13. *Examination of temporomandibular joints.* **A,** Maximum opening in midline. **B,** Lateral mandibular movement with teeth out of occlusion. **C,** Lateral mandibular movement with teeth in occlusion. **D,** Protrusive movement.

REFERENCES

Ash, M. M.: A handbook of differential oral diagnosis, St. Louis, 1961, The C. V. Mosby Co.

Ash, M. M., Hard, D., and Tondrowski, V. F.: The role of the hygienist in the detection of disease, J.A.D.A. **59**:546, 1959.

Broadman, K., Erdman, A. J., Lorge, I., and Wolff, H. G.: The Cornell Medical Index: An adjunct to medical interview, J.A.M.A. **140:** 530, 1949.

Feinstein, A. R.: Clinical judgment, Baltimore, 1967, The Williams & Wilkins Co.

SECTION IV

ELEMENTS OF THE DIAGNOSTIC METHOD AND TREATMENT PLANNING

The greatest stumbling block to students of diagnosis lies in the collection and evaluation of the facts. Collection of the facts is difficult because of the student's inadequacy in systematic observation and his failure to realize that the same disease may present itself in many forms. More often than not he is accused of poor judgment when the chief problem is a lack of training in interviewing and examination procedures. All too often he has forgotten his basic science and has little conception of its value in the practical solution of diagnostic problems.

The examiner should seek to select objective features that will serve to orient the analysis. The beginning student in oral diagnosis usually has difficulty in determining the significance and relative importance of some finding and is led up a blind alley. Normal variations, insignificant shadows in radiographs, minor complaints, and changes secondary to primary disease are frequently given undue consideration. It is only through trial and error that the student learns to arrange the facts in proper perspective.

Although many times the signs and symptoms may appear to be the same as those described for many diseases, this does not necessarily mean that more than one disease is present. Neither does it mean that the selection of the disease with the greatest number of signs and symptoms common to the disease in question will be the true diagnosis. Where several diseases are sus-

pected, the final diagnosis may ultimately be that of a disease that has the fewest number of signs and symptoms present that are common to the disease being evaluated. The signs and symptoms of many diseases usually indicate an alteration of an anatomic or physiologic system. For example, an alteration of the blood may reflect changes in the respiratory, neuromuscular, digestive, and cardiovascular systems. Further, an alteration of the digestive system may show ultimately the same signs and symptoms as those seen in the disturbance of the blood. More specifically, the symptoms of temporomandibular joint disease may be pain, restricted movements of the mandible, referred pain, and paresthesia. The same symptoms may be present in disease of the pulp of a mandibular molar tooth. Although the symptoms given are the same for both disturbances, the diagnosis is entirely different. These examples serve to point out that the relative importance of each symptom to the disease has to be fully evaluated and, in such instances, more facts are needed to make the correct diagnosis. One must remember that when dealing with a system or a group of systems that are as intimately related as those that comprise the body, a disturbance in one area or one system may be reflected on other areas or systems.

Facts obtained by interviewing and examining the patient are the primary requirements for making a diagnosis. Without adequate facts no progress toward a diagnosis can be made. During the examination the examiner must be constantly aware that additional supplementary procedures may be required. He will learn by experience when such procedures are necessary. An analysis of the facts collected as a result of the clinical examination serves to determine the reliability of the history so that proper significance can be placed on the signs and symptoms noted in the history.

The following is an outline of the diagnostic method:

1. Collecting the facts
   a. Clinical history
   b. Clinical examination
   c. Supplementary examinations when indicated by analysis of collected facts from (a) and (b)
2. Analysis of the facts
   a. Critical examination of the collected data
   b. Consideration of the alteration of anatomic and physiologic systems that may give rise to the signs and symptoms
   c. Determination of the relative importance of the findings
   d. Review of the positive and negative findings to determine if it is necessary to collect more information
3. Synthesis of examination facts and of descriptive features of disease
   a. Selection of the central features of the collected facts (those features most directly related to the disturbed physiologic processes responsible for the signs and symptoms of the disease)

   b. Correlation between collected facts and those diseases that may account for important significant findings
   c. Establishment of cause and effect relationship, where rational and practical
   d. Evaluation of the possibility of the presence of more than one disease
   e. Listing of diseases in which the same significant features are present
4. Making the diagnosis
   a. Selection of the disease that best explains the collected facts and the apparent and/or proved disturbed physiologic processes
   b. Significance of the diagnosis

The following is an outline for the treatment plan:

1. Systemic treatment
   a. Referral to a physician for systemic evaluation and treatment as indicated by history and clinical findings
   b. Appraisal of the influence of systemic treatment on the dental treatment plan
   c. Premedication with antibiotics or sedatives as indicated by the history
   d. Corrective therapy for oral infection
2. Preparatory treatment
   a. Oral surgery
   b. Endodontic therapy
   c. Caries control
   d. Periodontal therapy
   e. Orthodontic treatment
   f. Occlusal adjustment
3. Corrective treatment
   a. Operative dentistry
   b. Prosthetic dentistry
4. Periodic recall examinations and maintenance treatment

15

Diagnosis and treatment planning

DIAGNOSIS

The term "diagnosis" (from the Greek word meaning 'distinguishing' or 'discernment') means the identification of a disease by an investigation of the signs and symptoms. The exact meaning is obscured by the many ways in which the term is used: clinical diagnosis, laboratory diagnosis, physical diagnosis, radiographic diagnosis, deductive diagnosis, exclusion diagnosis, and so on. Use of the word "diagnosis" with a qualifying adjective connotes an awareness of the meaning of observations made by particular methods. It does not necessarily signify identification of a disease by these methods. The term "diagnosis," without a qualifying adjective, is used in this discussion to mean identification of a disease by a systematic synthesis of all its manifestations. This identification not only signifies the identification of the disease but the process by which the identification is derived.

"Differential diagnosis" is a determination of the one of several diseases from which a patient is suffering by systematic comparison and contrast of their symptoms. In the final analysis all diagnosis is probably differential diagnosis. It is easy to enumerate the symptoms of an acute pulpitis, but to present a system of diagnosis whereby the conditions that simulate pulpitis may be excluded easily is difficult. Specialists in oral diagnosis sometimes find it difficult to commit their methods of reasoning to writing. Teachers of oral diagnosis usually rely on two methods of teaching differential diagnosis: the chair side or demonstration clinic and the clinical pathologic conference. These methods are not without drawbacks. Usually the student will hear little of the reasoning or methods involved in arriving at a diagnosis. Such demonstrations should not become mere deductive diagnostic clinics, but rather times for teaching methods of reasoning. Neither a perusal of lists of symptoms of disease nor referrals to treatises that enumerate the various diseases that give rise to a specific sign or symptom can develop an adequate concept of the process of synthesis that must be used in solving diagnostic problems.

Collecting the facts

The history and clinical examination will provide the essential facts necessary to make a diagnosis. The procedures for interviewing and for making a clinical examination have been presented in the foregoing chapters. Also, the value of laboratory diagnostic aids has been pointed out. If the results of laboratory tests do not correlate with the facts obtained from the history and examination, they should be considered as subsidiary in importance. When collecting the facts, one must bear in mind that they may well represent the natural history of a disease whose manifestations are being recorded. The examiner should be alert to the usual pattern of development of diseases as well as to their manifestations. If a pattern of disease appears to be unfolding during the history and examination, all the facts pertaining to the natural history of the disease should be positively or negatively correlated.

375

Frequently the dentist is called upon to render a diagnosis after the disease has been in progress for variable lengths of time and after treatment of one form or another has been rendered. He should attempt to analyze the facts in light of the passage of time and the treatment rendered. He must also remember that he may be called on to make a diagnosis before all the facts have become apparent in the course of the disease. In most instances it is necessary to make an early diagnosis to prevent further inroads of the disease. In a few instances a period of observation may be necessary before the final diagnosis can be made and correct therapy instituted. An example will serve to illustrate this point. Upon the initial examination of a lesion of the oral mucosa that has no particular orienting features, a presumptive diagnosis of traumatic ulcer is rendered with reservations on the possibility of its being of neoplastic origin, and the patient is requested to return in a week or two for reexamination and evaluation, since a lesion of traumatic origin will have had time to heal whereas one of neoplastic origin will not heal. If the lesion heals, the diagnosis of traumatic ulcer is confirmed by exclusion. However, if the lesion fails to heal and begins to show some signs of a neoplastic growth, biopsy should be considered. In this example the facts necessary to render a final diagnosis could not be collected before more information was available.

Analysis of the facts

The examiner should begin his analysis by determining the reliability and significance of the information obtained from the history and examination. For example, a negative serologic test in a patient with a lesion suggestive of syphilis may be of no significance if carried out before dissemination of the organisms. The negative test does not constitute valid grounds for ruling out syphilis. By the same reasoning, occlusal interference in itself is not sufficient evidence to warrant the assumption that occlusal trauma is present and a toothache cannot always be attributed to the presence of a carious lesion. In analyzing the information regarding a toothache, the examiner should be aware that pulpitis may be primary or secondary in origin and may, for example, result from sinusitis. Recording the fact that the patient has a toothache is not a significant finding unless additional information about the cause is brought out. Thus a critical evaluation of the collected facts in relation to the overall picture of the complaint is necessary to arrive at the correct diagnosis.

An attempt should be made to analyze the findings in terms of disturbed physiologic processes. This will aid in correlating seemingly unrelated symptoms. For example, an inability to carry out certain mandibular movements should be analyzed in terms of the known normal functions of the components of the masticatory system. Inability to perform certain movements may be a result of disturbances in occlusion, joints, or the neuromuscular system. Positive or negative correlative data should be collected and analyzed with regard to the function of all the components of the system. If the abnormality is considered to be neuromuscular, the facts should include information relative to the status of the nerves and muscles usually concerned with the movement that cannot be performed. In analyzing gingival bleeding the examiner must relate it to the state of the blood and vascular system if possible. Though such bleeding is most often the result of local factors and inflammation, it is occasionally associated with a hemorrhagic diathesis. Gingival bleeding and positive findings from screening blood tests do not constitute an adequate collection of the facts if the information that the patient is on Dicumarol therapy is overlooked in the history. Thus, an analysis of the completeness of the collected facts should also be considered. Similarly the method whereby the information is collected should be analyzed; for example, a blood glucose analysis is of little value if the patient is not in the prepared fasting state before the test is done.

Importance of findings. One of the difficult features of analyzing the information obtained from the history and examination lies in determining the relative importance of each fact. As mentioned previously, the beginning student has difficulty in separating the wheat from the chaff, and only through practice in assessing the importance of signs and symptoms can their proper perspective be determined. For practice the student can list his signs and symptoms in the order in which they are found in the history and examination. To illustrate, assume that a 9-year-old girl has been referred to a dentist by a physician and the following list of symptoms is forwarded to the dentist: sore mouth, high fever, anorexia, dysphagia, lymphadenopathy, sialorrhea, ulceration of gingiva, fetor ex ore, coated tongue, dental caries, and poor oral hygiene.

The problem of assessing the importance of each of these may be reduced by placing those symptoms that occur rather frequently in most individuals low on the list of importance. Another consideration in establishing the importance of a sign or symptom is the correlation between the degree of the subjective complaint and the extent of the objective sign of disease. Thus, mild localized tissue destruction does not generally produce pronounced constitutional reactions unless the disease is infectious in nature. On the other hand, pronounced tissue destruction is accompanied by a rather pronounced constitutional reaction in many individuals. Those related facts that give a good degree of correlation between themselves should be placed high on the list. Still another means of determining the relative importance of the collected facts is the grouping together of signs and symptoms that are usually associated with each other in a disease. These findings may

be placed under one heading: for example, sialorrhea, poor oral hygiene, coated tongue, and fetor ex ore might accompany any disease of the mouth; high fever and anorexia usually occur together; sore mouth and ulceration might be expected to be associated; and lymphadenopathy might be expected to be found secondary to infection in the mouth. Finally lesions should always be placed high in importance. Revision of the foregoing list in order of importance might appear as follows:

> Ulceration (an expression of sore mouth)
> Lymphadenopathy (frequently associated with extensive oral lesions)
> High fever (anorexia to be expected with fever and sore mouth)
> Dysphagia (possibly related to lymphadenopathy)
> Sialorrhea
> Fetor ex ore (commonly related to poor oral hygiene)
> Dental caries

It is apparent that these are the symptoms of more than one disease and that additional information is necessary before a diagnosis can be made. The ulcerative lesions and lymphadenopathy are important symptoms and require detailed evaluation.

The evaluation of soft tissue lesions should follow a systematic procedure. Lesions of the mouth may be primary or secondary in nature and may be the manifestation of local or systemic disease. The following outline suggests the facts that should be collected in the history and examination to relate lesions of the soft tissues to a descriptive knowledge of disease.

1. Case history
   a. Inquiry into the general health of the patient and a review of the body systems whose altered function may be related to the lesions present
   b. Inquiry into the subjective symptoms associated with the lesions
      (1) Cause
      (2) Manner of onset
      (3) Duration
      (4) Constitutional symptoms
      (5) Treatment, if any
2. Clinical examination of the lesions
   a. Location

b. Arrangement—coalescing, discrete, irregular, grouped, linear, circinate, etc.
c. Elevated or depressed
d. Consistency—firm, soft, hard, etc.
e. Character of base—broad, infiltrated, narrow, pedunculated, stalked, indurated, depth of involvement
f. Involution—ulceration, resorption, atrophy
g. Color of lesion and surrounding mucosa and/or skin
h. Sequelae—pigmentation, scarring, etc.
i. Cause

If these facts are known, it is then possible to extend the scope of the information regarding the disease in the hypothetical case mentioned:

Ulceration

Unknown cause; began as small vesicles but rapidly formed into ulcers; all the mucosa of the mouth affected, but gingival involvement most pronounced; few scattered ulcers elsewhere; sudden onset; duration—2 days; initial lesions described as small blisters by patient; few lesions present on the lips—termed "cold sores" by patient; latter dry with a crustlike surface exuding serum and yellowish white in color; ulcers in the mouth are shallow, present a ragged edge, a membranelike yellow base, and an erythematous halo; a few of the lesions show healing without scar formation.

Lymphadenopathy

Difficulty in swallowing and "sore throat" prior to lesions in mouth; lymph nodes in neck painfully swollen prior to lesions.

Fever

Fever preceded oral lesions; increased salivation, cachexia, and anorexia commenced with fever and became pronounced with the oral lesions; temperature 103° to 105° F.

Dysphagia

Difficulty in swallowing present early in course of the disease; throat not actually sore; dysphagia actually related to lymphadenopathy.

Sialorrhea and fetor ex ore are nonspecific findings and may accompany many forms of oral disease. Sialorrhea is of importance in metallic intoxications but never of a degree to be considered as an orienting or central finding. Dental caries resulting in sharp and badly broken teeth may be of significance in traumatic ulcers. The diffuse nature of the ulcers and the presence of fever and lymphadenopathy rule out this consideration.

After the facts have been evaluated and listed in the order of importance, it is desirable to select the central or outstanding features necessary to orient the examination.

Synthesis of examination facts and of descriptive features of disease

It is sometimes difficult to select the central and most important feature of a disease. It is best to select the symptom that logically explains the disturbed physiologic process. In the example used and in other instances, the selection of a single item will be impossible. In this case a summary of one or more features that are logically related should be listed. For the preceding case the following summary is suggested: Vesicular eruptions with secondary lesions (ulcerations) present; constitutional factors and lymphadenopathy occur prior to the eruptions. These are the central features of the disease and must be correlated with diseases that produce similar symptoms. The vesicular phase of the disease may well be overlooked, and for this reason it is generally best to select two features that have potential value. It is not wise to overlook the possibility that without the presence of vesicles being established, the oral manifestations presented and the lymphadenopathy might represent lesions secondary to a primary systemic disease.

At this time it is well to list the diseases that might account for the signs and symptoms collected. It would be impossible to list all the diseases that might produce ulcerations in the mouth. However, it is possible to list diseases that have this feature plus the other symptoms presented. To be brief, yet not overlook logical possibilities, only the most common diseases likely to produce the clinical impression given in the case presented will be considered.

Those diseases *most commonly* producing fever, lymphadenopathy, and ulcerations of the mouth are herpetic gingivostomatitis, necrotizing gingivitis (Vincent's infection), and erythema multiforme.

The same symptoms may also be secondary to leukemia and chickenpox, but far less frequently. The possibility that more than one disease is present must be evaluated, for example, Vincent's infection superimposed on leukemia.

There are several approaches to the problem of selecting the disease that best explains the facts collected: (1) select several diseases, each of which best explains some of the facts; (2) review all evidence with the most likely diagnosis that is in mind; (3) from a knowledge of the natural history of the diseases considered, determine what additional facts might be present that have been overlooked; (4) consider the possibility of more than one disease process being present; (5) give careful consideration to the negative findings in light of the usual positive findings attending certain diseases; (6) reevaluate the information that is considered to be the most significant; and (7) select an outstanding feature of the facts collected that may serve to orient the synthesis.

In making the differential diagnosis from the choices mentioned, the examiner will have little difficulty in separating herpetic gingivostomatitis from necrotizing gingivitis if the presence of *vesicles* has been recognized. From a practical standpoint, this orienting or central feature is frequently overlooked, and the disease is diagnosed as acute necrotizing gingivitis (Vincent's infection). However, even if the vesicles are not discovered, the natural history of the disease as well as the character of the ulceration will make the differential diagnosis possible. (See Chapters 2 and 5 for descriptions of the lesions of herpetic stomatitis and necrotizing gingivitis.) It should be noted that the natural history of herpetic gingivostomatitis is rather characteristic in that the constitutional symptoms, lymphadenopathy, and "sore throat" begin prior to the formation of the lesions. In

acute necrotizing gingivitis the constitutional symptoms and lymphadenopathy, when present, occur after the onset of the ulceration. Another feature of Vincent's infection is the age at which this disease is likely to occur. Vincent's infection rarely, if ever, occurs in a 9-year-old child; primary herpetic gingivostomatitis occurs frequently in young children.

A descriptive knowledge of erythema multiforme is necessary to evaluate this disease. No definite characteristic lesions are present. The multiplicity of lesions encountered assists in making the diagnosis. Erythema multiforme is an acute process with a sudden onset. The lesions may be macules, papules, nodules, vesicles, or bullae, may be vesicular in appearance, or may appear as hives and urticaria. They usually start as small macular or papular lesions but expand rapidly, with the center becoming blue and violaceous on an erythematous base—"bull's-eye type of lesion" (iris type). There is some tendency to undermine. In herpetic lesions the erythematous halo develops after rupture of vesicles, whereas the halo precedes the vesicle formation in erythematous lesions. The lesions subside in a 3- to 4-week period. There are exacerbations and remissions without cause. Severe acute manifestations last for 2 to 4 weeks.

Making the diagnosis

The diagnosis in the hypothetical case presented is evident from the facts collected and their identification with the symptoms of herpetic gingivostomatitis. Since this is a self-limiting disease, the diagnosis can be confirmed when the disease subsides. A bacteriologic smear should reveal the absence of overwhelming numbers of Vincent's organisms, which might be expected in acute necrotizing gingivitis. However, a bacteriologic smear presents little evidence of the etiology of the lesion. One must also remember that Vincent's organisms are present in most mouths, and a smear is of little positive diagnostic value. For those who wish to further substantiate the diagnosis by clinical laboratory methods, scrapings from the lesions can be used for intracerebral inoculation of mice or to show diagnosable corneal scarification of an inoculated rabbit. These tests are cumbersome, and the disease has usually abated by the time the results from the laboratory studies are known.

A tentative diagnosis is sometimes made on the basis of the facts available at the time of examination. Treatment can then be instituted before the final diagnosis is established. The tentative diagnosis need not be expressed in specific terminology. A description of the disease may be all that is possible. Students are frustrated many times because of an inability to call something by name. This implies that all disease processes have a specific name and that the ultimate in diagnosing ability is to be able to affix a name tag to a disease. This is unfortunate since the emphasis is in the improper place. A name of a disease is merely shorthand for the signs and symptoms of a diseased state. Emphasis should be placed on recognition of the facts collected and not on the name of the disease.

Diagnosis of neoplasms

The dentist in general practice assumes the responsibility for recognizing neoplasms that may arise in or about the mouth. The dentist must make the decision as to the malignant or benign nature of soft tissue lesions. The ability to recognize clinically the nature of a lesion of the mouth is usually directly proportional to the diagnostician's training and experience in the field of oral pathology. The diagnostician who has limited training and experience must rely on the most positive procedures available to diagnose soft tissue lesions. The uncertainty of the clinical nature of a soft tissue lesion of the mouth cannot be eliminated by observation of the lesion for a period of time. During prolonged observation, growth and extension can occur to the

extent that the lesion is untreatable and can prove fatal. Immediate determination of the histologic features of a soft tissue lesion may be ascertained by biopsy. This procedure will prevent delay in diagnosis and thus improve prognosis.

Soft tissue lesions have characteristics that are helpful in determining their nature. In general, they may be thought of as being developmental in origin, inflammatory, systemic in origin, or neoplastic. When a soft tissue lesion can be characterized unequivocally clinically as one of the three nonneoplastic lesions, biopsy is unnecessary. Since biopsy is impractical for every soft tissue lesion of the mouth, some clinical judgment must be exercised; it should be based on the recognition of tissue characteristics. Still, a safe rule is—when in doubt, biopsy.

Developmental lesions are limited in number and maintain rather constant characteristics. Fordyce's disease and median rhomboid glossitis are two developmental lesions that may vary in size or area of involvement; however, the location in which they occur and their general appearance are quite constant. Dermoid cysts and teratomas occur only rarely and usually produce a change in contour of normal tissue, that simulates neoplastic disease, and therefore they require biopsy.

Inflammatory lesions are most likely to be confused with neoplastic lesions. Blastomatoid lesions are reactive in nature; they are well named since they produce a clinical picture similar to neoplasia. Many times the diagnosis is not known until the lesion is seen microscopically. Blastomatoid lesions such as mandibular and palatal tori are common enough to be readily recognized even by dentists with limited experience. Traumatic fibromas and giant cell tumors, on the other hand, often simulate neoplasia by their persistence and growth characteristics. Traumatically induced ulcers of the tongue often present perplexing problems in diagnosis, particularly when an ulcer is deep, secondarily infected, and of long standing. Ulceration elsewhere in the mouth also requires close attention to tissue characteristics. The evidence of an inflammatory halo and tenderness is not always sufficient to permit the clinical diagnosis of inflammatory reaction.

White lesions in the mouth that are reactive in origin often simulate the premalignant process of leukoplakia. The chronicity and appearance of white lesions are seldom indicative of their true nature. Extensive clinical experience with white lesions of the mouth is helpful but not a positive means by which to decide the benign or malignant character of the lesion.

Systemic reactions in the mouth are secondary to a generalized process, and therefore their recognition is extremely important. The varied causes and appearances of these reactions make is impossible for anyone to immediately recognize them all. Since systemic reactions only occasionally simulate neoplasia, they are not a major consideration. The occasional appearance of leukemic lesions, amyloidosis, hyperparathyroid tumors, and multiple myeloma may be dealt with by referral to the proper specialists for diagnosis.

Neoplasms are commonly characterized by their persistence, continued growth, and increase in size. Benign neoplasia in the mouth is not extremely common, but its recognition is nonetheless important in differentiating a benign growth from a malignant growth. Benign lesions on soft tissue are frequently slow growing and noninvasive in character. Benign neoplasms of bone may be well demarcated, or, in the case of ameloblastomas, locally invasive in character.

The characteristics of malignant neoplasms vary according to the type of tissue undergoing neoplastic change. Carcinomas originating on the surface of the soft tissues should be evident to the careful examiner; however, early lesions are not infrequently overlooked by the casual examiner. Lip lesions are important when they have been present for a period of several weeks without signs of regression. Deformity of the lip, induration, ulceration, or extension to deeper structures should be considered signs of carcinoma until proved otherwise. The same characteristics may be stated for carcinomas on the mucous membrane; a white surface or granular base may be an additional finding. Salivary gland carcinomas arise beneath the mucous membrane and produce focal swelling that should not be interpreted clinically as primarily an inflammatory reaction although inflammation may accompany such swellings.

Sarcomas arise in connective tissues and present frequently as unexplained swelling of the jaws or focal swelling under the mucous membrane surface. Lymphomas are known to involve the mouth and may appear as innocent localized swellings that cannot be explained on the basis of trauma or infection. Focal swellings of the mucosa that tend to appear bluish and that have overlying telangiectases should be considered seriously as malignant connective tissue neoplasms or lymphomas on the basis of clinical findings. Giant cell tumors that recur may on rare occasion prove to be malignant neoplasms and may rapidly involve a wide area of jaw even though the histologic features are typical of benign giant cell tumors. This should not change one's confidence in histologic examination but should stimulate prompt treatment of all giant cell tumors.

Examination of lymph nodes of the neck and face that reveal evidence of lymphadenopathy should be investigated thoroughly for the causative factor. Positive intraoral findings must be related to lymphadenopathy to determine if lymph nodes are enlarged as the result of inflammation in the mouth or throat, neoplastic disease in the mouth and pharyngeal area, or a generalized neoplastic process primarily involving lymph nodes.

The detection and prompt diagnosis of neoplasms are two of the most important services a dentist offers to a patient even though malignant neoplasms may not be seen frequently in the average dental practice. The dentist should be able to recognize neoplasms in the mouth when they are in the early stages and while treatment can still be effective. Success in recognition of neoplasms is more a matter of developing a thorough examination procedure and inquisitive mind in regard to minor and major soft tissue abnormalities than it is a matter of learning to recognize specific types of neoplastic disease.

Prognosis

The prognosis of a disease should be expressed in terms of time and tissue response. It is not enough to state that the disease can be eliminated in a certain length of time; the degree of tissue damage, loss of function, and susceptibility to recurrence must be considered. All too frequently patients believe that the cure of Vincent's infection will restore their gingival tissues to normal. However, the tissue lost from extensive interdental necrosis will not and cannot be made to return to its original form. Furthermore, the altered form poses an added burden for the patient in maintaining adequate oral hygiene to prevent recurrence of the disease. The dentist is obligated to point out these facts in the prognosis of acute necrotizing gingivitis.

DIAGNOSIS IN DENTISTRY

An oral diagnosis is seldom the identification of a single disease process in the mouth; rather it is a statement of a set of circumstances of oral and systemic importance that require recognition, management or treatment. There are findings such as geographic tongue, Fordyce's disease, or median rhomboid glossitis, that have little practical significance with respect to requiring definitive treatment. Yet, these entities in the mouth must be identified and recorded for the purpose of establishing that their presence is recognized and that they have been differentiated from more important possibilities.

The term "management" may be applied to circumstances that require control or prevention rather than actual treatment. An especially important example is the control of bacteremia in patients susceptible to bacterial endocarditis. Other systemic problems requiring special precautions should be noted also. Local problems requiring control or prevention such as habits of a potentially harmful character are included here.

The statement of findings that require dental treatment constitutes the focal point of an oral diagnosis. This part of the statement consists of a complete list of specific problems and conditions found in the patient that will require definitive therapy or restoration. The obvious advantage of recording an oral diagnosis in detail is that the translation of the diagnosis into a plan for treatment and countinuing care is based on the total needs of the patient. It also brings into focus special precautions or limitations that may be imposed on the treatment plan.

TREATMENT PLANNING

Successful dental treatment is always based on careful planning. Regardless of how simple or complex therapy may be, it cannot be carried to a successful conclusion without a planned procedure. Dental treatment has become more complex with the development of specialties and with the improvement of technics. It is no longer possible for treatment to be planned at each appointment without denying the patient the possibility of receiving the benefits of long-range treatment planning and maintenance of oral health.

Rationale and outline for a treatment plan

Rational treatment is dependent on an accurate diagnosis. An accurate diagnosis in dentistry includes a consideration of all oral structures. Oral diagnoses are seldom concerned with one disease and one treatment; they frequently result in a series of various types of treatment for different areas of the mouth. For example, a dentist cannot proceed with gingival treatment in a patient who has a suspicious lesion on his lip nor place extensive fixed bridges on teeth that show evidence of periodontal disease. There are many examples that can be cited in which one type of treatment requires priority over another or in which one phase of treatment depends on completion of another phase.

A rational treatment plan is made with these considerations in mind: the urgency of treatment, the sequence of treatment, and the result expected from treatment. Diagnosis of a condition of an urgent nature compels the dentist to carry out treatment that, if not done first, may result in unnecessary discomfort to the patient or may even endanger his life. The sequence in which therapy progresses may mean the difference between success and failure of dental treatment. A well-organized sequence of treatment prevents many false starts, repetition of treatment, and, in some cases, waste of energy, time, and money. Dental treatment is never directed toward the cure of one disease; it should be directed toward the prevention and correction of all forms of oral disease. Unless the treatment plan is made with the end point visualized, therapy cannot progress to a satisfactory end point.

In developing a rational plan of treatment, even the most experienced dentists follow a pattern of organization of treatment. A pattern or outline, broad in scope, is essential in developing the sequence of treatment with the total needs of the patient in mind. An outline that is broad in scope serves as a reminder of the phases of treatment that must be considered (see p. 374).

Systemic treatment

The dental profession is well aware of the influence of systemic disease on dental treatment. Such disease may be suspected in the course of examining a patient, and a past history of systemic disease may influence the way in which a patient is cared for. A patient undergoing medical treatment who also needs dental treatment may present special problems in treatment planning. The interrelationship of dental and medical treatment should be fully appreciated by both physicians and dentists and a cooperative plan of treatment worked out for the benefit of the patient.

Significance of systemic disease in the treatment program. The importance of the recognition of the presence of systemic disease and the significance of systemic disease to the dental patient cannot be overemphasized. It is imperative that the individual outlining a program of treatment for a patient take into consideration all facets of the information obtained in the history and examination of the patient. The correct diagnosis and a rational therapy can be provided only when information regarding all aspects—biologic, physiologic, psychologic, and sociologic—of the patient has been obtained, correlated, and evaluated. Each facet provides something of importance in the proper plan of therapy.

All of the relationships of systemic factors to therapy cannot be discussed in this text, but some of the relationships between systemic disease and therapy will be considered.

Consider, for example, the patient who presents with a systemic disease that is terminal, but whose chief complaint concerns his oral symptoms. Some therapy is therefore indicated. This may be the patient with terminal cancer who has lost a restoration because of recurrent caries with resultant pulp exposure. Extraction without replacement is indicated, of course, because of the short life expectancy of the patient. On the other hand, the patient may be in the terminal stages of leukemia with gingival ulceration and bleeding and a periodontal abscess. In this instance, extensive dental therapy is not indicated because of the short life expectancy, the possibility of producing severe, uncontrollable hemorrhage, and the possibility of initiating septicemia. Nevertheless, the individual's chief complaint is oral and he must be provided with palliative therapy within the limits permitted by his systemic disease. It is necessary that the dentist recognize the limitations imposed by the systemic disease and develop an effective and palliative treatment plan for this patient. The dentist must be capable of evaluating the systemic status in relation to the treatment needs of the patient and must know the limitations imposed by the biologic state so that he can carry out a beneficial palliative therapy.

Another example of a patient with a systemic disease is the patient who presents with a history of rheumatic heart disease, sensitivity to penicillin, and a moderately advanced periodontitis with early bifurcation involvement of molar teeth and 5 to 6 mm. pockets on the anterior teeth. Because of the nature of the patient's systemic disease and his dental disease and the requirements for periodontal therapy, the patient may not be considered for periodontal therapy. The presence of periodontal disease that cannot be eliminated will leave residual areas of infection to produce intermittent bacteremia associated with oral physiotherapy or with vigorous chewing. This situation provides a precarious life for the patient, with subacute bacterial endocarditis existing as a constant hazard. Any program not providing adequate periodontal therapy would not give adequate consideration to the evaluation of the patient's history and the examination findings.

Another example of the effect of systemic disease on treatment is demonstrated by the "brittle" diabetic patient who presents with moderately advanced periodontitis and a history of recent frequent periodontal abscesses. It is well recognized that the effect of the dental infection may make stablization of blood glucose difficult and may be responsible for the patient's "brittle" character. The elimination of the infection is

therefore an important part of the treatment of the systemic disease. On the other hand, it may be difficult to alter the activity of the periodontitis while the patient has only limited control of blood glucose. The cooperation of physician and dentist to achieve optimum control of systemic disease and dental disease is significant, and the success of this initial therapy will determine the future course of treatment. If the patient's blood glucose level can be maintained at a normal level, he can be treated as a normal patient. Treatment of the periodontal disease must result in complete elimination so that recurrence will not rob the individual of his controlled blood glucose level. Although the patient with controlled diabetes responds normally to treatment and is a candidate for periodontal therapy, he must receive definitive, positive therapy that does not temporize with complete elimination of periodontal infection. The treatment for such a patient may be limited by his physiologic status.

In the patient with newly discovered diabetes there is no way to evaluate the nature of the patient's response to the periodontal disease or to predict the degree of success of medical treatment. In such instances it is necessary to eliminate the acute oral disease and then evaluate medical therapy. After full control of the systemic disease is achieved, the patient may then be adequately evaluated for dental therapy.

Another example of the effect of systemic disease on treatment plan may be observed in the patient who has scleroderma. The patient presents with moderately advanced periodontal disease and a history and evidence of advanced and progressive scleroderma with fixation of the face resulting in a small, inelastic oral orifice. The extent of periodontal disease indicates that treatment will be unsuccessful but not impossible. It is evident that if the disease progresses to any extent, the patient will be unable to insert or remove a denture. In this case the systemic disease dictates the temporizing dental therapy that is necessary to provide a temporary usable dentition for this patient. His systemic disease dictates the temporary type of therapy.

Finally, dental disease may dictate the nature of dental treatment. For example, a patient who presents with moderately advanced periodontal disease that would necessitate periodontal surgery with the resultant exposure of root surface and who also has evidence of moderate caries susceptibility, especially of exposed root surfaces, is not a candidate for periodontal therapy. Exposure of root surfaces is a condition that frequently results from chronic necrotizing ulcerative gingivitis. Restoration of extensive carious lesions on the roots of teeth under such circumstances may be impractical.

The situations proposed are only a few of the possible situations in which the total information about the patient is necessary to outline an effective, rational, healthful therapy. There is no substitute for total information with accurate correlation of all factors to determine the physiologic requirements for the achievement of a biologically acceptable therapy that will provide a status of total body health.

Referral to a physician. Whenever a patient's history or findings of the clinical examination are suggestive of systemic disease, the dentist should refer the patient to a physician.

This may be done by means of a letter of referral containing a precise statement of those symptoms or signs suggestive of systemic disease and a specific request for information from the physician relative to the dental aspects of the disease.

Systemic treatment already in progress. It may be necessary to consult the physician of a patient who is receiving medical treatment at the time dental treatment is being planned so that any forms of medical therapy that may be potentially hazardous to the patient can be discussed.

A patient receiving medical treatment for an illness that is expected to terminate fatally in a relatively short time will require special treatment planning by the dentist. In such a patient he may elect to plan treatment on an emergency basis. On the other hand, much can be done to avoid oral disease in such patients by carrying out preventive measures.

Preventive therapy. Premedication by antibiotics prior to oral procedures that cause bleeding is important in treatment planning when there is a history of rheumatic fever, rheumatic heart disease, or congenital heart disease. Insofar as possible, treatment that causes bleeding (such as scaling) should be carried out in one appointment rather than several to avoid the necessity for repeated premedication. In such instances the treatment plan may call for longer appointments than usual.

Apprehensive patients should be given a suitable sedative prior to treatment. This type of premedication should be freely discussed with the patient when his treatment plan is presented to him.

Corrective therapy. Systemic therapy with antibiotics and other drugs for oral infections is generally of an emergency nature. However, before such treatment is instituted, the patient should be questioned regarding a history of sensitivity to certain drugs.

Preparatory treatment

Preparatory treatment is the treatment employed in preparing the mouth for corrective treatment. Although many of the procedures presented in the following paragraphs may be considered corrective in nature, they nevertheless prepare the mouth for the final corrective restorative and reconstructive procedures. This portion of the treatment plan is discussed to emphasize the necessity for completion of certain phases of treatment before proceeding to the next phase.

Oral surgery. The surgical eradication of soft tissue lesions often receives priority in dental treatment planning. Small lesions that are amenable to excisional biopsy should be considered early in the plan. Larger lesions, particularly neoplasms, may take priority over any other form of oral treatment.

Extraction of teeth on an emergency basis because of infection or pain should be given early attention in treatment planning. Teeth that have advanced carious lesions or are impacted should also be given early consideration. Those that are hopelessly involved with periodontal disease may be extracted early, but in some instances extraction may be delayed so that function may continue until the treatment is further along. Sequence of extraction may be planned in certain types of periodontal disease in order to maintain as much edentulous ridge as possible. Extraction of maxillary teeth preparatory to the insertion of a complete maxillary denture may be delayed, pending completion of a partial mandibular denture that the complete maxillary denture is to oppose.

Correction of anatomic tissue defects must be completed prior to complete and partial denture construction.

Endodontic therapy. Endodontic therapy is carried out early in the treatment plan because of the emergency nature of the condition in many instances. However, the condition of the remaining teeth should be considered so that treatment is not carried out on teeth that are ultimately to be extracted. When there is any question concerning retention of a tooth, pain relief and control of infection should be instituted until the condition of the mouth is completely evaluated and the fate of the tooth determined.

It is desirable to remove carious dentin from deeply involved teeth early in the course of treatment so that the necessity

for endodontic treatment may be determined well in advance of corrective treatment.

The placement of temporary restorations is desirable when the carious involvement of a tooth has progressed to a point where the pulp might be involved if the process is not interrupted before other treatment is continued.

Caries control. An evaluation of the rate at which dental caries is likely to progress is an important part of every treatment plan short of complete dentures. Lactobacilli counts should be done when it is evident that some means for control of caries is necessary to preserve the teeth and the proposed restorations. Institution of a caries control diet should be considered seriously for patients who show a desire to cooperate and reduce the progress of caries.

Periodontal therapy. Periodontal therapy on a conservative basis and on a preventive basis is within the scope of the general practitioner of dentistry. More advanced periodontal treatment may require referral to a specialist. In any case, periodontal treatment should be done prior to corrective treatment. Only when periodontal therapy has been completed can there be any assurance that the supporting structures of the teeth will withstand the additional stress placed on them by prosthetic appliances. Not until periodontal treatment is completed is it possible to determine which teeth are to be retained and which will require replacement.

Orthodontic treatment. The orthodontist is best qualified to plan orthodontic treatment; nevertheless, the dentist in general practice must consider orthodontic treatment not only for young individuals, but also for certain adults. There are many instances in which a better result could be obtained in restoration of a dental arch if tooth position were more favorable. Orthodontic consultation should be obtained and should be indicated where it is best suited in the overall treatment plan.

gently prepared, the patient will find the plan of treatment a desirable procedure. However, if the examination is hasty and incomplete, the explanation of the oral condition vague, the treatment plan presented with uncertainty, and the prognosis indefinite, the patient will find it difficult to accept the treatment plan with confidence.

The dentist should make use of his diagnostic aids in presenting treatment plans. The patient is usually extremely interested in the radiographs and models because they represent his problem. The models and radiographs can be used to point out areas of both health and disease and the areas in need of special attention. The use of models to show the patient what the various types of restorations will look like when completed may be an important deciding factor in acceptance of the plan when anterior teeth are involved or when a removable prosthesis is contemplated.

A frank discussion of fees is in order when the treatment plan is presented. The patient should know the expense involved before he is allowed to accept a treatment plan; otherwise in the middle of treatment he may decide he is unable to meet the expense. With the payment plans available today for dental treatment, ideal dental therapy is within the reach of much of the population.

• • •

In the last analysis a diagnosis is but one of the components in an evaluation of a case. A diagnosis is only as accurate as the steps leading up to it. In dentistry the use of the term "diagnosis" may be used to indicate the recognition of a single disease or the result of an appraisal and summary of all the abnormalities concerning a patient. In the latter all the significant abnormal findings should be summarized. It is this summary, termed "the diagnosis," that is the basis for treatment planning. The following illustrative case is presented to show how a case should be evaluated.

ILLUSTRATIVE CASE (Figs. 15-1 to 15-3)

The patient is a female, 52 years of age.

Chief complaint

"I have a sore place on my gums."[1]

Present illness

The patient had no complaints[2] about her mouth until about three weeks ago[3] when a very painful, tender, swollen area occurred overnight on the gingival tissues adjacent to the lower lateral incisor.[4] It was intensely painful, especially during eating.[5] The pain was continuous, throbbing, and burning and radiated over the lower jaw; it was not related in any way to recumbency or exertion,[6] nor did it keep the patient awake or prevent her from eating. The tooth was not particularly sensitive to touch, but the gingiva was very tender.[7] After a day or so there was a remission of the acute pain, but a continuous feeling of discomfort persisted. The remission was associated with a decrease in the size of the swelling and the occurrence of a bad taste in the mouth.[8] The patient noted some mobility of the tooth but no fever, malaise, lethargy, or swelling under the chin or neck.[9] She did not recall having eaten any popcorn, nut meats, or food containing seeds, nor had she noted that her toothbrush was losing bristles

---

[1]This is the patient's chief complaint in her own words.

[2]It is apparent that the onset of this condition was abrupt. A statement of prior health is helpful in determining the type of onset. It also indicates the patient's attitude toward her oral health prior to the time of her chief complaint.

[3]This statement begins the chronology of the primary symptoms.

[4]This statement gives the location of the complaint and some associated symptoms.

[5]It is significant that the character of the symptom should change with a specific activity. It directs attention toward factors present during eating that could be contributing to the cause of the symptoms.

[6]This is negative correlative data and points out to some extent that the condition is not caused by pulpal disease.

[7]This serves also as a negative correlative fact to further emphasize that this is probably not pulpal disease.

[8]The sudden decrease in symptoms with an associated "bad taste" suggests the possibility of a draining abscess.

[9]The fact that there were no constitutional symptoms is significant and aids in determining the severity of the disease process. The presence of tooth mobility tends to point to the possibility of periodontal disease. The lack of swelling in the neck suggests the absence of lymph node involvement.

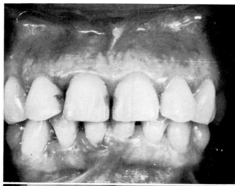

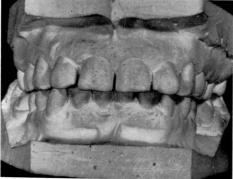

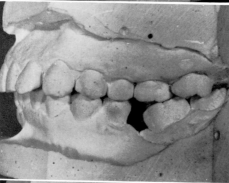

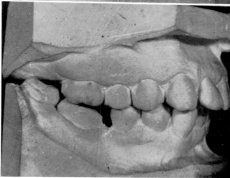

Fig. 15-1. *Illustrative case.*

prior to the onset of her complaint.[10] She had noticed that food frequently caught between the teeth in the area of the lower central incisors and that there had been a recession of the gum for the past several months.[11] She did not consult a dentist but treated herself by placing aspirin directly on the swelling for relief of the pain. She also though this medication would kill infection.[12]

The patient states that she has tried to go to the dentist once a year. On her present visit to the dental clinic she expected to "get her teeth cleaned, gone over, and fillings checked." She is concerned about her teeth because her husband recently had immediate dentures made and is experiencing difficulty with them.[13]

The patient complains of a pain in her back that has been present for some time—"possibly to the time of hysterectomy" that was done about 3 years ago. She also thinks that possibly her "bad teeth may be poisoning her system." The pain is localized to the neck and shoulders and is dull in character.[14] On further questioning she believes that the pain in her neck and shoulders might be associated with "overwork" since she is no longer

---

[10]These are the factors that may be initiating causes of periodontal abscess, especially in the presence of periodontal disease with periodontal pockets.

[11]Food impaction and gingival recession in the area of the chief complaint prior to the onset of the chief complaint are positive correlative data pertaining to the possibility of periodontal abscess.

[12]It is important to know what the patient did for treatment and what she excepted of her treatment. It is obvious in this case that her treatment was incorrect, and her premise as to the effect of the drug was wrong. In this particular case, we may know on later physical examination that there is a good possibility of an aspirin burn.

[13]This suggests that the patient's primary concern is not so much the pain but the thought of losing her teeth and the necessity for replacement with complete dentures, which she believes would probably be unsuccessful since her husband's were not successful.

[14]In discussing her general health and its relation to her teeth, the patient has assumed that poisons from her teeth may be responsible for the neck and shoulder pain. The duration and character of the pain and the fact that she can sleep at night gives some estimate of the actual severity of the complaint. One might wonder at this time if the hysterectomy has any connection with this complaint; since it is not logical to assume teeth have anything to do with complaints relative to the neck and shoulders aside from possible muscle tensions, it becomes necessary to consider the reason for the hysterectomy and, if it were for a neoplastic disease, whether or not the presence of these associated symptoms might be referable to metastatic lesions.

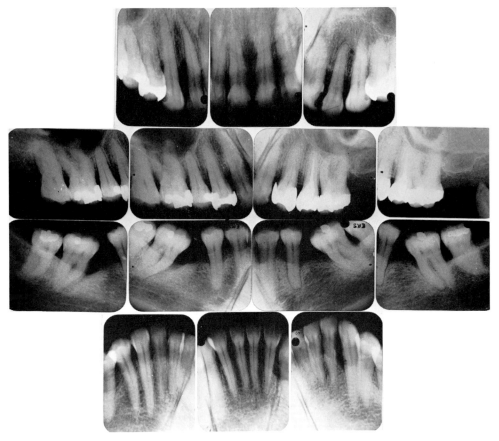

Fig. 15-2. *Illustrative case.*

able to do things she likes—like being out of doors, gathering wood, etc.[15] She has a lump in her throat when her back aches.[16]

The patient consulted a chiropractor who indicated that she had "overdone" since her son had been in the Army. She commented that the chiropractor said she had a "tricky back" and she believes he is the only one that can put it back.[17]

She believes she is developing a case of arthritis or something.[18]

She has recently gained 8 pounds, which she attributes to eating too much. She has had no fever and complains of some fatigue associated with "overdoing."[19]

---

[15]An associated complaint suggests that she might have some limitation of former capacity.

[16]This associated symptom gives the impression of being psychogenic in origin rather than organic.

[17]In questioning the patient as to her last visit to her physician she disclosed she has seen a chiropractor in addition to her family physician. This is significant since her physician has not considered her complaints organically important.

---

[18]It is well established what the patient believes the cause of her complaint to be. Upon inquiry as to why she thought she was getting arthritis, she gave very vague answers that strongly imply that she has a desire to get some argument for her diagnosis.

[19]The patient has given what she considers to be a true answer, and without further contributory evidence to the contrary it must be accepted. However, further questioning relative to possible causes are in order at this time.

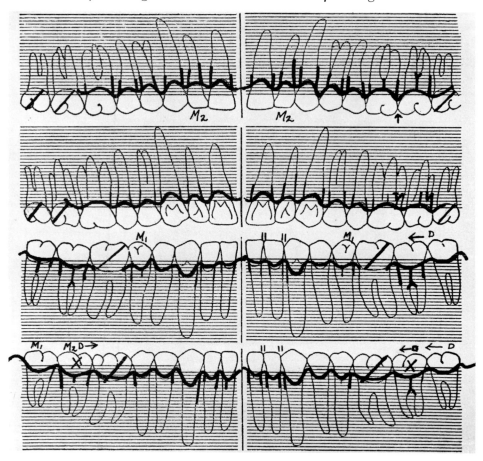

Fig. 15-3. *Illustrative case.* Periodontal charting completed.

Past history

The patient had "severe" measles, with a temperature of "105.5°," at about 18 or 19 years of age. She lost most of her hair at the time but does not remember any other complications. She does not remember having had any other childhood diseases[20] nor any severe toothaches or premature losses of primary dentition.[21] The patient denies any history of typhoid fever, malaria, asthma, eczema, pneumonia, or pleurisy. She has a "little hay fever and cannot take aspirin."[22]

There is no history of tuberculosis, weak heart, nervous breakdowns, stomach ulcers, anemia, or kidney trouble,[23] nor a history of herpetic gingivostomatitis.[24] The patient states that her upper right and left third molars were extracted because of discomfort associated with their eruption. Her "lower stomach teeth" were extracted "many years ago." She had never been injured.[25] She had her tonsils removed 15 years ago because of frequent sore throats. None of these episodes was severe

[20]Although the patient seems to have had severe measles, there does not appear to be any contributory history in reply to questions concerning possible sequelae.

[21]In relation to childhood diseases, the premature loss of deciduous dentition is of significance in the development of malocclusion. There appears to be no contributory evidence here.

[22]No doubt this is based upon her experience of using aspirin locally on her gums; in any event do not prescribe aspirin.

[23]These are additional illnesses with possible associated sequelae that are significant to dental procedures.

[24]This may at times be confused with Vincent's disease, and detailed questioning may be needed to bring out the differences.

[25]This category is not limited to major injuries. All injuries should be noted. Patients tend to forget small but sometimes significant injuries.

enough to confine her to bed.[26] A mastectomy was done when she was 38 years of age and a hysterectomy when she was 46 years of age because of neoplastic disease.[27] No complications have been recognized, and she last saw her physician about 6 months ago.[28]

Family history

The patient's mother and father are deceased. Her father died at the age of 73 as a result of cardiovascular disease and her mother at the age of 73 as a result of postoperative complications occurring after gallbladder removal.[29] The patient does not recall any history of diabetes, cancer, tuberculosis, allergy, or nervous or mental disease in her immediate family.[30] She does not remember any significant information regarding the status of her parents' dentition.[31]

Personal and social history

The patient is happily married and has one living child. She lost a set of twins during the first pregnancy but does not remember the cause.[32] She is a housewife, and her duties are fairly light. Her son is in the army in Korea and this has been of considerable concern. Although the family income seems to be adequate, it is not so good as it could be because her husband has not been

---

[26]This gives an estimate of how severe "sore throats" may have been. It is well to determine, when possible, why the tonsils were removed. The patient should be questioned regarding the possibility of an association with rheumatic fever.

[27]The time of occurrence and reason for operations should be listed. The patient's operations are significant because they indicate the possibility of further neoplastic disease by metastases.

[28]The patient should be questioned at this time to explore the possibility of recurrence of disease by asking about her last visit to her physician and about what he had to say concerning her present status. Associated complaints indicated the necessity for eliminating possibility of metastases.

[29]By inference this may suggest the possibility of gallbladder disease; however, the patient was able to state that her physician had already eliminated this possibility.

[30]The patient was not positive in her knowledge; so under such circumstances it is best to state that she does not recall any history of these diseases.

[31]Even though a patient may remember this information, the correlation between a patient's condition and that of the parents is no greater than the correlation in most other diseases except in malocclusion, where there seems to be a somewhat higher rate of correlation. Remember also that histories are for the collection of data for the study of such problems.

[32]It is important to know about recent severe illnesses during pregnancy because they may have a direct reflection on the care and conditions of the gingival tissues.

able to work because of glaucoma.[33] She appears to be apprehensive about her condition but not overly so. She does not use tobacco in any form but likes "to eat, especially candy."

Systems review[34]

Head. The patient does not have headaches.

Eyes. She wears spectacles because of failing vision. She has not noticed any changes in vision recently, and there is no history of pain, inflammation, burning, or diplopia.

Ears. Hearing is good. There is no history of deafness, discharge, vertigo, or tinnitus.

Nose. No history of epistaxis. The patient has frequent colds and is bothered with hay fever and "sinus trouble." She states that she has no difficulty in breathing through her nose.

Throat. Tonsils were removed 15 years ago as indicated under past history.[35] She has a "lump in her throat" when she has neck and back pains.[36]

Cardiorespiratory. The patient complains of shortness of breath[37] when she is nervous, and her heart "pounds" at such times. She has not noticed any recent change in her ability to climb stairs or any undue shortness of breath.[38] "I have pressure on the heart sometimes and can't take a deep breath and I believe indigestion causes it."[39] The patient complains of pain in the substernal and epigastric regions.[40] This pain is related to the time she experiences pressure on the heart and not to exercise. She complains of edema of her lower

---

[33]Financial status of the patient indicates that she may be unable to assume the expense of ideal treatment if too extensive in nature.

[34]The systems review may be carried out at a later date if necessary, and at times it is well to obtain this part of the history at a later appointment since many times a patient may recall some of the information desired after the initial reminder and can give a better account at the next appointment.

[35]It is permissible to refer to items previously reviewed. History of sore throat, dysphagia, hoarseness, and other symptoms should be reviewed to remind the patient of any symptoms missed previously.

[36]There seems to be no indication that the associating complaint is organic in nature.

[37]This is an important complaint and should be given considered attention in the clinical examination.

[38]This information serves to give some quantitative evaluation to her complaint of shortness of breath.

[39]This information seems to indicate that her complaint of shortness of breath may be referable to cardiorespiratory disease.

[40]Complaints of substernal pain and pain in the epigastric region are significant. Substernal pain should be evaluated in relationship to the patient's complaint of shortness of breath, and the epigastric pain should be evaluated in reference to her examination by her physician for gallbladder disease. It is also possible that her complaints may be poorly localized and caused by flatulence.

extremities on standing and walking and attributes this to tight shoes. She does not think the swelling is very noticeable. She has night sweats that occur fairly frequently, but they are not drenching in character.[41] She does not give a history of cough or hemoptysis.

Gastrointestinal. The patient complains of "gas" on her stomach and also of constipation. Her appetite is good. Up to 4 or 5 months ago she complained of pain in the epigastric region that frequently lasted about 2 hours. It did not seem to be associated with eating or exercise. The patient got some relief from nausea by "stretching out on her stomach."[42]

A gastrointestinal series was done recently with no significant findings, and the patient's physician ruled out gallbladder disease.[43] She was treated 25 years ago for "very, very red, inflamed, and sore gums that felt like they were drawing up."[44] She was treated three times with a "greenlike solution that seemed to shrink the gums."[45] This took place during her first pregnancy. Two of her lower "stomach teeth" were extracted at about the age of 16 years because of abscesses.[46] No excessive hemorrhage occurred with the extractions.

Neuromuscular. The patient complains of insomnia and nervousness and sometimes uses phenobarbital to sleep. Her hands and fingers are frequently "asleep" in the morning irrespective of

---

[41]The description of the night sweats and the lack of associated symptoms suggest that the patient does not have tuberculosis. The possibility of other diseases should also be ruled out. Those diseases in which night sweats occur should be remembered and their symptoms reviewed.

[42]In many instances methods of gaining relief and whether the relief is gained are of significance in evaluations of a complaint.

[43]The suggestion that the patient may be suffering from gallbladder disease has been ruled out by her physician. The information that she had a "G.I. series" indicates that she had been examined for these complaints by her physician. This serves to relieve the dentist of any responsibility for further evaluation of this phase of the patient's health status.

[44]This description is highly suggestive of Vincent's infection. It is of considerable significance in reviewing the oral health and the etiology of her present condition.

[45]The medication used is helpful in establishing the disease. This is positive correlative data for establishing a history of Vincent's infection.

[46]The reasons for dates of extractions are important because of their relation to the etiology of oral conditions. At times it is important to determine the contributing factor in subacute bacterial endocarditis, actinomycosis, abscesses, and so on.

her sleeping position.[47] She has pain in the back as described under present illness. There is no history of syncope, convulsions, paralysis, or ataxia and no mental confusion.[48] The patient has had some changes of temperament; she is more irritable lately. She has no particular loss of memory except that it "does not seem to be as good as it used to be."

Bone and joint. The patient complains of pain along the right and left sides since her hysterectomy. She had pain and swelling of one knee joint during her second pregnancy. Otherwise there is no past history of pain, limitation of motion, or swelling of any joints, including the temporomandibular joint; lately, however, she has had some stiffness of the finger joints.

Genitourinary. The patient has no history of hematuria, dysuria, or nocturia and urinates with a normal frequency of three or four times per day.

Catamenia. The patient complains of "hot flushes," palpitation of the heart, flatulence, some nausea, constipation, and occasionally dizziness. The "hot flushes" are localized over the upper portion of the body and produce a sensation of warmth. This patient is in menopause.[49]

Clinical physical examination

The patient is a well-developed, heavyset, white female weighing 150 pounds, of about her stated age, and appears to be in good health.

Head. The external features of the cranium are normal.

Skin. The hair shows greying commensurate with the patient's age.[50] The texture and quantity of the hair are normal. An increased amount of hair on the upper lip has forced the patient to shave.[51] The skin is of normal consistency for her age. There is no evidence of drying, pigmentation,

---

[47]Anesthesia of the hands may be seen in many diseases. Although it is not uncommon for it to occur in one extremity as a result of sleeping on that extremity, it is uncommon for it to occur bilaterally and so regularly.

[48]This is a minimum review of this system. Other history should be listed when indicated.

[49]This should be suspected in view of her hysterectomy. The menopause must be proved in this particular case by the symptoms since no menstrual bleeding is possible. In view of the fact that this patient is in the menopause, all of her many symptoms must be evaluated in light of this.

[50]Greying of the hair in older people is of little significance but may be of considerable importance in younger age groups.

[51]This may well relate to symptoms of menopause and can be considered as positive correlative data to this effect.

or discoloration. There is no evidence of flushing.[52] The lips are of normal color and are not chapped or fissured. The nails appear to have good care, and the hands are normal.

Eyes. The patient has difficulty seeing anything close up without her spectacles, and she does not have photophobia. Both accommodation and light reflection appear to be normal. There is no discharge, inflammation, or restriction in the movements of the eyeballs.

Nose. The patient has a postnasal drip, and there is no obvious sign of obstruction of the nose nor inability to breathe through the nose.

Neck. Palpation of the thyroid gland does not indicate any obvious abnormality as to its size, shape, or attachment. There appears to be no apparent enlargement of the lymph nodes in the neck and preauricular region. The salivary glands appear to be of normal size and consistency. The veins of the neck do not show any distention or pulsation when the patient is seated in the dental chair.[53]

Mouth. The transition between the skin and the oral mucosa is fairly uniform with the exception of a few ectopic sebaceous glands on the inner aspects of the lips near the commissure. The mucous glands on the inner surface of the lower lip are fairly prominent but of normal consistency. The labial frenulum is attached high on the gingiva and is red. It is attached in an area of inflammation associated with the periodontal pocket and gingival recession.[54]

The buccal mucosa has no scarring and is not particularly prominent. The orifices of the parotid duct are prominent but show no inflammation.[55] The mucosa is pink and shows no obvious pigmentation. The vestibular fornix is shallow in the posterior region and in the lower anterior region.[56] There is no evidence of abnormality except in the area of "aspirin burn" adjacent to the lower right incisors. There is a change in the normal red coloration of the mucosa in the fornix and of the pink color of the attached gingiva in the region of the lower right lateral incisor. The latter is associated with the area of swelling of the patient's chief complaint. The hard palate is pale pink from the rugae to the junction of the hard and soft

palates. In the anterior region the rugae adjacent to the teeth are red, swollen, and spongy. There are no changes in the orifices of the mucous glands of the palate. The soft palate is reddish in color and shows no evidence of any inflammation, lesions, or induration on inspection and palpation. The tongue is coated. The circumvallate papillae are not particularly prominent. The filiform papillae are not atropic, and the fungiform papillae are normal. There are no lesions on the dorsal or inferior surfaces of the tongue. There is no prominent fissuring of the tongue, and the median rhomboid area is not conspicuous. The orifices of the glands in the floor of the mouth are normal. The color of the gingival margin is bluish pink in all areas except adjacent to the mandibular right central and lateral incisors. The rest of the gingiva is bright red. The attached gingiva is bluish pink but does not have the same intensity of blue that the free gingival margin does. The attached gingiva in the area of the mandibular lateral incisor is bright red, with a central area of white discoloration extending to the labial vestibule and labial mucosa.

The form of the free gingiva is abnormal. The margin is blunted and rolled in all areas and is nowhere closely adapted to the surfaces of the teeth. The interdental papillae do not fill the interproximal areas, and in some areas they are bulbous and have no functional contour. There is no stippling of the free or attached gingiva. The density of the papillae and free gingiva is characterized by being soft, spongy, and flabby. The attached gingiva is soft and is not firm or dense.

The depth of the gingival crevice is everywhere more than 3 mm.[57] The level of attachment is nowhere on the enamel, and the lowering of the attachment measures from 5 to 9 mm.[58] There is a swelling and light discoloration on the labial gingiva of the mandibular right lateral incisor. Pus may be expressed from the crevicular area adjacent to the swelling. The area is painful to touch. There are distal trifurcation exposures of the maxillary left first and second molars and a bifurcation exposure on the lingual side of the mandibular left second molar.[59]

There are considerable supragingival and subgingival calculus deposits in all areas of the mouth. Pockets of 8 to 9 mm. in depth are present on the distal side of the maxillary lateral incisors and on the mesial side of the mandibular right cuspid.

During swallowing, the floor of the mouth adjacent to the alveolar ridge containing the sublingual gland rises to a level higher than the height

---

[52]Although this may be negative correlative data regarding the menopause, "flushing" may not be a consistent finding or occur at the time of the examination.

[53]This is negative correlative data regarding cardiac insufficiency but does not rule out cardiac disease.

[54]The labial frenulum may contribute to the maintenance of a periodontal pocket when the attachment is high on the gingiva and the free margin of the gingiva is low on the tooth.

[55]Large parotid papillae are not uncommon and are usually of no clinical significance.

[56]This is of importance in determining periodontal therapy, toothbrushing instruction, and placing of prosthetic appliances.

[57]Any crevice over 2 mm. in depth can be considered as abnormal.

[58]This information is also placed on the periodontal chart.

[59]The treatment plan is dependent to a large extent on the status of these areas. The fact that these areas are involved with disease is an indication for removal of the teeth so involved.

of the crest of the alveolar process at the site of the extraction of the lower permanent molars.[60]

Radiographic examination

There is a discontinuity of the lamina dura at the alveolar crest between all the teeth.[61] There is extensive loss of 7 to 8 mm. of bone support between the upper right and left lateral incisors and the cuspids.[62] There is a widened periodontal space about the upper left second bicuspid as well as an irregular lamina dura.[63] There is an extensive loss of bone on the mesial side of the lower left and right-tipped permanent second molars.[64] The loss of bone support ranges from one-third to one-half the length of the root, and in some instances (lateral incisors and lower right cuspids) there is a greater loss of bone support.[65]

In those areas of interradicular bone loss, there is a loss of lingual and labial cortical plate bone, but this is not extensive. There are overhanging margins present on the mesial surface of the maxillary right and left bicuspids. The lamina dura is continuous about the apex of the roots of all teeth. The upper right second molar has a root canal filling present.

Examination of the teeth

The teeth show spacing caused by loss of teeth, extrusion, and occlusal changes. There are areas of

---

[60]This is of considerable importance in the placing of partial or full dentures since this mass of tissue tends to displace the denture saddles.

[61]This gives some indication as to the severity of the condition and is helpful in calling attention to particular areas that may occur as in traumatic occlusion, apical abscesses, and overhanging margins.

[62]This points out particular areas of bone loss and should call attention to possible causes such as food impaction, occlusal trauma, malposition of teeth, and inadequate toothbrushing technic.

[63]The width of the periodontal space is some indication of the amount of function of the tooth. Very narrow width indicates a loss of function, whereas wide periodontal membrane spaces indicate heavy function. If the function exceeds the physiologic limit of the teeth or a sustained orthodontic type of force is placed upon the tooth, there may be a crushing of the periodontal membrane between the tooth and the bone so that there is a very narrow periodontal membrane space. Where there is any irregularity of the width of the periodontal membrane space, the possibility of occlusal trauma should be evaluated.

[64]Loss of first molars has contributed to this area of disease.

[65]The loss of bone as evidenced by radiographs does not necessarily indicate that there is a pocket of the same depth present. This should be correlated with actual measurements of the pockets with a thin probe. The measurements should be recorded on a periodontal chart.

pronounced occlusal wear, and some teeth are without centric stops or functional contacts. There are many restorations; some have faulty margins and overhangs and have become broken. There is evidence of dental decay throughout the mouth, and there are a few instances of cervical decay.[66] There is No. 2 to 3 mobility of the upper right and lateral incisors and No. 3 to 4 mobility of the lower left and right second bicuspids. There is No. 1 to 2 mobility of the lower right second and third molars but not so pronounced as in the other teeth mentioned.[67] There is a discrepancy between centric relation and centric occlusion.[68] The patient has limited functional efficiency because of loss of teeth and loss of occlusal contact. The patient has an abnormal pattern of mastication characterized by anterior chewing and chopping action. There are balancing interferences in both right and left working excursions of the mandible. The interocclusal space is about 4 mm. when the patient is at tonus or rest position.

Diagnosis

This patient has extensive periodontal disease involving supporting structures of all the teeth. She has an *acute periodontal abscess associated with periodontitis.*[69] She appears to be in the climacterium.[70] Most of her complaints appear to be referable to this or to her concern over her son being in the army. There appears to be no real evidence of heart disease or other systemic disease.

Significance of the diagnosis. The patient has mentioned that she expects to see her physician in the near future. Because of previous neoplastic disease, her complaints referable to her back, and so on, should be evaluated for the presence of metastatic lesions. In view of the appraisal of her

---

[66]Cervical decay makes periodontal therapy difficult. The presence of unrestored cervical cavities makes it difficult to decrease gingivitis. When gingivectomy is anticipated in the presence of cervical decay, the possibility of rapid decay of the exposed surfaces of the roots should be taken into consideration. A lactobacilli count is indicated under these circumstances.

[67]Mobility may be indicated in terms of relative movements such as No. 1, 2, 3, 4 or in terms of millimeters and is incorporated in the periodontal charting.

[68]This is a slide in centric relation and is an important factor in occlusal trauma. When possible, gross premature contacts should be indicated and an estimate of the functional efficiency in lateral excursions should also be made. The presence of balancing interferences should be recorded.

[69]This is the diagnosis of the chief complaint referable to the oral cavity.

[70]This is the impression obtained from the complaints referable to her status of health.

medical status, a report from her physician should be requested.[71]

The presence of deep periodontal pockets with the entrapment of bacteria and debris has led to the formation of an abscess on the labial aspect of the mandibular right lateral incisor.

The patient's oral condition is the result of poor oral hygiene, migration of teeth, occlusal trauma, loss of teeth, faulty restorations, previous gingival disease, and chronic inflammation. The menopause factor (less inclination for home care) could only add to the already present local factors sufficient in themselves to produce the present condition. This condition has been present many years and was present before the onset of the menopause. Scientific evidence available at this time precludes the possibility that the patient's teeth per se or the complaint per se is responsible for her arthritis or neck and back complaints.

Prognosis

The prognosis depends to a large extent upon her ability and desire to cooperate in home care. Though her temperament is not the best at present, one may assume that it will be better when the menopausal symptoms have subsided. Her son's arrival home in May of this year should also contribute to her well-being. Her husband's attitude regarding dental service may be a handicap; however, her cooperation is expected in view of her concern over losing any teeth.

In view of the patient's previous neoplastic disease, it is well to consider the prognosis of this disease. The undertaking of extensive rehabilitation in the presence of metastatic neoplasm is contraindicated. Medical consultation is indicated here before any extensive therapy is considered.

The quantity of restorative dentistry necessary and the number of periodontal treatments necessary indicate that the time required for treatment will be extensive. Patient cooperation and tissue response cannot be fully evaluated at this time. The completed treatment should present a favorable term of service provided that adequate maintenance is carried out. Certain deviations from the ideal treatment plan may have to be carried out for economic reasons.

Treatment plan

The following treatment plan has been suggested for this patient in view of the diagnosis and

significance of the diagnosis. It is not to be considered as a completed or detailed treatment plan nor a final treatment plan. Modifications may be instituted as response of the patient and the tissues is evaluated.

1. Systemic treatment
   a. A consideration of the patient's constitutional status relative to nutrition, metabolism, and hormonal balance indicates that she has a hormonal imbalance related to menopause.
   b. A review of the patient's health history indicates the possibility of the presence of neoplastic disease metastases; consultation with her physician should be requested.[72] If the disease is present, the periodontal therapy plan outlined here should be modified.
2. Preparatory treatment
   a. Treatment of periodontal abscess[73]
      (1) Establish drainage
      (2) Scale the teeth
      (3) Irrigate with iodine lotion
      (4) Place tetracycline ointment in the periodontal pocket
   b. Scaling and polishing of all teeth
   c. Home-care instructions[74]
   d. Removal of overhangs[75]
   e. Extractions of teeth 18, 15, and 31[76]
   f. Observation of tooth 14; observation of patient cooperation and tissue response
3. Corrective treatment
   a. Occlusal adjustment and reduction of the lingual cusp of tooth 14 for oc-

---

[71]The information gained from the case history and clinical examination makes possible an intelligent request for a medical consultation that is based on sound principles. It indicates that there are no oustanding contraindications to dental therapy in this patient. However, it does indicate the possibility of systemic disease of importance to the patient. In the event that the patient is in menopause, certain factors such as temperament complaints and inadequate cooperation should be carefully weighed.

[72]Referral of a patient or a request for information relative to a patient should be by written inquiry with patient's permission.

[73]Treatment of periodontal abscess should be carried out as soon as a preliminary examination has been made. Sufficient history should be acquired to determine whether or not there are contraindications for this form of therapy.

[74]Home-care instructions should be given the patient regarding irrigation with warm saline solution at time of treatment of the abscess.

[75]This includes the removal of gross overhangs. In some instances replacement of the restoration may be necessary. However, as much as possible of the overhang must be removed at this time for the most effective results of the scaling and polishing procedures.

[76]Extraction of tooth 15 is necessary because of trifurcation involvement and extraction of tooth 31 because there is a bifurcation involvement. Removal of tooth 15 should only be done prior to the placing of the lower fixed appliance because of the possibility of extrusion of the opposing teeth.

clusion with lower fixed prosthesis[77]
b. Gingivectomy and gingivoplasty[78]
  (1) Subgingival curettage of upper lateral incisors
  (2) Combined subgingival curettage and gingivectomy of the lower anteriors
  (3) Gingivectomy of bicuspids and molar region
c. Operative dentistry
d. Prosthetic dentistry
  (1) Splinting of teeth 20 and 21 with attachment to tooth 17, replacing teeth 18 and 19
  (2) Splinting of teeth 28 and 29 with attachment to tooth 32, replacing teeth 30 and 31

---

[77]There is a beginning distal trifurcation involvement of tooth 14. Because of this position and the possibility of treatment by gingivectomy, this tooth will be treated and observed since its removal does not basically alter the treatment plan at this time.
[78]Because of the irregularity of loss of supporting structures in the lower anterior region (area of periodontal abscess), elimination of the residual pocket must be modified to establish a more favorable gingival contour of this area. Subgingival curettage is carried out at the time of gingivectomy. In this instance the surgical removal of the gingiva does not extend to the complete depth of the periodontal pocket. In this manner, part of the pocket is removed by gingivectomy and part by an attempt at reattachment through subgingival curettage.

4. Maintenance phase

At the completion of the corrective phase of treatment, periodontal tissues should be in a physiologic state of health that can be maintained by adequate home care. The patient should be instructed to return for periodic prophylaxis as needed. This will be determined at the time of each visit and will be based upon the patient's oral hygiene. The patient should be examined at least two or three times a year to evaluate the condition of her oral hygiene. A thorough examination of her mouth, including oral hygiene, dental caries, and dental appliances, should be carried out often enough to prevent further disease.

If it is determined that this patient is in the final phases of metastatic carcinoma, only limited and palliative periodontal therapy should be considered. Although it is recognized that only complete dental service and periodontal therapy can prevent the progressive loss of her teeth, palliative therapy may be the treatment of choice.

REFERENCES

Bush, J. B.: Teaching integrated treatment planning in oral diagnosis as it relates to periodontics, J. Dent. Educ. **29**:379-381, 1965.

Davidson, G. B.: Diagnosis and treatment planning in operative dentistry and in crown and bridge prosthesis, Dent. Clin. N. Amer. 201-212, Mar., 1963.

Mann, A. W.: Examination; diagnosis and treatment planning in occlusal rehabilitation, J. Prosth. Dent. **17**:73-78, 1967.

Index

A

Acromegaly, 90, 124
Acrylic resin sensitivity, 52
Actinomycosis, bacteriologic examination, 306, 307
Addison's disease, 105, 134-135, 168
Adenoid facies, 89-90, 218
Adenopathy, 109
Adrenocorticosteroids, 71
Age
  dentin and, 193
  enamel and, 193
  gingiva and, 162, 165, 166
  gingival form and, 171-172
  mandible rest position and, 250
  occlusion and, 227-228
  patient's complaint and, 40-41
  pigmentation and, 134
  tooth color and, 193
Agranulocytosis, 71, 72, 73, 75, 314
Alcohol intake, 54
Alkaline phosphatase determination, 316
Allergy, 50-53; see also specific agents and diagnoses
  contact sensitivity tests, 319-322
  to drugs, 50-53, 352, 354, 355
  history of, 354
  nasal, 56
Alveolar abscess, 152
Alveolar bone, radiography, 265
Alveolar crest
  buccal and lingual bone levels, 269-270, 272
  –cementoenamel junction relation, radiography, 269-272
  horizontal bone loss, 272
  lamina dura, 266
    radiography, 291
  radiography, 265
  vertical bone loss, 272
Alveolar crest level, radiography, 291
Alveolar process, radiography, 265
Amalgam
  abnormal sounds, 83
  deposition, radiography, 288
  gingival impregnation, 170
Ameloblastoma, radiography, 282-283
Amelogenesis imperfecta, 196, 199-200
Aminopyrine, 71
Amphetamine, 73

Analgesics, 71-72
  ataractics and, 53
  potentiation, 71-72, 73
Anaphylactic shock, 51
Anemia, 72, 100-101, 106, 134, 168
  drug-induced, 75
  hematologic diagnosis, 308-309
  hemolytic, 104
  history of, 359
  tongue in, 159-160
Anesthesia; see also Local anesthesia
  reactions to, 355
Anesthesias, 67, 359
Angina pectoris, 58, 72, 75, 357-358
Angle classification, 227
Angle of convexity, 220
Anhidrotic ectodermal dysplasia, 201
Ankle swelling, 358
Anodontia, 201
Anomalies, 195-201
  treatment plan and, 390
Anorexia, 61
Anterior teeth inclination, 216, 218, 221
Antianemic compounds, 72
Antianginal drugs, 72
Antianxiety drugs; see Ataractics
Antiarrhythmic drugs, 72
Antibiotics, 72-73
  allergy to, 50-52
  inhibition in cultures, 306
  sensitivity tests, 304
Anticoagulants, 23, 47, 73, 310, 312, 353, 354
Anticonvulsants, 73
Antidepressants, 73
Antigout drugs, 73
Antihistamines, 73, 124
  reactions to, 53
Antihypertensive drugs, 74
Antineoplastics, 73-74
Antisialagogues, 356
Antispasmodics, 74
Antituberculosis drugs, 74
Anxiety, 351, 359
  blood pressure and, 48, 353
Appetite, 358
Appliances, 387; see also Dentures
  alveolar crest–cementoenamel junction relation and, 270, 272
  examination of, 254
  history of use, 45, 64

Appliances—cont'd
 insertion and removal, 344-345
 surveying for, 344
Argyll Robertson pupil, 97
Arrhythmias, 21, 22, 72, 75, 87
Arteriosclerosis, 86
Arthritis, 69; *see also* Temporomandibular joint
  arthritis
 gonorrheal, 234
Aspiration biopsy, 323, 325, 328
Aspirin
 allergy to, 50, 51, 53, 354
 antigout drugs and, 73
 eschars, 33
 hemostasis and, 71
Asthenia, 20-21
Asthma, 51, 74, 86
 aspirin and, 53
 history of, 354
Atabrine, 104
Ataractics, 72
 analgesics and, 53
Ataxia, 67, 85
Atropine, 74
Attrition, 228-229, 244
 functional factors, 228, 229-230
 radiography, 276
 stresses and, 229
Auricular fibrillation, 87
Auscultation, 83

B

Bacteriologic examination, 304-308
 cultures, 304, 305, 306-308
  media, 305, 306
 fresh moist preparations, 306-308
 smears, 305, 306-308
 specimen collection, 304, 305, 306
Barbiturates, 74
 reactions to, 354
Behçet's syndrome, 97
Belladonna, 74
Bell's palsy, 90, 96
Bicuspid eruption, 222, 224
Biochemical profiles, 319
Biopsy, 135, 136, 152, 322-326, 380
 armamentarium, 322
 aspiration, 323, 325, 328
 contraindications, 322-323
 excisional, 323-324
 exfoliative cytology and, 327
 incisional, 323, 324-325
 indications, 322
 medicolegal factor, 326
 precautions, 322-323
 punch, 323
 specimen handling, 325-326
 specimen selection, 323
 tissue removal, 323-325
Bishydroxycoumarin (Dicumarol), 310, 312
Bite, edge-to-edge, 228-229
Bite fork, 337-339
Bite-raising procedure, 244
Bitot's spots, 97

Blandin and Nuhn's gland, 154
Blastomatoid lesions, 380
Bleeding, 22-23
 anticoagulants and, 47, 73
 hematologic diagnosis and, 309-313
 history of, 355
Bleeding time, 311
Blood clotting, 47, 73
Blood cultures, 305
Blood dyscrasias, 22-23, 56
 from drugs, 53
 history of, 359
Blood examination, 23, 308-318
 indications, 308
Blood glucose, 319
Blood pressure, 22, 87, 353
Blood transfusion, 352
Body build, 85
Body temperature, 85-86
Bone; *see also* osseous entries
 biopsy, 325
 palpation, 81
 percussion, 83
 radiotherapy and, 49, 50
 in systems review, 68-70
Bone disease, serologic tests, 316-317
Bone dysplasia
 endocrinopathic, 284
 radiography, 288, 289-290
Bone marrow, depression, 72, 73
Bone whorls, radiography, 287
Bradycardia, 87
Branchial cleft cyst, 110
Breath, 119
Bronchial dilators, 74
Bruising, 359
Bruxism, 67-68, 235-236
Buccal fat pad, 130-131, 137
Buccal mucosa, 125-139; *see also* Cheek
Bullae (blebs), 26-27
Burton Vitalometer, 331-332

C

Cacogeusia, 63-64
Calcification, in odontogenic neoplasms, 289
Calcium determinations, 316
Calculus
 -decalcification differentiation, 209
 radiography, 276, 293
Caliculus angularis, 131
Cancer phobia, 41, 144, 154, 326
Cancrum oris (noma), 307
Candidiasis
 antibiotics and, 72
 bacteriologic examination, 306, 307
Canker sores, 26, 58, 160, 357
Capillary fragility, 311-312, 359
Carbohydrate intake, caries and, 204, 205, 306
Carcinoma, 381
 case, 298-301
 radiography, 284
Cardiac insufficiency, 64
Cardiorespiratory system, 58-59
Cardiovascular disorders, 21-23

Caries, 204-209
  areas involved, 205
  carbohydrate intake and, 204, 205, 306
  charting, 212
  in children, 208
  clinical exploration, 205-206
  control, 386
  examination for, 8, 207-209
    instruments, 206-207, 208, 209
  incipient lesion, 206
  occlusal, 274-275
  periodic examination for, 204
  radiography, 205-206, 208, 274-276, 293
  rate of development, 204-205
  at restoration margins, 275-276
  treatment plan, 390
Caries activity tests, 205, 305-306
Carotene, 104
Case history; *see* History
Catamenia, 65-66
Cavity preparation, radiography, 292
Cementoenamel junction–alveolar crest relation, radiography, 269-272
Cementoma, 272-273
  radiography, 287, 289
Cementum-enamel differentiation, 209
Centric occlusion, 236, 239
Centric relations, 236, 239
Cephalometry, 297
Cerebrovascular accident, 67, 354
Chancre, 315
Charting, 211-213
Checklist, 37
Cheek, palpation, 131
Cheek biting, 137
Chemotherapy
  oral manifestations, 314
  hematologic diagnosis and, 314
Cherubism (familial fibrous dysplasia), 90
Chest pain, 58
  history of, 357-358
Childhood diseases, 45-47
Children
  caries detection in, 208
  growth and development, 84-85
  history taking, 38
  radiography for, 297-298
Chloasma gravidarum, 105
Chloramphenicol, 72
Chvostek's sign, 83
Cleft palate, 145-146
Cleidocranial dysostosis, 201
Climacteric; *see* Menopause
Clinical examination, 77-258, 348
  general, 84-117
  negative findings, 77
  outline, 78
  principles, 77, 79-83
Closed-bite, 244
  anterior, 245
Clot retraction time, 311
Coagulation factors, 22, 23
Coagulation (clotting) time, 311

Cold (common), 56
  history of, 356
Cold sores, 357
Complement fixation test, in syphilis, 315-316
Congenital heart disease, 46, 47
Conjunctivitis, 51
Constipation, 62
Contact dermatitis, 52, 53
Contact relationships, examination of, 209-211
Contact sensitivity tests, 319-322
Contrast media, iodism from, 51
Convulsions, 67, 73, 359
Coronary thrombosis, 47
Coronoid process, radiography, 263
Corrigan's (water-hammer) pulse, 87
Cortical bone, radiography, 267-268
Corticosteroids, 71
Corticotropin, 71
Cough, 58, 63, 358
Coumarin derivatives, 73
Cretinism, 90, 124
Cross-bite, unilateral, 230
Crown
  fracture, 203
  radiography, 291-292
Crusts, 33-34
Curettage, 323
Cushing's disease, 90
Cuspids
  eruption, 222, 223-224, 226
  primary, premature loss, 223, 224
Cyanosis, 103, 122, 168
Cyst
  mucous retention, 125
  radiography, 281-282
Cytology, exfoliative; *see* Exfoliative cytology

D

Deafness, 56
Decalcification-calculus differentiation, 209
Dehydration, 90
Dental arch(es), 220
  examination of, 248-251
  in primary dentition, 221, 222
  space prediction, 224
Dental floss, 209
Dental practice, 3-4
Dental pulp; *see* Pulp
Dentin
  age and, 193
  sensitivity, 18
Dentin dysplasia, 200, 279
  radiography, 200, 279
Dentinogenesis imperfecta, 200
  radiography, 279
Dentist
  -physician relationship, 302, 303, 308, 310-311, 351, 385, 388
  radiation hazards, 298
Denture(s); *see also* Appliances
  adjustment to, 251-252
  anteroposterior ridge relationship, 250
  border, palatine foveas and, 249
  border estimation, 251

Dentures—cont'd
buccal fat pad and, 137
buccal flange, 250
complaints about, 252
esthetic result, 42
examination for, 247
examination of, 247
frenula and, 138
gastrointestinal disturbances and, 63
gingivopalatal groove and, 141, 142
hard-soft palate junction and, 142-143
history of use, 45
impressions for; *see* Impressions
incisive papilla and, 249
indigestion and, 61
learning to wear, 252
lingual flange, 251
looseness, 253
mouth preparation, 247
palatal hyperemia and, 143
palatal hyperplasia and, 144
palatal papillomatosis and, 144
palatal reflex and, 145
palatal tissues and, 141
palatine torus and, 249
partial
abutment teeth for, 254-255
anteroposterior relationships and, 257
appliance examination, 254
classification system for, 255
complaints about, 258
crown form and, 257
edentulous arch–teeth relationship and, 257
fixed versus removable, 255
gingival margin and, 257
intermaxillary space and, 256
malposed teeth and, 255
occlusal relationships and, 255-256
oral hygiene and, 256-257
preparation for, 253
root form and, 257
tissue tone and, 257
pterygomandibular ligament and, 250
rebasing, 45
sensitivity to, 52, 63
stability, 252-253
supporting tissues for, 251
tongue and, 155
torus palatinus and, 144
vertical dimensions, 250-251
Denture-bearing areas
cortical bone resorption in, 267-268
examination, 247, 251-253
in partially edentulous mouth, 253-258
tissue response, 251
Denture-sore mouth, 52, 63, 252-253
Depression, 73
Dermatitis medicamentosa, 354
Dermoid cyst, 380
Description, 3
Desquamation, 33
Developmental defects; *see* Anomalies
Diabetes mellitus, 48-49, 63, 318-319
appointment time and, 353

Diabetes mellitus—cont'd
history of, 353
periodontitis and, 384
Diagnosis
definition, 375
determination of, 379-380
differential, 373, 375
early, 376
facts in, 373-374
analysis of, 376-378
collection of, 375-376
disease features correlation, 378-379
physiologic process correlation, 376
importance of findings, 377-378
method in, 373-382
outline, 374
of neoplasms, 380-382
oral; *see* Oral diagnosis
perspective in, 373
of soft tissue lesions, 377-378
tentative, 380
Diagnosis synopsis, 348-372
Diarrhea, 62
Diastema, 164-165
Dicumarol, 310, 312
Dilaceration, radiography, 278
Diphenylhydantoin (Dilantin Sodium), 21, 173
in gingival hyperplasia, 178
Disclosing solution, 345-346
Disease; *see* Systemic disease; specific diagnoses
Dish face, 220
Diuretics, 74
Dizziness, 56
Drug addiction, 72, 75, 97
Drug-induced diseases, 75
Drug(s), 71-75
allergy, to, 352, 354, 355
blood dyscrasias and, 53
history of use, 45, 53
incompatibility, 71
side effects, 71
for systemic disease, 351
tooth stains and, 194
Drug reactions, 50-53
diagnosis, 53
fixed, 52
Dry mouth, 64, 74, 136
Dysentery, 62
Dyskinesia, tardive, 75
Dysphagia, 61-62
Dyspnea, 21, 58, 358

E

Ears, 56, 356
Ecchymoses, 22, 24, 25, 135
Ectodermal dysplasia, anhidrotic, 201
Edema, 64, 90
history of, 358
Edentulous arch, cortical bone radiography, 267-268
Edentulous mouth examination, 247-258
alveolar ridges, 247-250
alveololingual sulcus, 251
lingual frenulum, 251

Edentulous mouth examination—cont'd
  mandibular arch, 249-251
  mandibular buccal fornix, 249-250
  mandibular buccal shelf, 250
  mandibular lingual tubercule, 251
  mandibular postmylohyoid fossa, 251
  mandibular tori, 251
  maxillary arch, 248-249
  mylohyoid ridge, 251
  palatal tissues, 249
  posterior palatal seal, 248-249
  procedure, 247-251
  tissue evaluation, 251
Edge-to-edge bite, 228-229
Electrocardiogram, 58-59
Emergency (incomplete) examination, 6-7, 10, 77, 348
Emotional factor
  anesthesia reactions and, 355
  in asthma, 74
  in bruxism, 235
  in dyspnea, 58
  in headache, 55
  in indigestion, 61
  with menopause, 66
  in nail biting, 107
  in oral habits, 107
  in pain perception, 15-16, 18
  in patient's complaints, 39, 40, 42
  in syncope, 67
  in temporomandibular joint disorders, 70, 234
  in tongue pain, 158-159
  in weakness, 21-22
Emotional illness, drug therapy, 72
Emphysema, 74
Enamel
  age and, 193
  -cementum differentiation, 209
  dysplasia, 195-196, 199
    radiography, 278
  hypomaturation, 195-196
  hypoplasia, 195-196
  mottling, 197
  opacity, 196-197
Enamel pearl, radiography, 287
Endocarditis, subacute bacterial, 46-47, 97, 135, 352, 354
  prophylaxis, 47
Endocrinopathy, 105-106
  radiography, 284
Endodontic treatment, 278, 386
  tooth stains and, 194, 195
Enostoses, radiography, 287
Eosinophilic granuloma, radiography, 284
Epilepsy, 21, 67, 73
  history of, 359
Epinephrine, 48, 72
Epistaxis, 22, 56
  history of, 356
Erosions (excoriations), 29-30
Erythema, 102
  ninth-day, 51
Erythema multiforme, 52, 379
Erythematous macules, 24-25

Eschars, 31-33
Esthetic factor, 42
Estrogens, 74
Examinations
  radiographic; *see* Radiography
  supplementary, 259-260, 302-347; *see also* specific procedures
  types of, 5-10
Exfoliative cytology, 326-328
  advantages, 327
  biopsy and, 327
  disadvantages, 327
  materials, 327
  method, 327-328
Exophthalmos, 96-97
Exostoses, radiography, 287
Explorers, 206-207, 208, 209
External oblique line, radiography, 265
Extractions, 386
  bleeding in, 23, 44
  nerve impulses and, 56
  neurologic effects, 56, 67
  prothrombin concentration and, 310, 312
  radiotherapy and, 49, 355
  subacute bacterial endocarditis and, 46, 47
Eyes
  clinical examination, 96-97
  history of complaints, 356
  in systems review, 55-56
  vascular disease, 47

F
Face, vertical dimensions, 218, 244, 245
  dentures and, 250-251
Face-bow, 337, 338-339
Facial angle, 220
Facial angulations, 218
Facial form
  -malocclusion relation, 218
  normal range, 216
Facial form analysis, 215-221
  method, 218-220
Facial growth, 215
Facial injuries, 49, 355
Facial neuralgia, 19
Facial planes, 216
  anterior, 216
  Frankfort horizontal (eye-ear), 216
  occlusal, 220
Facial profile, 216-218
  facial planes and, 216
  points of reference, 216-217
Facial symmetry, 90, 96, 216
  examination for, 216
  in midsagittal plane, 216, 218, 220
Facies, 89-90
Fainting, 359
Familial fibrous dysplasia, 90
Fatigue, 360
Fees, 261, 391
Fever, 86
  hematologic diagnosis and, 313
Fibroma, traumatic, 380
Fibrosarcoma, radiography, 284

Fibrous dysplasia, radiography, 290
Fingernails, 106
Fissures, 30
Flocculation test, in syphilis, 315-316
Fluorosis, 197, 208
Food avoidance, 358
Fordyce's disease, 380
Foreign bodies, radiography, 287-288, 290, 296
Fracture, radiography, 294
Frenulum (frenula), 128, 137-138, 154
    lingual, 148, 154, 251
    persistent, 138
Fungal disease, 72-73

G

Gagging, 145
Gait, 85
Gastrointestinal disturbances, dentures and, 63
Gastrointestinal system, 59-64
Genetic factor
    in dentin defects, 279
    in enamel defects, 279
    in history, 53-54
    in tooth form, 195-196, 199-200
Genial tubercles, radiography, 264
Genitourinary system, 64-65
Giant cell tumor, 303, 317, 380, 381
Gingiva
    age and, 162, 165, 166
    biopsy, 174, 324
    bullae, 174
    charting, 184-192
    clinical examination, 162-192, 211
    color, 162, 164, 166, 167-168, 169-170, 182
    contour (form), 164-165, 166, 170-173, 182
        age and, 171-172
    density, 165, 166
    in disease, 167-182
    ectopic sebaceous glands, 174
    edema, 174
    epithelial attachment, 166-167, 175, 176, 184, 187
    examination procedure, 182-184
    exostoses, 174
    fluctuance, 174
    free margin measurement, 187
    granulation tissue, 169
    healthy, 167
    hyperkeratotic, 175
    hyperplasia, 173, 174
    hypertrophy, 182
    impregnated amalgam, 170
    inflammation, 168-169, 171-172, 174
    inspection, 182
    keratinization, 165
    McCall's festoons, 172
    melanosis, 170
    metallic pigmentation, 170
    in neoplasms, 174
    normal, 166-167
    palpation, 165-166, 173-174, 184
    pigmentation, 162, 170
    plaques, 169
    pseudomembrane, 169

Gingiva—cont'd
    Stillman's clefts, 172
    stippling, 165
    texture, 165, 173-175
    tissue loss, 172-173
    ulceration, 169
    vascular bed alterations, 168
    vesicles, 174
Gingival bleeding, 22, 72, 313, 314
    history of, 357
Gingival crevice (sulcus) depth, 166, 167, 175-176, 187
Gingival enlargement, 313, 314
    diphenylhydantoin and, 21
Gingival fibromatosis, hereditary, 178
Gingival margin, 166
Gingival probe, 187
Gingival probing, 187
    of bifurcation area, 187
    of trifurcation area, 187, 191
Gingival recession, 173
    abrasion and, 203
Gingivectomy, 173
Gingivitis, 175
    from anticonvulsants, 73
    atrophic, 180-181
    desquamative, 102, 175, 180
    hormonal, 180-181
    hyperplastic, 57, 177-178
    infective, 177
    lymphadenopathy in, 109
    with menopause, 66
    mouth breathing and, 57, 98
    necrotizing ulcerative, 14, 31, 47, 58, 86, 169, 172, 173, 177, 307, 308, 379, 382
    pregnancy, 65, 178, 360
    pubertal, 178
    simple, 176-177
    systemic factors in, 178, 180
Gingivostomatitis, herpetic; *see* Herpetic gingivostomatitis
Glaucoma, 356
Glossitis
    deficiency, 102
    median rhomboid, 155, 157, 380
Glossitis migrans, 160-161
Glycosuria, 319
Goiter, 90
Gonorrhea, 48, 65, 234
Gout, 73
Grand mal, 73
Granuloma, eosinophilic, radiography, 284

H

Hair texture, 105-106
Halitosis, 119
Hamulus, radiography, 263
Hanau bite fork, 337
Hanau face-bow, 337
Hand-Schüller-Christian disease, radiography, 284
Hatchet face, 220
Hay fever, 354
Head
    clinical examination, 88-98

Head—cont'd
  injury, 55
  in systems review, 54-55
  wounds, 89
Headache, 20, 55, 56
  history of, 355
  local anesthesia in diagnosis, 20, 55
Health questionnaire, 8, 37, 348-360
  significance of questions, 351-360
Heart, valvular prosthesis, 46
Heart attack, 353
Heart disease, 58-59, 86, 87-88
  congenital, 46, 47
Heart failure, 358
  congestive, 48, 58, 109
  left ventricular, 86
Heart murmur, 354
Heart rate, 87
Heat intolerance, 359
Hematemesis, 62
Hematocrit, 309
Hematologic diagnosis; *see* Blood examination;
    specific diagnoses
Hemoglobin, 309
Hemoptysis, 58, 358
Hemorrhage; *see* Bleeding
Hemorrhagic disease, 22, 23, 308
  hematologic diagnosis, 309-313
  history of, 355
  screening examination, 310-312
Hemosiderin, 105
Hemostasis, 71
Heparin, 73
Hepatitis, viral, 48, 353
Hereditary brown teeth, 200
Herpes, 26
  simplex, 124, 357
Herpetic gingivostomatitis, 47, 86, 177, 379
  lymphadenopathy in, 109
  therapy in, 14
Herpetic stomatitis, 26, 58, 160, 357
Herpetic ulcers, 31
Hirsutism, 105-106
History, 3, 8, 12, 36-70
  of allergy, 50-53
  checklist, 37
  chief complaint, 39-42
  of child patients, 38
  of childhood diseases, 45-47
  complaint shaping, 39-42
  of drug reaction, 50-53
  examiner's attitude, 37-38, 41
  family, 53-54
  health questionnaire for; *see* Health question-
    naire
  of injuries, 49
  objectives, 36-37
  outline, 38-39
  past dental, 43-45, 64
    treatment plan and, 389
  past medical, 45-53
  of patient's attitude toward prior treatment, 43-
    44
  personal, 54

History—cont'd
  of present illness, 42-43
  scope, 36
  of serious illness, 47-49
  social, 54
  of surgery, 49
  systems review in, 54-70
Hives, 354
Hoarseness, 58, 61, 86
Hodgkin's disease, 108
Hospitalization, 352
Hot flash, 65
Hutchinson's incisors, 197-199
  radiography, 279
Hutchinson's triad, 97, 199
Hydantoin drugs, 73
Hyperalgesia, 17
Hypercementosis, radiography, 277-278
Hyperkeratinization, 29
Hyperkeratosis, 33
Hyperparathyroidism, 284
Hypertension, 22, 48, 56, 74, 87
  history of, 353
Hyperthyroidism, 96-97, 359
Hyperventilation, 67
Hypnotics, 74-75
Hypotensive drugs, 74

I

Id reactions, 52
Immunosuppressants, 73
Impacted teeth, radiography, 290, 296
Impressions
  floor of mouth and, 251
  soft tissue displacement and, 247
  tissue landmarks, 247
  tray flange, 250, 251
Incisive foramen, radiography, 263
Incisive fossa, radiography, 263
Incisive papilla, 139, 144
  cyst, 144
  dentures and, 249
Incisor eruption, 222, 223
Inclinations of anterior teeth, 216, 218, 221
Indigestion, 60-61, 358
Infection, 86
  cultures, 305
  diabetes mellitus and, 48, 49, 353
  hematologic diagnosis in, 313
  lymphadenopathy in, 108, 109
Injuries, 49
Inspection, 79
Insulin shock, 48-49, 353
Interdental papillae, 164-165, 173, 211
Interocclusal (freeway) space, 242-243, 244, 245
Interproximal space, 164
Intestinal polyposis, 105
Iodine, allergy to, 354
Iodism, 51
Iron therapy, 72
Irradiation; *see* Radiotherapy

J

Jaundice, 48, 62-63, 97, 104, 134
  history of, 352-353

Jaw(s)
    clinical examination, 114-117
    injury, 355
    inspection, 115-117
    palpation, 117
    percussion, 117
    radiography, 279-291, 296
    radiopacity, 288
    serologic tests in bone disease, 316-317
Jaw click, 357
Joints, 68-70, 358-359; *see also* Temporomandibular joint

K

Kahn test, 316
Keratitis, interstitial, 97
Keratosis, 29
Kidney disease, 358
Koilonychia, 106

L

Labial frenula, 128, 138
Labial mucosa, 125-139; *see also* Lips
Labiomarginal sulcus, 121, 124
Laboratory examinations, 259-260, 375
    indications, 303-304
    practicability, 302-303
Lactobacillus counts, 204, 205, 305-306, 386
Lamina dura
    in bifurcation area, 267
    radiography, 265
        of continuity, 266-268, 291
        of thickness, 268
    in trifurcation area, 267
Lassitude, 20, 21
Lesions; *see* Morphology
Leukemia, 135
    acute, 314
    chronic lymphocytic, 314
    chronic myelocytic, 314
    hematologic diagnosis, 313-314
Leukemic gingivitis, 180
Leukocytosis, 313, 314
Leukopenia, 312
Leukoplakia, 29, 33, 175, 381
Lichen planus, 25, 29, 175
Lid lag, 96
Linea alba (torus) buccalis, 131
Lingual foramen, radiography, 263-264
Lingual frenula, 148, 154, 251
Lingual gland, 154
Lingual tonsils, 152
Lip(s)
    allergic reactions, 124
    clinical examination, 120-125
    color, 122
    in disease, 124-125
    ectopic sebaceous glands, 123
    exposure effects, 122
    fissuring, 124
    inspection, 120, 121-122
    palpation, 121, 123
    pigmentation, 124
    position, 218

Lip(s)—cont'd
    second, 123
    -teeth relationship, 121
Lip chewing, 122
Lip habits, 218
Lisping, 86
Liver disease, 48
Local anesthesia, 72
    with bronchial dilators, 74
    contact dermatitis from, 52
    cross-reactions, 52
    in headache diagnosis, 20, 55
    reactions to, 44, 52-53, 355
    with vasoconstrictors, 48
Lung disease, 58-59
Lymph nodes
    cervical, 111
    enlargement, 313, 314
    of neck, 107-109
    submaxillary, 111
    submental, 111
Lymphadenopathy, 107-109, 313, 381
Lymphoid hyperplasia, 109
Lymphoid tissue, pharyngeal, 146, 147
Lymphoma, 313, 381

M

McCall's festoons, 172
Macroglossia, 155, 157
Macules, 24-25
Malar bone, radiography, 263
Malocclusion; *see also* Occlusion
    Class I, 220, 227
    Class II, 220, 223, 227
        Division 1, 227
        Division 2, 227
    Class III, 220, 227
    classification, 226-227
    developmental factors, 226
    facial angles and, 220
    facial form and, 96, 218
    facial planes and, 216
    functional factors, 226
    incipient, 215
    mouth breathing and, 57
    radiography, 223
    sequence of eruption and, 222-224
    in temporomandibular joint disorders, 68-69
Mandible
    centric relation, 236, 239
    deviation, 96
    examination for slide in centric, 236-240
    radiographic landmarks, 263-265
    relative size, 218
    in senile osteoporosis, 66
    tonus (rest) position, 242-245
        age and, 250
Mandibular displacement, 217-218
Mandibular lingual tubercle, 251
Mandibular movement, 116-117, 232, 233, 234, 240-242
    limitation, 357
    palpation, 117

Mandibular tori, 251, 380
  radiography, 285, 287
Mastication, 64
  attrition and, 228, 229-230
  difficulty, 351
Masticatory system, 68
  function in occlusal development, 226
  functional analysis, 231
Maxilla
  radiographic landmarks, 263
  relative size, 218
Maxillary sinus, raidography, 263
Median lingual sulcus, 154
Medication; *see* Drug(s)
Medicolegal record
  biopsy and, 326
  history as, 37
Melanin, 102, 103, 134
Melanoplakia, 105
Melanosis, 104-105, 168, 170
Melena, 62
Melituria, 319
Ménière's disease, 56
Menopause, 65-66, 106
  denture-supporting tissues and, 251
  estrogen therapy, 74
Menstruation, 65, 66
Mental foramen, radiography, 264-265
Mental ridge, radiography, 265
Metallic foreign bodies, radiography, 287, 288
Metallic pigments, 105
Metals intoxication, 63, 64, 135, 136
Metastasis, 49, 108, 109
Mixed dentition
  arch space prediction, 224
  bicuspid eruption, 222, 224
  cuspid eruption, 223-224, 226
  eruption sequence, 222-224, 226
  incisor eruption, 222, 223
  molar eruption, 222, 223, 224
  tooth crowding, 222
  tooth migration, 224, 226
  tooth size prediction, 224
Mixed dentition analysis, 222, 226
Molar
  pericoronal flap, 138-139
  primary, premature loss, 224, 226
Molar eruption, 222, 223, 224
Mongolism, 90
Moniliasis; *see* Candidiasis
Morphology
  lesion examination, 34
  primary lesions, 24-29
    versus secondary lesions, 13, 23-24, 34
  secondary lesions, 29-34
Mouth
  clinical examination, 77
  ectopic sebaceous glands, 130
  general appraisal, 118-120
Mouth breathing, 56-58, 97-98, 147
  facial form and, 218
  history of, 356
  lips and, 122, 123

Mouth floor
  clinical examination, 148-152
  cysts, 151-152
  in disease, 150-152
  impressions and, 251
  inspection, 148, 150
  neoplastic disease, 151, 152
  palpation, 150
Mouth soreness, 357
  from dentures, 52, 63, 252-253
Mucous glands, 128
Mucous membrane; *see* Oral mucosa; Soft tissues;
    specific structures
Mucous patches, 315
Mucous retention cyst, 125
Mulberry molars, 197, 199
  radiography, 279
Multiple myeloma, 317
  radiography, 284
Mumps, 47, 64
Muscle
  palpation, 81
  percussion, 82, 83
Muscle contraction, in headache, 55

N

Nail biting, 106-107
Nails, 106-107
Nasal obstruction, 57, 97-98
Nasal septum, radiography, 263
Nasmyth's membrane, 182
Nausea, 60
Neck
  clinical examination, 107-114
    patient position, 112
    procedure, 111-114
  inspection, 112
  lesions, 114; *see also* specific lesions
  neoplasms, 110
  palpation, 107-108, 112
  swellings, 107-108, 110
Neck veins, 109
Needle puncture, 18
Neoplasms, 86; *see also* Tumors; specific sites and
    diagnoses
  benign
    versus malignant, 381-382
    radiography, 282-283, 289
  biopsy, 322, 323
  chemotherapy, 314
  diagnosis, 380-382
  drug therapy, 73-74
  gingiva in, 174
  lymphadenopathy in, 108, 109
  malignant
    primary, 283-284, 289
    radiography, 283-284, 289
    secondary, 284
  nonodontogenic radiography, 283, 289
  odontogenic, radiography, 282-283, 289
  periapical radiolucency in, 272-273
  radiography, 282-283, 289
  surgery for, 49

Nerves
  seventh cranial (facial), 122
  trigeminal, 16, 19
Nervous system, in pain perception, 16-17
Nervousness, 359-360
Neuralgia, 19-20, 67
  classification, 19
Neuritis, 19, 20
Neuromuscular system, 66-68
Neutropenia, 314
Nevi, vascular, 102
Nicotine stomatitis, 29, 143
Nikolsky's sign, 27
Nitroglycerin, 358
Nodules, 26
Nose, 56-58, 97-98
Nosebleed; *see* Epistaxis
Nutritional status, 85

O

Observation, 3
Occlusion; *see also* Malocclusion
  adjustment of, 387
  adult, 227-245
    changes in, 228
  age and, 227-228
  balancing interferences, 241
  centric, 236, 239
  centric interference, 236
  edge-to-edge bite, 228-229
  examination for slide in centric, 236-240
  premature contacts, 236, 239-240
  protrusive movements, 241
  temporomandibular joint in, 232-235
  traumatic; *see* Traumatic occlusion
  working position, 240-241
Occlusion analysis, 343-344
Occlusion development, 214-227
  facial form and, 215-221
  factors influencing, 215
  mixed dentition analysis, 222-226
  primary dentition analysis, 221-222
  stages of, 221-226
Occlusion examination, 214-246
  screening, 215
Occupational factor
  in pigmentation, 105, 135
  in tooth stains, 194, 195
Odontalgia, 68
Odontogenesis imperfecta, 97
Odontoma, radiography, 286, 289
Onychophagia, 106-107
Operations; *see* Surgery
Operative dentistry, 387
Oral contraceptives, 74
Oral diagnosis, 382; *see also* Diagnosis
  case report, 391-400
  definition, 1
  history in, 36-37
  principles, 1
  scope, 3-12
  system in, 3
Oral habits, 54, 107, 221, 222; *see also* specific
    habits

Oral hygiene, 54, 388
  partial dentures and, 256-257
Oral mucosa
  color, 128, 130
  ecchymoses, 135
  keratinization, 134
  labial and buccal
    clinical examination, 125, 128-129
    color alteration, 133-134
    in disease, 133-139
  pallor, 134
  petechiae, 135
  pigmentation, 134-135
  –skin relation, 24, 98-99
  traumatic lesions, 135-136
Oropharynx
  clinical examination, 146-147
  in disease, 147
Orthodontic treatment, 386
  history of, 44-45, 64
  tooth movement, 173
Osseous radiolucency, 279-285
  evaluation, 280
  with radiopacity, 288-290
Osseous radiopacity, 280, 285-288
  evaluation, 285-286
  with radiolucency, 288-290
Osteitis deformans, 89
  radiography, 289-290
Osteoarthropathy, hypertrophic, 106
Osteogenesis imperfecta, 97
Osteolytic lesions, radiography, 281-284
Osteomyelitis, radiography, 284-285, 290
Osteoporosis, senile, 66
Osteoradionecrosis, 355
Overbite, 229
  deep, 244-245
Overjet, 229
Ovulatory agents, 74

P

Paget's disease, 89, 317
  radiography, 289-290
Pain, 11, 15-20
  central, 18
  deep versus superficial, 17-18
  localization, 17-18
  psychogenic, 18
  qualities, 17
  referred, 17, 18-19, 68
  as subjective symptom, 16
Pain impulses, 16-17
Pain threshold, 15-16
  of teeth, 328-329
Palatal papillomatosis, 144
Palatal reflex, 145
Palate
  clinical examination, 139-146
  color, 143
  in disease, 143-146
  gingivopalatal groove, 141-142
  hard, 139-142
  -soft junction, 142-143
  hyperemia, 143

Palate—cont'd
hyperkeratinization, 143
hyperplasia, 144
polypoid, 52
soft, 142
paralysis, 145
traumatic ulceration, 144
Palatine foveas, 140
denture borders and, 249
Palatine glands, 140-141
Palatine raphe, 139-140, 143-144
Palatine rugae, 140
Palatine tori, 380
dentures and, 249
Palliation, 383-384
Pallor, 100-102, 134
Palpation, 79-81
bidigital, 79
bilateral, 79, 81
bimanual, 79
tissue differentiation, 81
Palpitation, 21-22, 87
Papilloma, 28, 29
Papillomatous (papillomatoid) mass, 28
Papules, 25-26
Paracentesis, 323
Paralysis, 67, 85
Paresis, 67
Paresthesias, 67, 359
Parkell Dentotest Vitalometer, 332
Paronychia, 106
Parotid ducts, 136
Parotid gland
neoplasm, 109
palpation, 111, 136
Parotid papilla, 132, 136
Passavant's bar, 146
Patch tests, 53, 319-322
Patient
-dentist relationship, 36, 37-38, 41, 119
evaluation, 84-88
interview, 37-38
radiation hazards, 298
Pellagra, 105
tongue in, 160
Pemphigus, 26-27
Penicillin, allergy to, 50-52, 354
Percussion, 81-83
Periapical abscess, 272, 273
Periapical granuloma, 272, 273
Periapical inflammation, 266-267
Periapical radiolucency, 272-273
Periarteritis nodosa, 52
Periodic health-maintenance examination, 4, 5, 6-8,
36, 205, 351
frequency, 6, 44
survey findings, 7
Periodontal abscess, 63, 174, 176, 267
Periodontal chart, 162
Periodontal disease, 63, 175-176, 192
alveolar crest–cementoenamel junction relation
in, 269
chart, 192
classification, 176-182

Periodontal disease—cont'd
gingivopalatal groove in, 141-142
history of, 64
palatal hyperplasia and, 144
periodontal space and, 269
radiography, 176, 266, 267
retromolar papilla and, 138-139
root surface exposure in, 385
tooth mobility and, 176
in trifurcation areas, radiography, 272
Periodontal pockets, 176, 187, 191, 267
radiography, 191
Periodontal space
in bifurcation areas, 269
radiography, 265-266
width variations, 268-269
in trifurcation areas, 269
Periodontal therapy, 386
history of, 44
Periodontitis, 175, 176, 181-182
chronic, 172, 173
diabetes mellitus and, 384
laboratory examination in, 318
rheumatic heart disease and, 384
Periodontium
charting, 211
clinical examination, 162-192
Petechiae, 22, 24, 25, 135
Petit mal, 67, 73
Pharyngeal lymphoid tissue, 57
Pharynx, 147
Phenol eschars, 33
Phlebectasia linguae, 154-155
Phosphorus determinations, 316
Photophobia, 56
Pigmentation, 25, 100, 104, 105
of gingiva, 162, 170
of lips, 124
of oral mucosa, 134-135
of teeth, 193-194, 203
Pituitary disease, 105
Plaques, 205
disclosing solution for, 345-346
Plummer-Vinson syndrome, 61-62, 106
appliances and, 257
Polycythemia, 168
hematologic diagnosis, 308-309
vera, 102
Polyp, 28
Polypoid mass, 28
Polyuria, 64
Postnasal drip, 56
Postoperative defects, radiography, 285
Pregnancy, 65, 105, 360
gingivitis and, 178
Premenstrual tension, 65, 66
Preventive dentistry, 3-5
in malocclusion, 214, 215
Primary dentition
occlusion analysis, 221-222
premature loss, 221, 222
retention of, 222
Procaine, cross-reactions, 355
Profile (facial), 90

Progestogens, 74
Prognathism, 217, 220
    functional, 241-242
Prognosis, 382
Prophylaxis, 193
    subacute bacterial endocarditis and, 46, 47
Prosthesis; *see* Appliances; Dentures
Prosthetic dentistry, 387
Prothrombin, 48, 73, 310, 312, 353
Pseudomembrane, 31
Psychalgia, 19
Psychogenic factor; *see* Emotional factor
Pterygomandibular ligament, dentures and, 250
Ptosis, 96
Public education, 4
    patient's complaint and, 41
Pulp
    calcification, radiography, 274, 292-293
    devital, 194, 272, 273, 336
        lamina dura in, 266-267
        radiography, 269
    radiography, 269, 292-293
    sensitivity, 18
Pulp disease, 151, 152
    with lymphadenopathy, 108
Pulp polyp, 336
Pulp stones, 274
Pulp test(s), 6, 194, 203, 328-336
    electrical, 328, 332-334
        electrode placement, 333-334
        leakage, 333, 334
        of multirooted teeth, 334
        problems, 329-330
        rubber dam isolation for, 334
    in facial injury, 49
    interpretation, 335-336
    pain perception threshold, 329
    periodontal membrane–pulp response differenti-
        ation, 329
    stimulation methods, 328
    stimulation requirements, 329
    thermal, 334-335
        with cold, 335
        with heat, 334-335
    threshold stimulus, 328-329, 330, 331, 336
    tooth damage from, 330
Pulp testers, electric, 329-332
    types, 331-332
Pulpitis
    after fracture, 203
    hyperplastic, 336
    pain in, 18, 19
Pulse, 86-87
Purpura, 22, 23, 72, 97, 135
    allergic, 75
Pustules, 26

Q

Questionnaire, health; *see* Health questionnaire
Quinacrine (Atabrine), 104
Quinidine, 72

R

Radial artery palpation, 86-87

Radiation badges, 298
Radiation hazards, 298
Radicular cysts, 273
Radiography (radiographs), 162, 259-301; *see also*
        specific diagnoses
    case, 298-301
    charting, 212
    for children, 297-298
    complete mouth, 266-291
    in facial injury, 49
    fee for, 261
    general landmarks, 265-266
    interpretation, 261-266
    intraoral alternatives, 296
    method, 266
    minimum requirements, 261, 266
    normal landmarks, 261
    panographic, 296-297
    periapical, normal landmarks, 261-266
    posterior bite-wing, 6, 8-9, 205, 291-293
    requirements, 259
    scheduling, 118
    supplemental, 293-297
        types, 294
Radiotherapy, 49-50, 102
    history of, 355
Red blood cell count, 309
Referrals, 385; *see also* Dentist-physician relation-
        ship
Regurgitation, 60
Respiration, 86
    abnormal sounds, 83
Restorations, 387
    abbreviations for materials, 213
    caries and, 206, 208, 275-276
    examination of, 210-211
    overhanging, radiography, 277
    radiography, 277, 293
    silicate, 275, 276
    tooth stains and, 194, 195
Retainer, 45
Retrocuspid papilla, 165
Retrognathism, 217, 218, 220
Retromolar pad, 133
Retromolar papillae, 132-133, 138-139
Rheumatic fever, 45-46, 47, 352
Rheumatic heart disease, 384
Rheumatism, inflammatory, 352
Riboflavin deficiency, 97
Rickets, 89
Ritter pulp tester, 332
Root(s)
    dilaceration, 278
    form abnormalities, radiography, 278
    fracture, 203
    hypercementosis, 277-278
    neoplasms, 277, 280
        radiography, 267
    resorption, 176, 280
        radiography, 277
Root canal
    cultures, 306
    fillings, radiography, 291
    therapy, 274

Root cyst, lateral, 267
Root tips, retained, radiography, 285, 287-288, 290

S

Saddle nose, 97
Saliva, lactobacillus count, 305-306
Salivary calculus, radiography, 294-296
Salivary glands
  neoplasms, 152
  palpation, 81
  radiotherapy and, 49-50
Salivation, 64, 136
Sarcoidosis, 317
Sarcoma, 381
  osteogenic, radiography, 289, 290
Scleroderma, 384
Scratch tests, 321
Screening examination, 6, 7, 8-10, 77, 348
  in hemorrhagic disease, 310, 312
  indications, 10
  for occlusion development, 215
Scurvy, 312-313
Sebaceous glands, ectopic, 123, 130, 174
Sedatives, 74-75
Serologic tests, 314-318
Serum protein determinations, 316
Serum sickness, 50-51, 52
Sialography, 297
Sialorrhea, 136
Silicate restorations, 275, 276
Sinusitis, 56, 356
Sjögren's syndrome, 97
Skeletal displacement, 220
Skin
  allergic drug reactions, 52
  clinical examination, 98-107
  color, 99-105
  -oral mucosa relation, 24, 98-99
  palpation, 81
  texture, 99
  -tongue relation, 157, 158
Skin rash, 354
Skin tests, 53, 320-321
Skull, 88-96
Sleeping pills, sensitivity to, 354
SMA 12/60 analyzer, 319
Smoker's patch, 143
Smoking, 106
  palatal hyperkeratinization and, 143
  Snyder test, 305-306
Socioeconomic factor, 54, 388-389
Soft tissues
  clinical examination, 118-161
    equipment, 119-120
  lesions, 377-378, 380, 389
Sore mouth; *see also* Denture-sore mouth
  radiotherapy and, 49
Sore throat, 58, 356
Speech, 83, 86
Spoon nails, 106
Stensen's duct, 132
  calculus, 294, 296
  palpation, 136

Steroids, 73
Stevens-Johnson syndrome, 51, 97
Stillman's clefts, 172
Stomatitis, contact, 319-320
Stomatitis medicamentosa, 321-322
Stomatomicroscope, 345
Stroke, 48, 354
Study, casts, 336-344
  advantages, 336-337
  articulation, 337-344
  centric occlusion, 343
  centric relation, 343
  centric relation registration, 339-341, 343
    correct wax bite determination, 340
    wax versus plaster, 339-340
  condylar guidance adjustment, 342-343
  conventional hinge axis, 337, 339
  incorrect mountings, 343
  mounting mandibular cast, 341-342
  mounting maxillary cast, 339
  occlusal contacts, 343
  in occlusion analysis, 343-344
  protrusive registration, 341
  slide in centric, 343
Sublingual caruncle, 148
Sublingual glands, 148
Submaxillary fossa, radiography, 265
Sucking habits, 221, 222
Sugar intake, 204, 205, 306
Sulfonamides, allergy to, 354
Sulfur granule, 307
Supernumerary teeth, 201
  radiography, 290-291
Surgery
  in denture preparation, 247
  history of, 49, 352, 355
  oral, 386
Surveyor, 344-345
Swallowing, 358
Symptomatology, 13-35
  age factor, 40-41
  classification, 13
  duration of, 42
  in history, 39-43
  negative findings, 43
  objective, 14
  psychic component, 39, 40, 42
  quantitative evaluation, 42
  subjective, 13-14, 16, 39
Syncope, 21, 67, 75, 359
Syphilis, 48, 65, 106, 313
  chancre, 315
  congenital, 43, 89, 97, 197, 199
  lymph nodes, 108
  mucous patches, 157, 315
  serologic diagnosis, 314-316
  tertiary, 67
  tongue, 157
Systemic disease, 351-352; *see also* specific diagnoses
  cardinal manifestations, 11, 14-35
  drugs for, 351
  evaluation, 15
  history, 37

Systemic disease—cont'd
  mouth symptoms, 381
  natural history of, 375
  osseous radiolucency in, 284
  patient's complaint and, 43
  serious, 352
  treatment, 385
  treatment plan and, 383-385
Systems review, 54-70

T

Tabes dorsalis, 97
Tachycardia, 87
Taste, 63-64
Telangiectasis, hereditary hemorrhagic, 155
Temporomandibular joint
  in bruxism, 235
  examination, 232-233
  function, 357
  in occlusion, 232-235
  palpation, 117
  radiography, 296
  sounds, 83, 117
Temporomandibular joint arthritis, 48, 49, 65, 66, 69, 359
  acute suppurative, 234
  pain in, 19
  traumatic, 233-234, 235, 355
Temporomandibular joint disease, 11, 64, 68-69, 233-235, 356, 387
Temporomandibular joint-pain-dysfunction syndrome, 234
Teratoma, 380
Tetany, 83
Thielemann's law, 230-231
Thirst, 358
Throat, 58
Thrombocytopenia, 72
Thromboembolism, 73, 310, 312
Thrombophlebitis, 47
Thromboplastin time, partial, 311
Thrush; see Candidiasis
Thyroid gland, 106, 112, 114
Tissue smears, 323
Tobacco, 54, 106
  tooth stains and, 183-184, 194
Tongue
  in anemia, 159-160
  black hairy, 52, 161
  clinical examination, 152-161
  coated, 152
  in dermatologic disease, 157, 158
  developmental disturbances, 157, 158
  in disease, 155-161
  in drug reactions, 158
  fissures, 30
  foramen cecum, 152
  furrowed, 154, 157
  geographic, 160-161
  infective granulomas, 157, 158
  inspection, 152
  lymphoid tissue, 152, 154
  movements, 155
  neoplasms, 158

Tongue—cont'd
  pain, 158-159
  palpation, 155
  papillae, 152
  in pellagra, 160
  position, 155
  sensitivity changes, 158-159
  -skin relation, 157, 158
  soreness, 152, 154
  trauma, 157, 158, 159
  ulcers, 380-381
    traumatic, 160
  varices, 154-155
  wandering rash of, 160-161
Tongue depressor application, 146
Tongue thrust, 147
Tongue-tie, 154
Tonsillitis, 58
Tonsils, 146, 147
  lingual, 152, 155
Tooth (teeth)
  abrasion, 202-203
  absence, 201
  appearance, 351
  black stain, 182-183
  color, 193-195, 196-197, 203
    age and, 193
  crowding, 223
    in mixed dentition, 222
  devital; see Pulp, devital
  discoloration, 182
  erosion, 202, 203
  form, 195-200
  fracture, 203
    radiography, 203
  functional contours, 204
  general health and, 351
  green stains, 182
  in headache, 55
  -lips relationships, 121
  loss, 63
    mastication and, 64
    primary cuspids, 223, 224
    in primary dentition, 221, 222
    primary molar, 224, 226
  mobility, 176, 191-192
    charting, 191
    in occlusal trauma, 231
  number, 200-201
  orange stains, 183
  pain threshold, 328-329
  palpation, 81
  percussion, 81-83
  pigmentation, 193-194, 203
  resorption, 209
  sensitivity, 356-357
  size, 195
  sounds, 83
  spacing, 221, 223
  stains, 193-195
  structure, 195-200
  supernumerary, 201, 290-291
  tenderness, 81
  thermal sensitivity, 334

Tooth (teeth)—cont'd
  tobacco stains, 183-184
  vitality; *see* Pulp tests; Vitality
Tooth (teeth) charting, 211-213
Tooth (teeth) examination, 182, 193-213
  preparation for, 193
Tooth numbering system, 212-213
Tooth pathology, radiography, 274-279
Toothache, 63, 357
  headache and, 20
Toothbrushing, 54, 173
  frenulum attachment and, 138
Torus palatinus, 144
Tourniquet test, 23, 311-312
Tranquilizers; *see* Ataractics
Trauma
  pulp calcification and, 274
  in root resorption, 277
  treatment plan, 390
Traumatic devitalization, 273
Traumatic occlusion, 68, 172, 173, 176, 231-232
  bruxism, 235
  in headache, 55
  lamina dura in, 268
  pain in, 19
  periodontal space in, 269
Treatment
  rationale for, 15
  symptom relief in, 14
Treatment plan, 382-391
  for caries, 390
  case report, 391-400
  chief complaint in, 388
  corrective treatment, 387
  dental history in, 389
  in developmental disturbances, 390
  etiology and, 389-390
  maintenance treatment, 387-388
  modification, 390
  oral hygiene and, 388
  outline, 374, 382-383
  periodic examinations, 387-388
  preparatory treatment, 385-387
  presentation to patient, 390-391
  preventive therapy, 385
  principles for outlining, 388-391
  rationale, 382-383
  socioeconomic factor, 388-389
  for soft tissue lesions, 389
  surveying in, 344-345
  systemic disease in, 383-385, 388
  for trauma, 390
  work sheet for, 212, 213

Trigeminal nerve, 16
Trigeminal neuralgia, 19
Tuberculosis, 47, 74, 108, 353
  bacteriologic examination, 306, 308
Tumescence, 27
Tumors, 27-29; *see also* Neoplasms
  radiography, 286-287
  surgery for, 355
Turner's teeth, radiography, 279

U

Ulcers, 31
  traumatic, 135-136, 144, 160
Unconsciousness, 67
Urinalysis, 318-319
Urinary frequency, 358
Urticaria, 51, 52
Uvula, 146

V

Vasoconstrictors, 48, 72
Venereal disease, 64-65; *see also* specific diagnoses
  in history, 41, 353
Vertigo, 56
Vesicles, 26, 34-35
Vestibule of mouth, 132
Vincent's infection; *see* Gingivitis, necrotizing ulcerative
Virus infection, 34-35
Vitality, 203-204; *see also* Pulp tests
  of abutment tooth, 255
Vitamin A deficiency, 97
Vitamin K therapy, 312
Vitapulp pulp tester, 332
Vomiting, 60, 358

W

Waldeyer's ring, 147
Warthin's tumor, 110
Wassermann test, 316
Weakness, 20-21
Weight, 23, 85, 352
Wharton's duct, 151
  calculus, 294, 296
White blood cell count, 312, 313
  chemotherapy and, 314
Wound healing, 44

X

Xerostomia, 64, 74, 136
X-ray therapy; *see* Radiotherapy